Case Studies in Neuroanesthesia and Neurocritical Care

Case Studies in Neuroanesthesia and Neurocritical Care

Edited by

George A. Mashour
University of Michigan

Ehab Farag
Cleveland Clinic

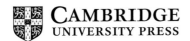

CAMBRIDGE UNIVERSITY PRESS
Cambridge, New York, Melbourne, Madrid, Cape Town, Singapore,
São Paulo, Delhi, Dubai, Tokyo, Mexico City

Cambridge University Press
The Edinburg Building, Cambridge CB2 8RU, UK

Published in the United States of America by
Cambridge University Press, New York

www.cambridge.org
Information on this title: www.cambridge.org/
9780521193801

First published 2011

Printed in the United Kingdom
at the University Press, Cambridge

*A catalog record for this publication is available from the
British Library*

Library of Congress Cataloging in Publication data
Case studies in neuroanesthesia and neurocritical care / edited by
George A. Mashour, Ehab Farag.
   p. ; cm.
Includes bibliographical references and index.
ISBN 978-0-521-19380-1 (pbk.)
1. Anesthesia in neurology – Case studies.   2. Nervous system –
Surgery – Case studies.   3. Neurological intensive care – Case
studies.   I. Mashour, George A. (George Alexander), 1969–
II. Farag, Ehab.

[DNLM: 1. Anesthesia – methods – Case Reports.
2. Neurosurgical Procedures – methods – Case Reports.
3. Critical Care – methods – Case Reports.   4. Nervous System
Diseases – surgery – Case Reports.
5. Perioperative Care – methods – Case Reports.   WL 368]
RD87.3.N47C37   2011
617.9′6748 – dc22   2010041507

ISBN 978-0-521-19380-1 Paperback

Contents

Contents

Neurocritical care

Part VIII – General topics in neurocritical care

Part IX – Subarachnoid hemorrhage

Part X – Stroke

Part XI – Intraparenchymal hemorrhage

Contributors

Basem Abdelmalak
Outcomes Research
Cleveland Clinic
Cleveland, OH
USA

Joseph Abdelmalak
Outcomes Research
Cleveland Clinic
Cleveland, OH
USA

Alaa A. Abd-Elsayed
Outcomes Research
Cleveland Clinic
Cleveland, OH
USA

David L. Adams
Department of Anesthesiology
University of Michigan Medical School
Ann Arbor, MI
USA

Eric E. Adelman
Department of Neurology
University of Michigan Medical School
Ann Arbor, MI
USA

Maged Argalious
Anesthesia Institute
Cleveland Clinic
Cleveland, OH
USA

Endrit Bala
Outcomes Research
Cleveland Clinic
Cleveland, OH
USA

Gene H. Barnett
Taussig Cancer Center
Cleveland Clinic
Cleveland, OH
USA

Sheron Beltran
Department of Anesthesiology
University of Michigan Medical School
Ann Arbor, MI
USA

Andrew Bielaczyc
Department of Anesthesiology
University of Michigan Medical School
Ann Arbor, MI
USA

William Bingaman
Epilepsy Center
Cleveland Clinic
Cleveland, OH
USA

James M. Blum
Department of Anesthesiology
University of Michigan Medical School
Ann Arbor, MI
USA

Alina Bodas
Anesthesia Institute
Cleveland Clinic
Cleveland, OH
USA

Vera Borzova
Anesthesia Institute
Cleveland Clinic
Cleveland, OH
USA

Richard Bowers
Department of Anesthesiology
University of Michigan Medical School
Ann Arbor, MI
USA

Adam Brown
Department of Anesthesiology
University of Michigan Medical School
Ann Arbor, MI
USA

Chad M. Brummett
Department of Anesthesiology
University of Michigan Medical School
Ann Arbor, MI
USA

Alexandra S. Bullough
Department of Anesthesiology
University of Michigan Medical School
Ann Arbor, MI
USA

James F. Burke
Department of Neurology
University of Michigan Medical School
Ann Arbor, MI
USA

Juan P. Cata
Anesthesia Institute
Cleveland Clinic
Cleveland, OH
USA

Neeraj Chaudhary
Department of Radiology
University of Michigan
Ann Arbor, MI
USA

Michael J. Claybon
Department of Anesthesiology
University of Michigan Medical School
Ann Arbor, MI
USA

Miguel Cruz
Anesthesia Institute
Cleveland Clinic
Cleveland, OH
USA

Milind Deogaonkar
Center for Neurological Restoration
Cleveland Clinic
Cleveland, OH
USA

Vikram Dhawan
Department of Neurology
University Hospitals – Case Medical Center
Cleveland, OH
USA

Thomas Didier
Department of Anesthesiology
University of Michigan Medical School
Ann Arbor, MI
USA

D. John Doyle
Anesthesia Institute
Cleveland Clinic
Cleveland, OH
USA

Zeyd Ebrahim
Anesthesia Institute
Cleveland Clinic
Cleveland, OH
USA

Hesham Elsharkawy
Cleveland Clinic
Cleveland, OH
USA

Wael Ali Sakr Esa
Anesthesia Institute
Cleveland Clinic
Cleveland, OH
USA

Ehab Farag
Anesthesia Institute
Cleveland Clinic
Cleveland, OH
USA

Ryen D. Fons
Department of Anesthesiology
University of Michigan Medical School
Ann Arbor, MI
USA

Joseph J. Gemmete
Department of Radiology
University of Michigan Medical School
Ann Arbor, MI
USA

Matt Giles
Department of Anesthesiology
University of Michigan Medical School
Ann Arbor, MI
USA

Phil Gillen
Department of Anesthesiology
University of Michigan Medical School
Ann Arbor, MI
USA

Goodarz Golmirzaie
Department of Anesthesiology
University of Michigan Medical School
Ann Arbor, MI
USA

Marcos Gomes
Cleveland Clinic
Cleveland, OH
USA

Lisa Grilly
Department of Anesthesiology
University of Michigan Medical School
Ann Arbor, MI
USA

Maged Guirguis
Anesthesia Institute
Cleveland Clinic
Cleveland, OH
USA

David W. Healy
Department of Anesthesiology
University of Michigan Medical School
Ann Arbor, MI
USA

Heather Hervey-Jumper
Department of Anesthesiology
University of Michigan Medical School
Ann Arbor, MI
USA

Shawn L. Hervey-Jumper
Department of Neurosurgery
University of Michigan Medical School
Ann Arbor, MI
USA

Paul E. Hilliard
Department of Anesthesiology
University of Michigan Medical School
Ann Arbor, MI
USA

Samuel A. Irefin
Anesthesia Institute
Cleveland Clinic
Cleveland, OH
USA

George K. Istaphanous
Cleveland Clinic
Cleveland, OH
USA

Teresa L. Jacobs
Department of Neurosurgery
University of Michigan Medical School
Ann Arbor, MI
USA

Ellen Janke
Department of Anesthesiology
University of Michigan Medical School
Ann Arbor, MI
USA

Greta Jo
Anesthesia Institute
Cleveland Clinic
Cleveland, OH
USA

James W. Jones
Cleveland Clinic
Cleveland, OH
USA

Rami Karroum
Anesthesia Institute
Cleveland Clinic
Cleveland, OH
USA

Allen Keebler
Anesthesia Institute
Cleveland Clinic
Cleveland, OH
USA

Stephen J. Kimatian
Anesthesia Institute
Cleveland Clinic
Cleveland, OH
USA

Colleen G. Koch
Anesthesia Institute
Cleveland Clinic
Cleveland, OH
USA

Robert Scott Kriss
Department of Anesthesiology
University of Michigan Medical School
Ann Arbor, MI
USA

Andrea Kurz
Outcomes Research
Cleveland Clinic
Cleveland, OH
USA

Jia Lin
Anesthesia Institute
Cleveland Clinic
Cleveland, OH
USA

Michael D. Maile
Department of Anesthesiology
University of Michigan Medical School
Ann Arbor, MI
USA

Negmeldeen F. Mamoun
Anesthesia Institute
Cleveland Clinic
Cleveland, OH
USA

Mariel Manlapaz
Anesthesia Institute
Cleveland Clinic
Cleveland, OH
USA

Edward Manno
Cerebrovascular Center, NICU
Cleveland Clinic
Cleveland, OH
USA

Donn Marciniak
Cleveland Clinic
Cleveland, OH
USA

Piyush Mathur
Cleveland Clinic
Cleveland, OH
USA

Nicholas F. Marko
Brain Tumor and Neuro-Oncology
Cleveland Clinic
Cleveland, OH
USA

Matthew Martin
Department of Anesthesiology
University of Michigan Medical School
Ann Arbor, MI
USA

George A. Mashour
Department of Anesthesiology and Department
of Neurosurgery
University of Michigan Medical School
Ann Arbor, MI
USA

Marco Maurtua
Anesthesia Institute
Cleveland Clinic
Cleveland, OH
USA

Scott T. McCardle
Department of Anesthesiology
University of Michigan Medical School
Ann Arbor, MI
USA

Julie McClelland
Department of Anesthesiology
University of Michigan Medical School
Ann Arbor, MI
USA

Uma Menon
Epilepsy Center, Neurological Institute
Cleveland Clinic
Cleveland, OH
USA

Paul S. Moor
Department of Anesthesiology
University of Michigan Medical School
Ann Arbor, MI
USA

Laurel E. Moore
Department of Anesthesiology
University of Michigan Medical School
Ann Arbor, MI
USA

Ruairi Moulding
Department of Anesthesiology
University of Michigan Medical School
Ann Arbor, MI
USA

Dileep R. Nair
Epilepsy Center, Neurological Institute
Cleveland Clinic
Cleveland, OH
USA

Todd Nelson
Department of Anesthesiology
University of Michigan Medical School
Ann Arbor, MI
USA

Julie Niezgoda
Anesthesia Institute
Cleveland Clinic
Cleveland, OH
USA

Edward Noguera
General Surgical ICU
Cleveland Clinic
Cleveland, OH
USA

Jerome O'Hara
Anesthesia Institute
Cleveland Clinic
Cleveland, OH
USA

Aditya S. Pandey
Department of Neurosurgery
University of Michigan Medical School
Ann Arbor, MI
USA

Mauricio Perilla
Anesthesia Institute
Cleveland Clinic
Cleveland, OH
USA

Paul Picton
Department of Anesthesiology
University of Michigan Medical School
Ann Arbor, MI
USA

Marc J. Popovich
Department of General Anesthesiology
Cleveland Clinic
Cleveland, OH
USA

J. Javier Provencio
Cerebrovascular Center, NICU
Cleveland Clinic
Cleveland, OH
USA

Venkatakrishna Rajajee
Department of Neurosurgery
University of Michigan Medical School
Ann Arbor, MI
USA

Mohit Rastogi
Department of Anesthesiology
University of Michigan Medical School
Ann Arbor, MI
USA

Stacy Ritzman
Anesthesia Institute
Cleveland Clinic
Cleveland, OH
USA

Lauryn R. Rochlen
Department of Anesthesiology
University of Michigan Medical School
Ann Arbor, MI
USA

Leif Saager
Anesthesia Institute
Cleveland Clinic
Cleveland, OH
USA

Vivek Sabharwal
General Surgical ICU
Cleveland Clinic
Cleveland, OH
USA

Oren Sagher
Department of Neurosurgery
University of Michigan Medical School
Ann Arbor, MI
USA

Kenneth Saliba
Anesthesia Institute
Cleveland Clinic
Cleveland, OH
USA

Milad Sharifpour
Department of Anesthesiology
University of Michigan Medical School
Ann Arbor, MI
USA

Lesli E. Skolarus
Department of Neurology
University of Michigan Medical School
Ann Arbor, MI
USA

Paul Smythe
Department of Anesthesiology
University of Michigan Medical School
Ann Arbor, MI
USA

Wolf H. Stapelfeldt
Anesthesia Institute
Cleveland Clinic
Cleveland, OH
USA

William R. Stetler, Jr.
Department of Neurosurgery
University of Michigan Medical School
Ann Arbor, MI
USA

Peter Stiles
Department of Anesthesiology
University of Michigan Medical School
Ann Arbor, MI
USA

Vijay Tarnal
Department of Anesthesiology
University of Michigan Medical School
Ann Arbor, MI
USA

Khoi D. Than
Department of Neurosurgery
University of Michigan Medical School
Ann Arbor, MI
USA

B. Gregory Thompson
Department of Neurosurgery
University of Michigan Medical School
Ann Arbor, MI
USA

Alparslan Turan
Anesthesia Institute
Cleveland Clinic
Cleveland, OH
USA

Christopher R. Turner
Department of Anesthesiology
University of Michigan Medical School
Ann Arbor, MI
USA

Justin Upp
Department of Anesthesiology
University of Michigan Medical School
Ann Arbor, MI
USA

Sumeet Vadera
Cleveland Clinic
Cleveland, OH
USA

Jennifer Vance
Department of Anesthesiology
University of Michigan Medical School
Ann Arbor, MI
USA

Anthony C. Wang
Department of Neurosurgery
University of Michigan Medical School
Ann Arbor, MI
USA

Robert J. Weil
Brain Tumor and Neuro-Oncology
Cleveland Clinic
Cleveland, OH
USA

Marnie B. Welch
Department of Anesthesiology
University of Michigan Medical School
Ann Arbor, MI
USA

Karen K. Wilkins
Department of Anesthesiology
University of Michigan Medical School
Ann Arbor, MI
USA

Erin S. Williams
Anesthesia Institute
Cleveland Clinic
Cleveland, OH
USA

George N. Youssef
Anesthesia Institute
Cleveland Clinic
Cleveland, OH
USA

Asma Zakaria
Neurointensive Care Unit
University of Texas Health Science Center
at Houston
Houston, TX
USA

Sherif S. Zaky
Anesthesia Institute
Cleveland Clinic
Cleveland, OH
USA

Andrew Zura
Anesthesia Institute
Cleveland Clinic
Cleveland, OH
USA

Preface

Neuroanesthesia and neurocritical care encompass the perioperative management of patients suffering from neurologic disease. There have been numerous textbooks on this subject that are generally organized according to basic physiology and pharmacology, neurosurgical procedure, postoperative neurocritical care, and the various techniques and monitoring modalities particular to the field. What has not been available is a comprehensive, case-based approach to the perioperative care of the neurologic patient that allows for an *integrated* discussion of management principles. This was the motivation behind *Case Studies in Neuroanesthesia and Neurocritical Care*, which is organized around compelling and realistic clinical scenarios followed by a concise discussion that is practically oriented but nonetheless informed by the current literature. Each brief but high-yield chapter highlights basic principles of neuroanesthesia and neurocritical care (e.g., management of elevated intracranial pressure), as well as classic complications (e.g., venous air embolism or the intraoperative rupture of an aneurysm). Tables, neuroimaging and other visual aids are abundant. *Case Studies* facilitates clinical preparation, scholarly review, and board examination study. Although written primarily for residents and fellows, the book will be a helpful aid for attending physicians, medical students, nurses and ancillary staff. *Case Studies* also serves as a quick reference guide for virtually any neuroanesthetic procedure, which is especially helpful for junior residents or student nurse anesthetists that are rotating through neuroanesthesia. The educational philosophy is consistent with the "problem-based learning" approach implemented in numerous medical schools and we hope it will serve as a valuable complement to more traditional textbooks in neuroanesthesia and neurocritical care.

Craniotomy. Supratentorial craniotomy

Preoperative evaluation

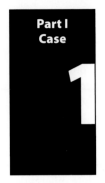

Paul Smythe and Mohit Rastogi

Supratentorial craniotomy is a common neurosurgical procedure, which may be emergent (e.g., evacuation of an expanding hematoma) or routine (e.g., scheduled resection of a mass lesion). Although the core preoperative evaluation is similar to that of the non-neurosurgical population, there are special considerations for patients with neurologic disease.

Case description

The patient was a 61-year-old female who presented with new-onset seizures, which were preceded by several weeks of bilateral frontal headaches described as "dull and achy." The headaches had become nearly continuous and were more recently accompanied by vertigo and nausea. The morning of admission, she had a witnessed generalized seizure. The seizure terminated and she presented to the emergency room where she was treated with benzodiazepines and supportive care; reversible physiologic and pharmacologic derangements were ruled out. Computed tomography (CT) and magnetic resonance imaging (MRI) were performed, which revealed a large left temporal fossa mass suggestive of a meningioma. She was admitted to the neurosurgical intensive care unit, where dexamethasone and a loading dose of phenytoin were administered. The patient was scheduled for tumor excision via stealth-guided craniotomy.

Prior to the headaches and seizure, the patient was otherwise healthy except for a history of asthma. She used an albuterol inhaler several times each week and had been taking ibuprofen for her headaches. On the morning of surgery, the patient was visibly anxious, but was alert and oriented to person, place, and time. Her cranial nerve examination was normal, pupils were equal and reactive to light, she demonstrated normal strength bilaterally and showed no pronator drift. Heart sounds were normal, but wheezing was appreciated on auscultation. Her blood pressure during the examination was 175/92, considerably elevated from

her usual baseline. Electrocardiogram and laboratory values were normal, including a therapeutic phenytoin level.

The patient's anxiety, increased blood pressure, and bronchospasm were addressed immediately. The anesthesiologist had a reassuring conversation with the patient and midazolam was administered, followed by an albuterol breathing treatment. Oxygen was delivered through a nasal cannula and she was monitored continuously with a blood pressure cuff, pulse oximeter, and by direct visualization to assure she did not experience somnolence or respiratory depression due to the benzodiazepine.

Anesthetic concerns for this patient included: (1) vigilance for any signs or symptoms of increased intracranial pressure (ICP), (2) keeping the patient as comfortable as possible during an emotionally difficult preoperative period, (3) history of asthma, (4) recent history of seizures and consequent phenytoin use, (5) maintaining proper fluid status during a procedure that could include fluid shifts both planned (diuretics) and unplanned (bleeding), and (6), the need for a timely, hemodynamically stable, and thorough awakening.

Once in the operating room induction of anesthesia was initiated with fentanyl, sodium pentothal and vecuronium; great care was taken to maintain the patient's blood pressure within 20% of baseline. The trachea was intubated with a 7.5 mm LITA (Laryngotracheal Instillation of Topical Anesthesia) endotracheal tube. An arterial catheter and two large-bore intravenous catheters were placed. General anesthesia was maintained with isoflurane and a total of approximately 10 mcg/kg of fentanyl was administered throughout the case for analgesia. The surgeons reported swelling of the brain and so the patient was hyperventilated to a $PaCO_2$ of 30 mmHg. Mannitol was administered to reduce brain volume and dexamethasone was given for the prevention of cerebral edema. There was an estimated blood loss of 1300 mL, and the patient was resuscitated with 2 liters of crystalloid, 500 mL of 5% albumin and one unit packed red blood cells. As surgical closure began, isoflurane was discontinued and infusions of propofol and remifentanil were initiated. After the surgical drapes were removed, the LITA tube was dosed with 4% lidocaine and albuterol was delivered via the endotracheal tube. The patient emerged within several minutes of the head dressing being applied, without bucking or coughing. She was neurologically intact.

Discussion

As with other complex cases, the patient presenting for supratentorial craniotomy is best served by an organized and systematic approach. Below is one strategy for the preoperative evaluation of these neurosurgical patients.

1. Stratify the case

It is first important to distinguish between the "elective" or scheduled resection of a supratentorial mass lesion and the patient presenting for emergent decompression due to intracranial hypertension. The former situation allows time for a full evaluation process [1] while the latter demands immediate attention to the "ABCs" of airway, breathing, and circulation, as well as management of increased intracranial pressure (ICP; discussed in the next chapter) [2].

2. Assess the patient

Even during the introductory process, the anesthesiologist should be assessing the patient's mental status and gross neurologic function. Are they alert or somnolent? Do they have any obvious facial asymmetry? Do they respond appropriately and with intact language skills? If the patient is interactive, obtain any history possible. If not, assess for ABCs.

Next, assess the vital signs – significant hypertension and bradycardia could be a Cushing's reflex revealing poor intracranial elastance. The physical examination that follows should focus on neurologic status, including a cranial nerve examination, assessment of the pupils and their reflexes, and motor strength. It is imperative to establish a preoperative neurologic baseline to which the postoperative status can be compared.

3. Review the chart

For a non-emergent case, there is often valuable information that can be derived from the surgical evaluation and that can help guide the preoperative anesthetic assessment. Any available neuroimaging studies should also be reviewed, with particular attention to the size and location of the lesion as well as signs of increased ICP such as midline shift, effacement of sulci and gyri, loss of gray–white differentiation, and herniation. Laboratory values should also be reviewed with particular attention to hematocrit, coagulation studies (especially in patients with hemorrhage or hematoma), sodium irregularities (common in neurosurgical patients), and glucose (which, when high, can exacerbate neural injury) [3]. Cardiac studies such as electrocardiogram or echocardiogram can provide important information, especially if the patient has suffered a stroke [3]. Review all medications, especially any anticonvulsants that could affect drug metabolism.

4. Develop a plan

Based on (1) your stratification of the case, and (2) your assessment of the patient, develop an anesthetic plan that addresses any medical issues that might be manifested in the perioperative course of a craniotomy.

Preparation: In general, an arterial catheter and large-bore intravenous lines are recommended for these cases, but especially in those involving vascular lesions and tumors with high potential for hemorrhage (such as meningiomas). Invasive blood pressure monitoring allows beat-to-beat readings and the ability to regularly assess pH status and PaCO$_2$ levels with arterial blood gases. Depending on the co-morbidities and venous access, a central line may be required. The subclavian approach is more appropriate for the neurosurgical patient, as an internal jugular catheter can potentially compromise venous return from the brain and thus increase ICP.

Ensure that commonly used agents such as mannitol, dexamethasone, and furosemide are available. Discuss anticonvulsant administration with the neurosurgical team. Phenytoin is often administered, but fosphenytoin is preferable because of decreased cardiovascular side effects. In either case, the drug should be administered slowly, as the goal is prophylaxis rather than acute termination of seizures. An anti-emetic strategy should also be established [4].

Premedication: Neurologic disease and neurosurgical intervention is a highly stressful event for the patient and the family. The need for compassion and reassurance cannot be overemphasized. Pharmacologic support can be attained using any number of drugs – it must be noted, however, that any sedative can cause respiratory depression. The patient must be monitored continuously, since a decrease in ventilation can cause an increase in CO_2 and therefore an increase in ICP via cerebral vasodilation. Sedation may also unmask or exacerbate focal neurologic deficits [5].

Anesthetic regimen: The choice of anesthetics depends on the state of intracranial elastance. Induction with propofol or sodium pentothal is appropriate, with attention to cardiovascular status. Ketamine is typically avoided, as it increases cerebral metabolic rate. In terms of maintenance, inhalational anesthetics may be used if the patient has normal intracranial elastance [6]. If the patient has compromised elastance and intracranial hypertension, then these anesthetics should be avoided. Although inhalational anesthetics reduce cerebral metabolic rate, they dilate cerebral blood vessels (nitrous > desflurane > isoflurane > sevoflurane), which increases cerebral blood volume and thus ICP. Inhalational agents can also disrupt cerebral autoregulation, which normally maintains constant cerebral blood flow (50 mL/100 g tissue/min) in the face of changing mean arterial pressures. The classically taught range of autoregulation is a mean arterial pressure of 50–150 mmHg, but the lower limit may be as high as 70 mmHg. Chronic hypertension can shift the autoregulatory curve to the right, which means that higher pressures are needed to stay in the autoregulatory range. The intravenous agents propofol and pentothal decrease cerebral metabolic rate but do not dilate cerebral blood vessels – their use is therefore recommended in patients with poor intracranial elastance and they also have minimal effects on autoregulation.

Analgesia: Appropriate pain control is imperative for patient comfort and a smooth emergence [7]. Preoperative scalp block may help reduce intraoperative opioid requirements and postoperative pain (see Case 5). Major stimulating events include intubation, cranial pinning, incision, removal of bone flap, and durotomy. An early focus on analgesia during the case is important such that opioid-associated sedation and hypoventilation are not a problem during emergence.

Emergence: All physiologic parameters should be optimized prior to emergence. There are two main strategies for achieving an emergence that occurs directly after undraping and does so without the patient undergoing hemodynamic responses that might increase the chance of intracranial hemorrhage. The first is by using, or least switching to, short-acting anesthetics and analgesics. For example, isoflurane can be turned off 1–1.5 hours prior to wake-up and replaced with remifentanil, propofol, or both. With this strategy, less remifentanil or propofol is required to achieve general anesthesia since the offset of isoflurane anesthesia is relatively slow and the stimulus of closing is minor. Remifentanil, like most narcotics, tends to soothe the airway and is especially helpful. Another method of facilitating a smooth wake-up is to decrease the stimulus of the endotracheal tube, which can be accomplished with the use of a LITA tube. The LITA allows the easy administration of lidocaine both above and below the cuff, anesthetizing the airway and thereby minimizing the irritation during wake-up. If a LITA is not available, one can place lidocaine down the endotracheal tube or into the posterior pharynx. This strategy may be especially important in patients with a reactive airway, as the patient described above. Careful planning to minimize physiologic and pharmacologic confounds in the immediate postoperative period is essential for an effective neurosurgical evaluation [8].

Conclusion

In conclusion, supratentorial craniotomy is a common case in neurosurgery during which both the neurosurgeon and anesthesiologist are modulating the same organ. Thoughtful planning and clear communication between the teams is required for optimal patient care.

References

1. **A. Schiavi, A. Papangelou, M. Mirski**. Preoperative preparation of the surgical patient with neurologic disease. *Anesthesiol Clin* 2009; **27**: 779–86.

2. **L. Rangel-Castillo, S. Gopinath, C. S. Robertson**. Management of intracranial hypertension. *Neurol Clin* 2008; **26**: 521–41.

3. **K. Lieb, M. Selim**. Preoperative evaluation of patients with neurological disease. *Semin Neurol* 2008; **28**: 603–10.

4. **L. H. Eberhart, A. M. Morin, P. Kranke** et al. Prevention and control of postoperative nausea and vomiting in post-craniotomy patients. *Best Pract Res Clin Anaesthesiol* 2007; **21**: 575–93.

5. **G. D. Thal, M. D. Szabo, M. Lopez-Bresnahan** et al. Exacerbation or unmasking of focal neurologic deficits by sedatives. *Anesthesiology* 1996; **85**: 21–5.

6.   **K. Engelhard, C. Werner**. Inhalational or intravenous anesthetics for craniotomies? Pro inhalational. *Curr Opin Anaesthesiol* 2006; **19**: 504–8.

7.   **A. Gottschalk, L. C. Berkow, R. D. Stevens** *et al.* Prospective evaluation of pain and analgesic use following major elective intracranial surgery. *J Neurosurg* 2007; **106**: 210–16.

8.   **N. Fabregas, N. Bruder**. Recovery and neurological evaluation. *Best Pract Res Clin Anaesthesiol* 2007; **21**: 431–47.

2

Evaluation and anesthetic management of elevated intracranial pressure

Andrew Bielaczyc and Paul Smythe

Understanding the appropriate interventions to manage increased intracranial pressure (ICP) is an essential skill of a neuroanesthesiologist. Intracranial pressure is of paramount importance because the cranial vault is nondistensible and within it are contained three noncompressible substances: brain, blood, and cerebrospinal fluid (CSF).

Case description

The patient was a 75-year-old male who presented for emergent subdural hematoma evacuation. During a witnessed slip and fall accident with no associated loss of consciousness, the patient suffered a left temporal contusion. Shortly after the accident he became confused and lethargic. Noncontrast head computed tomography (CT) revealed an acute right temporal subdural hematoma with 5 mm of horizontal shift. Past medical history was significant for hypertension and atrial fibrillation; current medications included coumadin, metoprolol, and lisinopril. Neurologically the patient was oriented to person only and moved all four extremities equally with full strength. No cranial nerve deficits were appreciated. The patient's blood pressure upon presentation was 155/85.

The immediate anesthetic goal was to minimize the rise in ICP while at the same time maintaining adequate cerebral perfusion pressure until the neurosurgeons could provide definitive treatment. In order to better monitor arterial pressure, a radial artery catheter was placed. Laboratory tests including type and screen, coagulation values, and complete blood count were drawn. After placement of standard monitoring and preoxygenation, general anesthesia was induced with propofol and care was taken to prevent precipitous increases in blood pressure during both laryngoscopy and placement of the head in a Mayfield frame. The patient was then positioned supine with the head of the bed elevated 30 degrees. A midline head alignment and unobstructed cervical venous drainage were ensured. Based on the patient's baseline blood pressure and estimated ICP, a mean arterial pressure (MAP) >80 mmHg was maintained in order to maintain cerebral perfusion pressure (CPP) >60 mmHg. Prior to the dura being opened, mannitol and furosemide were administered to decrease parenchymal volume. Definitive correction of intracranial hypertension was achieved with hematoma evacuation.

Discussion

The cranium is a nonexpandable bony structure with a fixed volume and therefore with only limited means of compensating for increased ICP. If pressure within that nonexpandable structure is allowed to rise the result is life-threatening neural injury. Normal ICP in the adult is <20 mmHg with a high degree of normal physiologic variability. A sustained ICP >20 mmHg should be considered pathologic and treatment should be initiated. Intracranial pressure along with MAP determine cerebral perfusion based on the equation CPP = MAP – ICP. Therefore, when managing patients with elevated ICP, adequate MAP must be achieved in order to maintain CPP >60 mm Hg. Below this threshold cerebral ischemia can occur.

The determinants of ICP are the contents of the cranium and include brain parenchyma (neurons, glia), blood (arterial and venous circulation), and fluid (interstitial and CSF). Increases in one of these volumes must be offset by decreases in the other constituent volumes or ICP will increase [1]. The magnitude of change in ICP is directly related to the intracranial elastance. As the volume of blood, fluid, or brain expands, physiologic mechanisms of compensation such as displacement of CSF out of the cranium or vasoconstriction result in relatively small increases in ICP. As intracranial elastance decreases, these mechanisms are eventually outstripped and further small increases in volume result in large increases in ICP

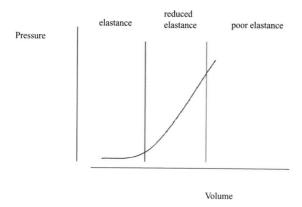

Figure 2.1. Intracranial elastance curve.

Table 2.1. Common causes of elevated intracranial pressure.

Substrate	Pathophysiology
Parenchyma	Malignancy 　Primary 　Metastatic Cerebral edema 　Cytogenic 　Vasogenic Eclampsia Fulminant hepatic failure
Blood	Subarachnoid hemorrhage Intraparenchymal hemorrhage Subdural hematoma Epidural hematoma Vasodilatation Venous outflow obstruction
Cerebrospinal fluid	Hydrocephalus CSF outflow obstruction

(Figure 2.1) [1]. A direct relationship exists between cerebral blood flow (CBF) and ICP, such that elevated ICP can be modified by decreases in CBF so long as cerebral perfusion is not compromised. If insufficient CBF results in brain ischemia, the associated cerebral edema will increase ICP, further compromising CBF and setting in motion a dangerous downward spiral.

Increased ICP is associated with many pathophysiologic states, each with the common mechanism of increasing the intracranial volume of CSF, blood, or brain tissue (Table 2.1). Increased tissue volume is caused by space-occupying lesions such as tumors, either primary or metastatic. Cerebral malignancies also increase ICP by obstructing absorption and outflow of CSF and producing cerebral edema. Cerebral edema is classified as cytogenic or vasogenic in origin. Cytogenic cerebral edema develops as the result of inadequate intracellular energy supplies resulting in failure of membrane integrity, increased cellular swelling and ultimately cell death. Vasogenic cerebral edema by comparison is the result of increased vascular permeability and the movement of protein-rich fluid into the cerebral interstitial space.

Increased intracranial blood volume elevates ICP and can present in varied forms. Subarachnoid hemorrhage is frequently caused by head trauma, disruption of aneurysms, and arteriovenous malformations. Blood in the subarachnoid space or in the ventricles impedes CSF outflow and results in ICP elevation. Intracranial hematomas, blood-filled space-occupying lesions, are classified by their location relative to the meningeal layers. Subdural hematomas are more frequently seen in elderly patients due to natural cerebral atrophy and the resulting fragility of cerebral bridging veins. Acute epidural hematomas are frequently the result of severe head trauma and produce a characteristic lenticular-shaped hemorrhage on CT scan.

Mental status can range from drowsiness to coma depending on ICP and the extent of brain tissue displacement. As ICP increases, signs and symptoms include headache, nausea, vomiting, and papilledema. Bradycardia, hypertension with widened pulse pressure, and Cheyne–Stokes breathing are referred to as Cushing's Triad, an ominous sign of decompensation. When intracranial elastance is low, further increases in ICP can result in brain tissue displacement and herniation of brain parenchyma across meningeal barriers, which heralds serious brain injury or death.

Intracranial pressure can be monitored in several ways. As described above, the clinical examination can indicate relative changes in ICP and therefore impact management. In addition, neuroimaging can be used to estimate intracranial elastance based on the degree of sulcal effacement and ventricular collapse. Invasive methods of ICP monitoring are routine; correct interpretation and management is critical. Ventricular catheters, parenchymal monitors, and subarachnoid bolts can all be placed at the bedside by trained neurosurgeons and neurointensivists. Ventricular catheters, which are considered the gold standard for ICP monitoring, can be used to drain CSF and therefore modulate ICP [1, 2]. Transduction of the ICP reveals a waveform composed of a larger P1, and smaller P2 deflections. This relationship becomes inverted as intracranial compliance decreases. The "A" wave or plateau wave is a sign of intracranial hypertension.

Numerous therapeutic maneuvers exist for lowering ICP, each with the common mechanism of decreasing the volume of one or more intracranial components. It cannot be overemphasized that all treatments of ICP carry risks and so each must be monitored closely. A rapid method of decreasing ICP is to raise the head as much as possible; this is not always possible, especially during surgery. Decreasing the size of a brain mass is not a job for the anesthesiologist; that can only be accomplished surgically or, if the mass is inoperable, perhaps by radiation or chemotherapy. Decreasing the amount of CSF can be accomplished using a ventriculostomy. Interstitial edema can be treated with corticosteroids but this is not an effective acute treatment. Reduction of cytogenic cerebral edema can be achieved with the administration of osmotic or loop diuretics. Hyperosmotic agents like mannitol increase plasma osmolarity and draw water out of tissues including across an intact blood–brain barrier. Mannitol is infused slowly at a dose of 0.25–1 g/kg and may transiently increase ICP due to increased cerebral blood volume. Maximal reduction in ICP is evident after 10–15 minutes and remains effective for two hours. Hypertonic saline, commonly used in 3% and 7.5% solution, has proved effective in decreasing ICP. However, no evidence of improved neurologic outcomes or survival has been shown [3]. The loop diuretic furosemide is used to decrease ICP by systemic diuresis and decreasing CSF production. Furosemide does not increase intravascular volume and therefore is a better choice in patients with impaired left ventricular function. Intravascular volume and electrolyte balance should be monitored closely during the administration of furosemide and diuretic therapy. Hyperventilation reduces CBF 1–2 mL/100 g/min for each 1 mmHg reduction in $PaCO_2$ and therefore reduces ICP. However, reducing end-tidal CO_2 ($ETCO_2$) below 30 mmHg is not recommended due to compromise of CBF and the development of cerebral ischemia. As discussed above, MAP, CBF, and ICP are intertwined and therefore stable hemodynamics are critical to preventing further increases in ICP. Ultimately the pathologic process underlying intracranial hypertension must be corrected.

Anesthetic management for patients with elevated ICP begins in the preoperative setting. Preoperative anxiolysis should consist of a calm environment free of unnecessary distractions and, when indicated, medication. However, administration of preoperative sedatives may cloud the neurologic examination and should be considered carefully in patients with decreased intracranial elastance as modest hypercarbia resulting from hypoventilation may dangerously increase ICP via cerebral vasodilation. Arterial and central venous catheters may need to be placed after induction of anesthesia to avoid additional patient stress.

The operating room should be a calm environment before induction, free from music, loud conversation, or undue distractions. After application of standard monitoring and thorough preoxygenation, anesthesia can be induced with a combination of agents. Succinylcholine can be used if a rapid sequence induction is required but the resulting defasciculations can produce a transient increase in ICP. Adequate depth of anesthesia should be achieved prior to tracheal intubation and a bolus of sedative hypnotic or lidocaine can be administered before laryngoscopy. After placement of the endotracheal tube and confirmation of $ETCO_2$, the patient can be modestly hyperventilated. The arterial/end-tidal CO_2 gradient should be investigated and an $ETCO_2$ of 30–35 mmHg targeted. The use of positive end-expiratory pressure to maintain oxygenation must be applied carefully. Increased intrathoracic pressures, transmitted through compliant lungs, can impede cerebral venous drainage and further increase ICP.

In order to assure a stable operative field, the patient's head may be placed in Mayfield pins. Prior to the application of pins, a bolus of sedative and or narcotic should be administered to blunt the response to this profound stimulation. Positioning for potentially lengthy neurosurgical procedures is of critical importance and should be carried out with the cooperation of members of the operative team. Patients with elevated ICP should be maintained in a neutral head position with slight reverse Trendelenburg bed tilt to ensure cerebral venous drainage [4].

Maintenance of anesthesia can be achieved with a variety of agents tailored to the patient's medical history and the presence of neurologic monitoring. All combinations should have the common traits of adequate depth, stable hemodynamics and lowered ICP. Volatile anesthetics are potent cerebral vasodilators and progressively abolish the cerebral autoregulatory curve at higher doses. However, volatile agents do decrease cerebral metabolic rate of oxygen and at modest doses do not produce significant elevations of ICP. By contrast, propofol and thiopental both reduce cerebral metabolism and decrease cerebral blood volume by vasoconstriction [5]. This combination produces a reduction in ICP. The use of neuromuscular blockers may also facilitate the management of ICP by preventing patient bucking or straining.

Conclusion

In conclusion, increased ICP can be a life-threatening condition, the definitive treatment of which is often in the hands of the neurosurgeon. It is the job of the anesthesiologist to effectively manage increased ICP until such treatment can be accomplished.

References

1. **L. A. Steiner, P. J. Andrews**. Monitoring the injured brain: ICP and CBF. *Br J Anaesth* 2006; **97**: 26–38.

2. **M. Smith**. Monitoring intracranial pressure in traumatic brain injury. *Anesth Analg* 2008; **106**: 240–8.

3. **G. F. Strandvik**. Hypertonic saline in critical care: a review of the literature and guidelines for use in hypotensive states and raised intracranial pressure. *Anaesthesia* 2009; **64**: 990–1003.

4. **I. Ng, J. Lim, H. B. Wong**. Effects of head posture on cerebral hemodynamics: its influences on intracranial pressure, cerebral perfusion pressure, and cerebral oxygenation. *Neurosurgery* 2004; **54**: 593–7.

5. **L. T. Dunn**. Raised intracranial pressure. *J Neurol Neurosurg Psychiatry* 2002, **73**: i23–7.

Craniotomy. Supratentorial craniotomy

Traumatic brain injury

Adam Brown and Paul S. Moor

Traumatic brain injury (TBI) is a leading cause of death and permanent disability in the western world and imparts a significant social burden. According to recent US statistics, of the reported annual TBI cases, approximately 50 000 patients die, 80 000 have permanent disability, and 235 000 are admitted to hospital [1]. With respect to mortality, 50% of patients who die from TBI do so within 2 hours of injury, and approximately 30% of patients admitted to a hospital with a Glasgow Coma Scale (GCS, Table 3.1) <13 will ultimately die.

The injury spectrum in TBI encompasses not only the initial insult, but includes the cascade of systemic responses and pathophysiology that occur after the focal or diffuse brain injury. Anesthesiologists are often involved throughout the care of TBI patients. It is through our effective physiologic manipulation of and pharmacologic intervention in elevated intracranial pressure (ICP), decreased cerebral perfusion pressure (CPP), secondary ischemic brain injury, and metabolic derangements, that we can positively influence patient outcome.

Case description

The patient was a 49-year-old male motorcyclist who was evaluated in the emergency room after a motor vehicle collision with an articulated truck ("Semi"). He was found prone 100 feet from the expressway with bilateral upper limb deformities, coarse respirations, and a GCS of 3. Endotracheal intubation was performed at the scene and transportation to our facility was complicated by five episodes of ventricular tachycardia, each requiring direct current cardioversion to sinus rhythm.

On arrival at the emergency room, primary survey revealed a normothermic intubated male with a patent size 7.0 mm endotracheal tube and cervical collar in place; breath sounds and chest excursion were equal bilaterally. Pulse oximetry revealed saturations of 100% on 15 liters oxygen, via nonrebreather mask. Five-lead EKG monitoring showed sinus tachycardia of 110 beats per minute without ectopy. Neurologically the patient was moving all four limbs spontaneously and purposefully, prior to anesthesia for computed tomography (CT) scan. Standard monitoring was applied and large bore intravenous access was obtained in two limbs; radial artery cannulation afforded invasive arterial blood pressure monitoring, as well as assessment of adequate gas exchange, balanced electrolytes and blood glucose. The patient was stabilized, sedated, and transferred for CT scanning.

Ongoing monitoring of pupillary size and reactivity was also maintained prior to direct ICP measurement. In the paralyzed and sedated patient, such clinical signs were indicative of tentorial herniation.

Noncontrast head CT revealed a right-sided epidural hematoma (Figure 3.1). Preliminary evaluation of the CT revealed no fractures or malalignments of the cervical spine. The preliminary review of the CT of the chest, abdomen, and pelvis revealed evidence of numerous, but stable, pelvic fractures and a right humeral fracture.

Around the time of CT scanning, the patient's right pupil became dilated and unreactive (6 mm unreactive right vs 3 mm reactive left). He was subsequently transported to the operating room for immediate craniotomy, evacuation of the extradural hematoma, and ventriculostomy insertion. The primary concern of the anesthesia team was poor intracranial elastance, increased ICP and potentially inadequate cerebral perfusion in the face of hemorrhagic hypovolemia. The team was also focused on the prevention of secondary brain injury [2, 3]. This required vigilance for and prevention of hypotension, hypoxia, hypercarbia, hyperthermia, and hyperglycemia, as these derangements contribute to enhanced parenchymal injury. A further concern, heightened by the mechanism of injury and polytrauma, was the suspicion of an accompanying

Table 3.1. Glasgow Coma Score.

Score	Infant <1 year	Child 1–4 years	Age 4–adult
Eyes			
4	Open spontaneously	Open spontaneously	Open spontaneously
3	To voice	To voice	To voice
2	To pain	To pain	To pain
1	No response	No response	No response
Verbal			
5	"Coos, babbles"	"Oriented, speaks, interacts, social"	Oriented and alert
4	"Irritable cry, consolable"	"Confused speech, disoriented, consolable"	Disoriented
3	Cries persistently to pain	"Inappropriate words, inconsolable"	Nonsensical speech
2	Moans to pain	"Incomprehensible, agitated"	"Moans, unintelligible"
1	No response	No response	No response
Motor			
6	"Normal, spontaneous movement"	"Normal, spontaneous movement"	Follows commands
5	Withdraws to touch	Localizes pain	Localizes pain
4	Withdraws to pain	Withdraws to pain	Withdraws to pain
3	Decorticate flexion	Decorticate flexion	Decorticate flexion
2	Decerebrate extension	Decerebrate extension	Decerebrate extension
1	No response	No response	No response

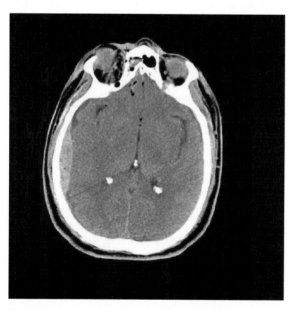

Figure 3.1. Head computed tomography demonstrating right epidural hematoma.

cervical spinal cord injury without radiologic abnormality and possibly unstable neck.

On arrival in the operating room, it was noted that despite adequate oxygen saturation by SpO$_2$, the endotracheal tube had migrated down the right main bronchus; this was corrected swiftly. Mannitol 1 g/kg was administered to acutely treat his increased ICP and tentorial herniation. Despite an apparently normal cervical CT scan, an occult injury could not be excluded

in our patient due to the mechanism of injury and the presence of an injury above the clavicle. As a result cervical immobilization continued throughout his course of care. Central venous access was obtained and after final confirmation of intended surgery, surgical anesthesia was carefully induced with propofol and fentanyl. Anesthesia was maintained with a propofol infusion, as well as vecuronium for paralysis. The goal for CPP was >60 mmHg. Initial arterial blood gas analysis demonstrated a metabolic acidemia and hyperglycemia (186 mg/dL). Compensatory efforts were thus made by increasing minute ventilation and an insulin infusion was started with a target blood glucose level of 120 mg/dL. Patient temperature was initially 34.2 °C rising through the procedure to 36.3 °C with forced air warming. On subsequent lavage of the epidural hematoma, bleeding from an epidural artery became evident and two units of packed red blood cells were transfused in response to a hematocrit of 22%. The remainder of the surgery was uneventful and the patient was transferred to a neurosurgical intensive care unit, still intubated and sedated.

Discussion

Traumatic brain injuries can be diffuse or focal, and result from multiple traumatic mechanisms. Diffuse brain injury includes diffuse axonal injury, hypoxic brain injury, brain swelling, and brain hemorrhages. Focal brain injury includes contusions, avulsions, hematomas, hemorrhages, infarctions, and infections. All of the above can lead to brain edema and all can increase ICP.

The severity of the initial injury, as defined by the GCS, is predictive of eventual outcome. For example, an admission GCS of 9–15 carries a low risk of developing intracranial hypertension. However, the relationship between GCS and survival is nonlinear, with a high rate of mortality for GCS 3–7, and a decline in mortality between GCS 8–15 [4].

Both military and civilian data support the correlation between initial (field) GCS and eventual outcome, despite them seeming disparate patient populations and mechanisms of injury. Mortality of American military service members with severe head trauma is 65% for GCS from 3–5, and 10% for GCS from 6–8. Of the survivors, progression to an independent living status is <10% for GCS from 3–5, and 60% for GCS from 6–8.

On completion of the ATLS primary survey the clinician's focus should remain on the provision of homeostasis for salvageable brain tissue. Such actions minimize secondary hypoxic brain damage and are essential in all phases of the patient's care. For our patient this began in the prehospital arena, with endotracheal intubation at the scene, rapid establishment of intravenous access, and fluid loading to resuscitate the hypovolemic polytrauma patient. Efforts should be directed at the treatment of increased ICP and the maintenance of adequate CPP (>60 mmHg), to drive perfusion to salvageable brain parenchyma and prevent secondary brain injury. Traumatic brain injury is often associated with polytrauma, which makes maintaining an adequate CPP difficult, especially in the face of concomitant traumatic hypovolemia and hemorrhage.

Efforts to re-establish and maintain normotension should be aggressive in head injury. It is well documented that just a single episode of systolic blood pressure <90 mmHg has a direct negative effect on patient outcome after TBI. Hypoxic cerebral damage, a common postmortem finding in TBI, is associated with arterial hypoxemia, decreased mean arterial pressure, or cerebral hypoperfusion, occurring as a consequence of shock, intracranial hypertension, or cerebral vasospasm. The vulnerability of TBI patients to cerebral ischemia (defined as inadequate cerebral oxygen delivery), hypotension, and reduced CPP most likely occurs due to many factors, including regions of brain tissue with precariously low cerebral blood flow and defective autoregulatory ability and underscores the need for maintenance of CPP. Such concerns over CPP maintenance should influence the choice of induction agent, a subject that has long been debated. The requirement for a cardiostable induction is clear; current opinion suggests the consideration of agents like ketamine, that have long been discouraged as a result of a transient rise in ICP. It is argued that the effects on ICP may well be attenuated by the subsequent cardiostability and reversal of hypoxia and hypercarbia [5].

The maintenance of oxygenation (maintain SpO_2 >90%), normocarbia or mild hypocarbia, normothermia (maintain temperature of 37 °C) and normoglycemia are vital actions. An increase in body (and thus brain) temperature is associated with an increase in metabolism, blood flow, and oxygen utilization, which can exacerbate potential brain ischemia. Current evidence for the role of hypothermia in TBI is inconclusive. Overall if hypothermia is initiated within 60 minutes of injury and maintained for 48 hours, it appears to confer some benefit on neurologic outcome in severe TBI patients.

As the brain is an obligate glucose user, hyperglycemia is associated with an increase in cerebral metabolism. Due to the decreased CBF subsequent to polytrauma and shock, hyperglycemia can result in increased anaerobic metabolism, changes in pH, and worse outcome [3]. As a result, glycemic control with insulin is often indicated. Additionally, all of the above pathologic processes interact synergistically, which ultimately can produce a greater deficit than could be attributed to the primary central nervous system injury alone.

In our patient, the epidural hematoma represented a neurosurgical emergency for hemorrhage control. Unchecked hematoma expansion led to elevated ICP and clinical signs such as an ipsilateral dilated pupil (due to herniation with dysfunction of cranial nerve III). These events could have led to further brain herniation and death in our patient without immediate pharmacologic intervention or decompression.

Given the mechanisms of injury that result in TBI, it is not surprising that spinal cord injuries often accompany TBI. With GCS < 8, a high index of suspicion for concomitant cervical spine injury must be maintained. Appropriate spinal stabilization techniques should be taken to help improve the chances of neurologic recovery.

Conclusion

The management of TBI patients requires swift physiologic and/or surgical manipulation in order to reduce the impact of primary injury on the remainder of the brain. Regardless of the apparent prognosis, resuscitation should proceed aggressively, keeping in mind the vulnerability of the acutely injured CNS to systemic insults. Definitive airway control, while maintaining a neutral cervical spine (due to the need for suspected concomitant spinal cord injury) should be instituted immediately. Hemodynamic resuscitation must be accomplished promptly, to maintain normal perfusion and normal CPP and because cerebral ischemia or intracranial hypertension may result from inadequately treated shock. Although a definitively effective neuroprotective therapy in CNS trauma remains elusive, through the skilled interactions of prehospital, emergency department, anesthesiology, and surgical personnel, the lives of many critically injured individuals can be saved and their neurologic function preserved.

References

1. **N. Badjatia, N. Carney, T. J. Crocco** et al. Guidelines for prehospital management of traumatic brain injury. 2nd edition. *Prehosp Emerg Care* 2008; **12**: S1–52.

2. **I. K. Moppett**. Traumatic brain injury: assessment, resuscitation and early management. *Br J Anaesth* 2007; **99**: 18–31.

3. **Brain Trauma Foundation**. American Association of Neurological Surgeons; Congress of Neurological Surgeons; Joint Section on Neurotrauma and Critical Care, AANS/CNS. Guidelines for the management of severe traumatic brain injury. *J Neurotrauma* 2007; **24** Suppl. 1: S1–95.

4. **P. Udekwu, S. Kromhout-Schiro, S. Vaslef** et al. Glasgow Coma Scale score, mortality, and functional outcome in head-injured patients. *J Trauma* 2004; **56**: 1084–9.

5. **C. Morris, A. Perris, J. Klein** et al. Anaesthesia in haemodynamically compromised emergency patients: does ketamine represent the best choice of induction agent? *Anaesthesia* 2009; **64**: 532–9.

4

Postoperative seizure

Allen Keebler

Postoperative seizures are a relatively common occurrence after surgery. They are very common in the intensive care unit, even in patients without a primary neurologic diagnosis. The incidence has been reported to be as high as 12% in this setting. In the postcraniotomy patient the causes are more likely related to the procedure itself, while in the general critical-care population without a primary neurologic diagnosis the most common cause is a metabolic disturbance [1].

Case description

A 56-year-old female presented for resection of a 2 cm by 2.5 cm mass in the right temporal lobe. She was brought to the emergency room after her first seizure three days prior, when the mass was discovered and she was scheduled for a craniotomy. She was started on phenytoin for seizure prophylaxis. Magnetic resonance imaging demonstrated the lesion in question and a mild decrease in ventricular size with no evidence of midline shift. Her past medical history included hypertension, which was well controlled with an angiotensin receptor blocker. Past surgical history showed a hysterectomy for dysfunctional uterine bleeding at age 46 that was uneventful. Laboratory testing showed only a mild anemia.

The patient was brought to the operating room for a scheduled resection of the tumor under general endotracheal anesthesia. After an uneventful induction with propofol and endotracheal intubation facilitated with rocuronium, anesthesia was maintained with isoflurane and fentanyl boluses. An arterial catheter and two large-bore intravenous catheters were inserted. The initial dissection was unremarkable, but during resection of the tumor the surgical team had difficulty with hemostasis. The acute blood loss was estimated at about 1.5 liters for which 2 units of packed red blood cells and 500 mL albumin 5% were infused for a final hematocrit of 28%. After an uneventful closure neuromuscular blockade was reversed and emergence was begun with 100 mg lidocaine administered through the endotracheal tube. Despite a gentle emergence the patient began to cough on the endotracheal tube and became hypertensive. Nitroglycerin boluses were given, the tube was removed and the patient normalized. The initial neurologic examination was favorable.

The patient was then transported to the postanesthesia care unit on 2 L nasal cannula where her neurologic exam was still unremarkable. After 20 minutes in the unit she had a grand mal seizure. Midazolam was administered and the seizure was terminated, but she was now lethargic and combative. Over the next 10 minutes her blood pressure began to rise and she became bradycardic with a heart rate of around 48.

Discussion

The causes of postoperative seizure are many. The most common causes seen in the postoperative period are listed in Table 4.1. Regardless of the cause, seizures need to be treated rapidly as they represent an acute imbalance between cerebral oxygen supply and demand and if uncorrected can lead to irreversible neuronal damage. Benzodiazepines, barbiturates, and propofol are all acceptable choices for seizure lysis [2].

The key to successful treatment is early seizure lysis as well as correct diagnosis and treatment of the underlying cause. The initial differential must include the most life-threatening possibilities. Adequate oxygenation and ventilation must first be confirmed. Bleeding within the cranial vault must be ruled out if the neurologic exam worsens or vital signs are ominous (i.e., Cushing reflex). In this case, hypertension and bradycardia represented worrisome signs of an uncompensated increase in intracranial pressure. This is a critical time because often there is a reflex reaction to treat the hypertension, which would be a grave mistake in this situation. The brain is an organ that autoregulates blood flow. In this case the brain requires the

Table 4.1. Causes of seizures in postoperative patients.

Physiologic factors	Hypoxia, hypercarbia, ischemia
Metabolic disorders	Eclampsia, sodium imbalance, phosphate imbalance, calcium imbalance, renal dysfunction, hepatic dysfunction
Medications	Antibiotics, antipsychotics, local anesthetics, cocaine, amphetamines, phencylidine
Drug withdrawal	Barbiturates, benzodiazepines, alcohol, opioids
Infection	Febrile seizures, abscess, encephalitis
Traumatic head injury	Hemorrhage or contusion
Surgical injury	Cortical irritation from craniotomy or endovascular cranial intervention

higher blood pressure to continue to perfuse because it is being opposed by the increase in the pressure within the cranial vault. Lowering this patient's blood pressure may result in brain ischemia and irreversible brain damage. If bleeding is indeed believed to be the issue such as in this case, surgical decompression with or without imaging can be employed. If imaging is used, computed tomography scan is the modality of choice as it can be obtained and performed quickly.

If imaging does not confirm the diagnosis of hemorrhage, other etiologies must be considered. Electrolytes should be measured. In cases of massive transfusion citrate toxicity may occur and cause hypocalcemia and seizures. Citrate is added to stored blood to bind calcium and prevent coagulation of the stored blood. If enough blood is given, serum calcium levels can fall low enough to cause a seizure. Sodium imbalance may also be present and serum/urine sodium levels are helpful. Should prophylactic antiepileptics have been given in the operating room? Depending on the dose and route of administration of the antiepileptic given, therapeutic levels may not have been achieved by the time of operation. This may simply be cortical irritation from the surgery because of nontherapeutic levels of the antiepileptic. A thorough medication review and discussion with the surgical team will help you decide on the prophylaxis to be given.

In this case, the cause was found to be a subdural hematoma at the surgical site and the patient returned to the operating room for decompression. The patient's emergence was less than desirable during the initial operation. Could we do anything different from an anesthesia perspective to make this emergence better? While administration of lidocaine intratracheally or intravenously may be of use, it may also lower the seizure threshold. Some advocate a remifentanil infusion be used intraoperatively as it can provide a smooth emergence and because of its short half life a quick return to neurologic baseline. One can also consider extubating the patient under deep anesthesia and emerging the patient without an entotracheal tube in place. This technique is not without risk. The risks include aspiration, laryngospasm if the patient is not deeply anesthetized, inability to ventilate and the need to reintubate along with its undesirable hemodynamic changes. These risks make this technique one to be considered only when the benefits truly outweigh the risks. These techniques can be used in an attempt to make the emergence smooth. However, there is no guarantee and emergence can still be unpredictable.

Conclusion

Postoperative seizures can have physiologic, pharmacologic, and pathologic causes. Immediate termination of the seizure should be followed by a rapid assessment of reversible physiologic causes and then a more extensive differential to identify the underlying source.

References

1. **M. A. Mirski**. Seizures and status epilepticus in the critically ill. *Critical Care Clinics* 2008; **24**: 115–47.

2. **T. P. Bleck**. Intensive care unit management of status epilepticus. *Epilepsia* 2007; **48**: 59–60.

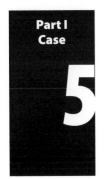

Pain management for craniotomies

Paul E. Hilliard and Chad M. Brummett

The perioperative pain management for craniotomies can be extremely challenging. Patients often present with other significant co-morbidities that can affect their anesthetic management and complicate postoperative pain therapy. While it is essential to keep patients comfortable and hemodynamically stable, it is often equally important that they be responsive to postoperative neurologic examination. In this chapter, we present a common clinical scenario and offer options for perioperative pain management.

Case description

A 52-year-old female American Society of Anesthesiologists class 3 patient presented for clipping of a cerebral aneurysm. She was morbidly obese (body mass index = 36) and carried diagnoses of obstructive sleep apnea and refractory gastroesophageal reflux disease. She had a history of postoperative nausea and vomiting requiring hospitalization after an elective surgical procedure. In addition, she had hypertension, with a baseline blood pressure of 140/80 and described shortness of breath after climbing one flight of stairs.

The primary concerns for the anesthesiology team in this case were (1) airway management in a morbidly obese patient with severe gastroesophageal reflux disease, (2) maintaining hemodynamic stability during laryngoscopy and incision in this patient with a cerebral aneurysm, and (3) pain management in a patient with sleep apnea, obesity and a history of postoperative nausea and vomiting.

In preparation for the stimulation associated with intubation, a radial arterial line was placed prior to induction. A rapid sequence intubation was performed with a bolus of esmolol prior to laryngoscopy to prevent hemodynamic derangement. After a smooth induction, an additional dose of fentanyl was given prior to performing a scalp nerve blockade (described below). Anesthesia was maintained with dexmedetomidine, propofol, and sufentanil infusions. The nerve

block was completed uneventfully and without hemodynamic compromise and adequate time was allowed for the block to take effect. The patient maintained a stable blood pressure during insertion of Mayfield pins and had no response to incision or calvarial contact. The case was completed without incident, multiple anti-emetics were administered, and the trachea was extubated in the operating room. The patient completed a normal neurologic examination. She had an uneventful recovery in the hospital with no nausea, and her pain was well controlled with minimal opioid medication.

Discussion

The case described above is a common example of the complexity frequently associated with neurosurgical patients. The combined regimen provided for analgesia and hemodynamic control, while allowing for an adequate neurologic examination. In addition, opioids were limited, thereby decreasing the risk of postoperative nausea and vomiting.

Intravenous analgesics

Opioids are a key component of intraoperative and postoperative pain management for craniotomies. Fentanyl is the most commonly used analgesic due to its rapid onset of action and hemodynamic stability. Morphine can cause histamine release, which can lead to venodilation and subsequent hypotension. Remifentanil has become a very popular option due to its ultra-short half life and ease of titration; however, longer-acting opioids must be given after the infusion is stopped. Sufentanil is more potent than fentanyl and has a duration of action between that of remifentanil and fentanyl.

Dexmedetomidine is an alpha-2-adrenoceptor agonist that is frequently used in neurosurgical anesthesia [1]. Whereas dexmedetomidine will not suffice as a sole anesthetic, it provides sedation, anxiolysis,

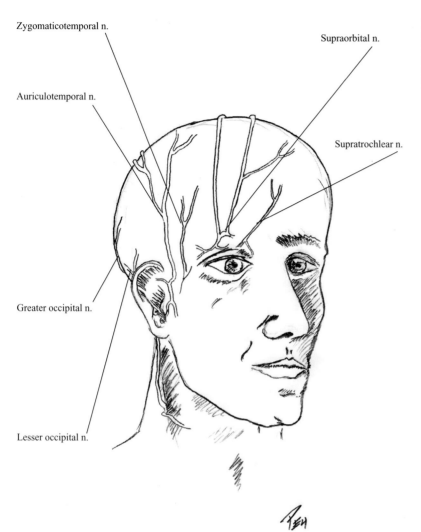

Zygomaticotemporal n.

Supraorbital n.

Auriculotemporal n.

Supratrochlear n.

Greater occipital n.

Lesser occipital n.

Figure 5.1. Innervation of the scalp. Blockade of the superficial nerves innervating the scalp can be easily accomplished with a small volume of local anesthetic using anatomic landmarks.

and analgesia with minimal respiratory depression. The sedation associated with dexmedetomidine has been termed "cooperative sedation." The calm and cooperative nature of patients on dexmedetomidine can be ideal for postoperative neurologic examination. Although it has not been demonstrated in humans, there are multiple laboratory studies demonstrating that it is also neuroprotective in animal models of cerebral and spinal cord ischemia.

Regional anesthesia

In 1918 Harvey Cushing used local infiltration for craniotomy in head-injury patients. He also mapped the sensory distribution of the trigeminal nerve and coined the term "regional anesthesia."$^\phi$ Since

that time the "scalp block" has continued to evolve. Approximately 60–80% of patients experience moderate to severe pain after craniotomy [2]. Blockade of the scalp is an effective, simple regional anesthetic technique that significantly improves patient comfort after craniotomy [3]. The use of regional anesthetic techniques for pain control is generally desirable when compared with opioid-based therapy, which can be associated with nausea and vomiting; such side effects are particularly problematic in neurosurgical patients. Additionally, a scalp block after induction of anesthesia and prior to placement of Mayfield head pins has been shown to significantly blunt hemodynamic response to pinning [4]. This is of obvious benefit in patients with an intracranial aneurysm, vascular anomaly or mass effect causing increased

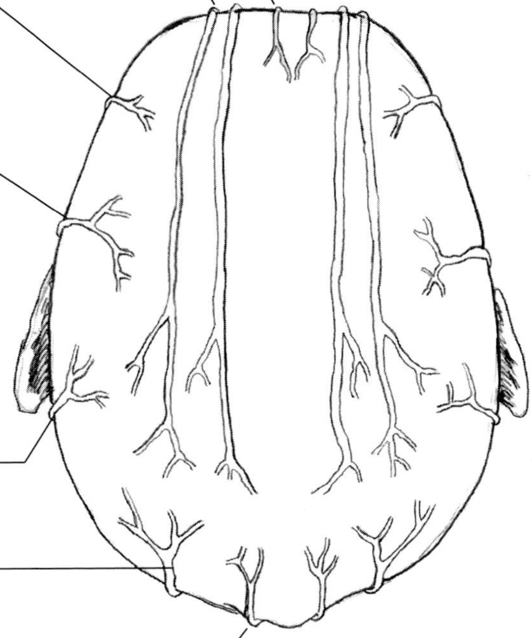

Supratrochlear n. —

Supraorbital n.

Zygomaticotemporal n.

Auriculo-
temporal n.

Lesser occipital n. —

Greater occipital n. —

Third occipital n. —

Figure 5.1. (cont.)

intracranial pressure. While regional anesthesia in this situation would appear to be an attractive option, it may not have significant impact on postoperative opioid requirements for pain control. Recently, a small prospective analysis of perioperative skull blockade failed to demonstrate significant benefit when compared with patients treated with a remifentanil infusion, which was titrated to blunt hemodynamic response during pin insertion [5].

Scalp blockade is generally performed after induction of anesthesia and preferably prior to noxious stimulation (placement of head in pins, incision, periostial-dural contact) and/or at the end of surgery, prior to awakening. This blockade provides anesthesia to the peripheral nerves that innervate the scalp. These include the greater and lesser occipital nerves, the supraorbital and supratrochlear nerves (from cranial nerve V, first division), the zygomaticotemporal nerves (from cranial nerve V, second division), the auriculotemporal nerves (from cranial nerve V, third divi-

sion), and the greater auricular nerves that arise from the superficial cervical plexus (Figure 5.1).

Blockade of the supraorbital and supratrochlear nerves are accomplished with 2 mL of local anesthetic solution as the nerves emerge from the orbit using a 23- or 25-gauge needle introduced above the eyebrow perpendicular to the skin. The auriculotemporal nerves are blocked with 5 mL of anesthetic injected 1.5 cm anterior to the ear at the level of the tragus by introducing the needle perpendicular to the skin and infiltrating along the deep and superficial fascia. The postauricular branches of the greater auricular nerve are blocked with 2 mL of local anesthetic between the skin and bone located 1.5 cm posterior to the ear at the level of the tragus. The greater and lesser occipital nerves can be blocked with 5 mL of local anesthetic introduced by infiltration technique along the superior nuchal line, approximately halfway between the occipital protruberance and mastoid process. The greater occipital nerve lies in a groove, the occipital notch, which can be palpated just lateral to the external occipital protuberance. Mild pressure should be applied at the site of injection for approximately 1 minute to decrease the risk of a hematoma.

Long-acting local anesthetics, such as bupivacaine or ropivacaine, should be used to maximize the duration of analgesia. If the speed of onset is important, as is needed to blunt hemodynamic response to head pinning, lidocaine can be added to the solution. Unlike other regional anesthesia techniques, motor stimulation is not required to complete the block. Therefore, in long cases, the nerve blocks can be repeated after surgery to maximize the duration of analgesia and improve the immediate postoperative course.

Regional anesthesia has a limited but important role in anesthetic management of the neurosurgical patient. These blocks are relatively simple to perform and may offer significant advantages, such as management of an awake patient, blunted hemodynamic response to pin insertion, and improved postoperative pain control with less need for opioid analgesics. The blocks described above are limited to superficial structures and are associated with a low rate of complications. The neuroanesthesiologist must weigh the risk and benefit of each block, but they are clearly a valuable asset.

Conclusion

In conclusion, craniotomies are often challenging cases with a number of important anesthetic consid-erations. A combination of intravenous analgesics and regional anesthesia can provide excellent pain relief and decrease the wide hemodynamic changes that can accompany anesthesia and surgery.

References

1. **A. Bekker, M. K. Sturaitis.** Dexmedetomidine for neurological surgery. *Neurosurgery* 2005; **57**: 1–10.

2. **G. De Benedittis, A. Lorenzetti, M. Migliore** *et al.* Postoperative pain in neurosurgery: a pilot study in brain surgery. *Neurosurgery* 1996; **38**: 466–9.

3. **A. Nguyen, F. Girard, D. Boudreault** *et al.* Scalp nerve blocks decrease the severity of pain after craniotomy. *Anesth Analg* 2001; **93**: 1272–6.

4. **M. L. Pinosky, R. L. Fishman, S. T. Reeves** *et al.* The effect of bupivacaine skull block on the hemodynamic response to craniotomy. *Anesth Analg* 1996; **83**: 1256–61.

5. **F. M. Gazoni, N. Pouratian, E. C. Nemergut.** Effect of ropivacaine skull block on perioperative outcomes in patients with supratentorial brain tumors and comparison with remifentanil: a pilot study. *J Neurosurg* 2008; **109**: 44–9.

Endnote

ɸ   http://www.scalpblock.com/, 2007, Irene P. Osborne, MD, Last accessed December 5, 2009.

Craniotomy. Posterior fossa craniotomy

Preoperative evaluation

George A. Mashour

The posterior fossa is an intracranial compartment that houses the cerebellum and the brainstem. Mass lesions and increased intracranial pressure (ICP) in this area can have profound consequences for neurologic, cardiac, and respiratory functions (Table 6.1).

Case description

The patient was a 54-year-old female who presented to her primary-care physician with complaints of headaches, progressive hearing loss and episodes of aspiration that were increasing in frequency. The patient was referred to a neurologist. Computed tomography and magnetic resonance imaging were performed, revealing bilateral acoustic neuromas. A diagnosis of neurofibromatosis type 2 was made and a posterior fossa craniotomy was scheduled. The patient's husband reported that her voice was hoarse and she had become increasingly somnolent in the preceding 24 hours. Physical examination revealed a somnolent but arousable patient who had difficulty hearing. The patient reported headaches when asked to extend her neck for an airway evaluation.

Immediate concerns for the anesthetic team included (1) a depressed level of consciousness, (2) the potential for increased ICP, and (3) aspiration on induction. Intravenous and arterial line access was obtained and the patient was transported to the operating room. The head of the bed was elevated to ensure adequate venous drainage and no premedication was given in order to avoid hypoventilation. A rapid sequence induction with propofol and succinylcholine was achieved without difficulty. Further large-bore intravenous access was obtained and sevoflurane was used for maintenance anesthesia. A remifentanil infusion was initiated because of the need to avoid neuromuscular blockade for cranial nerve monitoring.

With the exception of several episodes of transient vagal asystole, the case proceeded without difficulty.

Table 6.1. Diseases of the posterior fossa.

Extra-axial	Intra-axial
Schwannoma	Medulloblastoma
Nerve sheath tumors	Cerebellar astrocytoma
Clival tumors	Brainstem glioma
Arachnoid cysts	Ependymoma
Glomus jugulare tumors	Choroid plexus papilloma/Carcinoma
Epidermoid cysts	Dermoid tumors
Epidermoid tumors	Hemangioblastoma
Meningioma	Metastatic disease
Fatty lesions	Astrocytoma
Leptomeningeal diseases	Lymphoma
	Infection/inflammatory
	Vascular
	Metabolic

At the end of the case the sevoflurane and remifentanil were discontinued and no long-acting opioid had been administered for several hours. However, the patient failed to emerge. Irregular respiratory patterns were observed and the patient was not following commands. Laboratory values from 15 minutes prior to the end of the case revealed normal glucose and electrolytes. An arterial blood gas sample was analyzed, which demonstrated normal pH, CO_2, and O_2. After ruling out physiologic and pharmacologic causes, an emergent computed tomography scan was performed demonstrating hemorrhage in the posterior fossa. The patient was brought back to the operating room for re-exploration and hemostasis.

Discussion

Neurosurgical procedures involving the posterior fossa can be challenging for both the surgical and anesthetic teams. It is imperative to understand the vital

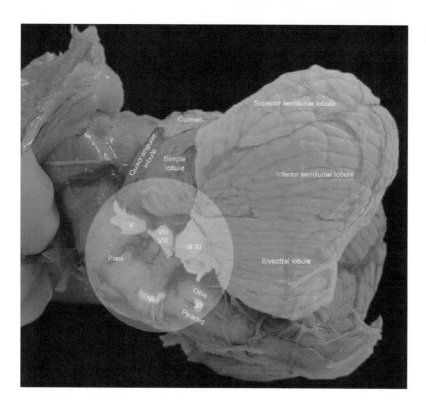

Figure 6.1. Structures of the cerebellopontine angle.

structures housed within this small compartment in order to best evaluate the patient in the preoperative setting.

Medulla

In addition to the ascending and descending fiber bundles that traverse the medulla, there are important cardiac and respiratory centers. Compression or dysfunction of the medulla can therefore have catastrophic consequences.

Pons

The pons contains several critical nuclei that serve to arouse the cerebral cortex [1] including the noradrenergic locus ceruleus, the serotonergic dorsal raphe, and the cholinergic laterodorsal and pedunculopontine tegmentum. Activity of these and other arousal centers is necessary for consciousness. Thus, compression or dysfunction of the pons can be associated with decreased levels of consciousness, as seen in our patient preoperatively.

Fourth ventricle

The fourth ventricle connects the spinal and cerebral subarachnoid compartments, across which cerebrospinal fluid normally communicates. Mass lesions in the posterior fossa may therefore lead to a noncommunicating hydrocephalus resulting in increased ICP.

Cerebellopontine angle

Lesions of the cerebellopontine angle (such as acoustic neuromas, which technically should be referred to as vestibular schwannomas) can compress the cranial nerves exiting from the brainstem (Figure 6.1). One of the most important of these nerves from the perspective of the anesthesiologist is the vagus or cranial nerve X. The significance is 2-fold. First, intraoperative compression or traction on the vagus can cause asystole, which is best terminated by cessation of surgery until the heart rate returns. The other point of significance relates to the superior and recurrent laryngeal nerves, which arise from the vagus. Since these innervate the glottis, dysfunction can result in difficulties with control of the airway, leading to chronic aspiration as well as aspiration pneumonia [2]. Impaired gag reflex during preoperative evaluation indicates dysfunction of cranial nerves IX or X.

Cerebellum

Disorders of the cerebellum will manifest as ataxia, dysmetria, intention tremor, and wide-based gait.

Vasculature

Aneurysms and arteriovenous malformations are also found in the posterior fossa; cerebellar infarctions and hematomas may occur.

In addition to the general preoperative evaluation, attention to level of consciousness, cardiorespiratory abnormalities, signs of intracranial hypertension, and airway control are of paramount importance with lesions in the posterior fossa. Complications of posterior fossa procedures include bleeding from venous sinuses, vagal asystole, venous air embolism, seizures, and delayed emergence [3]. Care should be taken to (1) obtain large-bore peripheral access or central venous access if necessary, (2) obtain arterial line for beat-to-beat blood pressure monitoring, (3) use appropriate monitors for air emboli, depending on the positioning, and (4) develop a strategy for prompt emergence from anesthesia such that any pathology can be rapidly identified. Brainstem auditory evoked potentials and facial nerve monitoring are common during posterior fossa procedures. Unlike somatosensory or motor evoked potentials, brainstem potentials are remarkably resistant to the effects of inhalational anesthetics [4]. As such, the only important modulation of the anesthetic plan relates to neuromuscular blockade, which should be avoided if the facial nerve is being monitored. Opioid infusions such as the remifentanil used in our case can aid in maintaining a quiescent surgical field.

Conclusion

In conclusion, the posterior fossa contains important neural structures that control essential functions such as cardiac and respiratory modulation, cortical arousal, and airway control. Preoperative assessment and preparation of these patients should focus on the consequences of posterior fossa abnormalities as well as the potentially life-threatening complications that may occur intraoperatively.

References

1. **N. P. Franks**. General anaesthesia: from molecular targets to neuronal pathways of sleep and arousal. *Nat Rev Neurosci* 2008; **9**: 370–86.

2. **S. N. Shenoy, A. Raja**. Acute aspiration pneumonia due to bulbar palsy: an initial manifestation of posterior fossa convexity meningioma. *J Neurol Neurosurg Psychiatry* 2005; **76**; 296–8.

3. **G. P. Rath, P. K. Bithal, A. Chaturvedi** *et al*. Complications related to positioning in posterior fossa craniectomy. *J Clin Neurosci* 2007; **14**: 520–5.

4. **M. Banoub, J. E. Tetzlaff, A. Schubert**. Pharmacologic and physiologic influences affecting sensory evoked potentials: implications for perioperative monitoring. *Anesthesiology* 2003; **99**: 716–37.

Craniotomy. Posterior fossa craniotomy

Air embolism

Jennifer Vance and Sheron Beltran

A venous air embolism (VAE) is a potentially life-threatening event caused by air in the vascular system. The entrainment of air from an operative site into the venous vasculature produces a wide array of systemic effects. The incidence is difficult to estimate due to the fact that many cases are subclinical. In addition, detection is dependent upon the sensitivity of the equipment used during the procedure.

Case description

The patient was a 37-year-old female with a right-sided acoustic neuroma presenting for a suboccipital approach to tumor resection. Her past medical history was positive for obstructive sleep apnea treated with a continuous positive airway pressure device, obesity with a body mass index of 35, and a history of a difficult airway with a previous Cormack–Lehane Grade IV view on laryngoscopy. Neurophysiologic monitoring of brainstem auditory evoked responses and cranial nerve function was planned.

The primary anesthetic concerns were (1) management of the known difficult laryngoscopy, (2) anesthetic maintenance consistent with successful neurophysiologic monitoring, and (3) prompt emergence to enable rapid assessment of any pathologic events in the cerebellopontine angle. In preparation for the awake fiberoptic intubation, glycopyrrolate was given as the antisialogogue. This was followed by nebulized and atomized 4% lidocaine for airway topicalization. A remifentanil infusion provided sedation for the procedure. After confirmation of endotracheal intubation, maintenance anesthesia was achieved by a remifentanil infusion, isoflurane and nitrous oxide each at 0.5 minimum alveolar concentration. The patient was placed in the lateral park bench position and the case proceeded without complication until 2 hours after surgical incision when the anesthesia team noticed a simultaneous fall in end-tidal carbon dioxide (ETCO$_2$), oxygen saturation, and blood pressure. The oxygen saturation dropped from 99% to a nadir of 68%, the ETCO$_2$ dropped from 30 to 18 mmHg, and the blood pressure fell from 110/60 to 75/40. Extra assistance was immediately called to the room, the patient was placed on 100% oxygen, and after the surgeons were notified of probable VAE they proceeded to flood the surgical field with normal saline. The patient was placed in the head down position and a valsalva maneuver was delivered. Phenylephrine was bolused for blood pressure support. The endotracheal tube was visualized and its position appeared unchanged. The patient remained easy to ventilate with no suspicion of airway obstruction. With the above maneuvers, the patient's condition rapidly improved and returned to baseline within 6 minutes. As the patient stabilized, the decision was made to proceed with a precordial Doppler in place for the rest of the case. The surgery continued without further complication and the trachea was uneventfully extubated at the end of the operation; the patient was neurologically intact.

Discussion

Venous air embolism was historically most often associated with craniotomies performed in the sitting position. It has been estimated that VAE occurs in up to 40% of sitting posterior fossa craniotomies, although the majority of these do not result in hemodynamic compromise [1]. A combination of factors results in the increased risk for air entrainment during neurosurgical procedures. Unlike most of the venous system, the dural sinuses and bridging epidural veins are noncollapsible structures that remain open to the surrounding atmosphere. The height of the surgical site above the right side of the heart also contributes to the likelihood of venous air embolism.

Despite this, venous air emboli have also been described with high frequency during neurosurgical operations performed in the supine, lateral, or prone positions, lumbar laminectomies, hip replacement surgeries, laparoscopic surgeries, and Cesarean sections, among others [2]. Morbidity and mortality associated with VAE are dependent upon the rate of air entrainment, the volume of air entrained, and the position of the patient. The lethal volume of air is unknown, however, injections of 100–300 mL have been reported to be fatal [2]. In large air emboli (5 mL/kg), there can be complete right ventricular outflow tract obstruction, which rapidly leads to right-sided heart failure and cardiovascular collapse. In more moderate-sized air emboli, there can be partial outflow tract obstruction leading to decreased cardiac output, hypotension, myocardial ischemia and, if untreated, death [3].

Clinical presentation depends on the severity of the air embolus. The use of nitrous oxide does not worsen the clinical severity of a VAE provided its use is discontinued upon detection of an air embolus [4]. Cardiovascular changes include tachyarrhythmias, evidence of right heart strain on EKG, and hypotension secondary to decreased cardiac output. Pulmonary artery pressures increase due to decreased cardiac output and spasm; central venous pressures increase due to right heart strain. Pulmonary changes depend on whether the patient is awake or under anesthesia. Awake patients will complain of dyspnea, coughing, and a sense of impending doom. In ventilated patients, one will see decreases in $ETCO_2$, arterial oxygen saturation, arterial oxygen tension, and hypercapnia [3]. Neurologic changes consist of altered mental status either due to cerebral hypoperfusion, cardiovascular collapse, or from direct cerebral air embolus through a patent foramen ovale.

There are several monitors that are capable of detecting venous air emboli. The most sensitive is transesophageal echocardiography (TEE). It is able to detect 0.02 mL/kg of air administered by bolus injection [2]. It also allows for detection of paradoxical arterial emboli via a patent foramen ovale. The presence of TEE also enables direct visualization of air aspiration through a central catheter if a VAE should occur. The downside is that it is expensive, invasive, and requires both expertise and constant surveillance [2]. Positioning a TEE during a sitting craniotomy in which the head is flexed can also prove difficult and there is little information on the safety of maintaining the TEE probe in this position for a prolonged period of time.

Table 7.1. Monitors used to detect venous air emboli.

Monitor	Sensitivity (ml/kg)	Comment
Transesophageal echocardiography	0.02	Can identify paradoxical embolus; invasive, requires training
Precordial Doppler	0.05	Most sensitive noninvasive monitor; difficult to use in obese patients and in lateral position
Pulmonary artery catheter	0.25	Increased pulmonary artery pressure correlates with amount of air entrained; invasive
End-tidal N_2	0.5	Affected by use of nitrous oxide; change occurs 30–90 s before end-tidal CO_2 change; not universally available
End-tidal CO_2	0.5	Standard monitor; less sensitive than above, nonspecific for VAE
Oxygen saturation	low	Late clinical sign requires severe physiologic disturbance
Direct observation	low	Look for back bleeding from bone or veins; no physiologic data

The most sensitive noninvasive monitor is the precordial Doppler ultrasound which can detect as little as 0.25 mL (0.05 mL/kg) of bolused air [3]. It is positioned along the right sternal border or between the right scapula and the spine. With small amounts of air entrainment a "washing machine" sound can be appreciated. With larger amounts of air, a classic "mill wheel" murmur can be heard. Pulmonary artery catheter, end-tidal nitrogen, $ETCO_2$, pulse oximetry, and direct observation can also be used to detect VAE (Table 7.1).

Upon detection of a VAE, several interventions can help prevent further air entrainment thus minimizing catastrophic hemodynamic changes. First, further air entrainment is prevented by notification of the surgeon to flood the field with normal saline. The operative site should also be lowered below the level of the right atrium. If the surgical procedure involves the cranium, then temporary occlusion of the bilateral jugular veins can be employed to prevent further entrainment, increase venous pressure, and promote retrograde flow. At the same time, the anesthesia provider should switch to 100% oxygen as nitrous oxide will increase the size of the air embolus.

Fluids should be administered judiciously in order to avoid further right heart strain. A valsalva maneuver can be performed to limit air entrainment. If a right atrial catheter is in place, aspiration of air can be attempted. However, there are no data to support emergent insertion of a venous catheter. As cardiovascular collapse can ensue, hemodynamic support with vasopressors and inotropes must be readily employed. One must also be prepared to initiate cardiopulmonary resuscitation, which may require patient repositioning. The application of positive end expiratory pressure is controversial in this scenario, as it may increase the risk for paradoxical air embolism or worsen cardiovascular disturbance; however, it may be beneficial for prevention of a VAE [3].

Conclusion

In conclusion, VAE is a potentially life-threatening event that can occur not only in neurosurgical procedures, but also in orthopedic, laparoscopic, and pelvic surgeries. Monitors for high-risk cases should be chosen depending on the expertise of the anesthesiologist, the surgery being performed, and the position of the patient.

References

1. **A. R. Fathi, P. Eshtehardi, B. Meier**. Patent foramen ovale and neurosurgery in sitting position: a systematic review. *Br J Anaesth* 2009; **102**: 588–96.

2. **S. C. Palmon, L. E. Moore, J. Lundberg** *et al.* Venous air embolism: a review. *J Clin Anesth* 1997; **9**: 251–57.

3. **M. A. Mirski, A. V. Lele, L. Fitzsimmons** *et al.* Diagnosis and treatment of vascular air embolism. *Anesthesiology* 2007; **106**: 164–77.

4. **T. J. Losasso, S. Black, D. A. Muzzi** *et al.* Detection and hemodynamic consequences of venous air embolism: does nitrous oxide make a difference? *Anesthesiology* 1992; **77**: 148–52.

Craniotomy. Posterior fossa craniotomy

8

Delayed emergence after posterior fossa surgery

Leif Saager and Alparslan Turan

Immediate emergence after neurosurgery is desirable to facilitate neurologic examination and early identification of complications. Awakening is determined by many factors including preoperative status, type of surgery, and intraoperative events.

Case description

A 58-year-old female with a body mass index of 32 complained about gradual hearing loss, increasing frequency of headaches and vertigo and subsequently was diagnosed with an acoustic neuroma. Her past medical history included type 2 diabetes, hypertension, seasonal allergies and 15 pack-years of smoking. Preoperative medications included metformin, enalapril, ibuprofen, atorvastatin, and diphenhydramine.

Preoperative magnetic resonance imaging was consistent with a 1.8-cm large left acoustic neuroma and the patient was scheduled for elective microsurgical tumor resection using a posterior fossa approach.

Anesthesia was induced with 150 mcg fentanyl, 200 mg propofol and 50 mg rocuronium and anesthesia was maintained with sevoflurane and 0.1–0.3 mcg/kg/min remifentanil. Throughout the surgery mean blood pressure was maintained between 70–85 mmHg and heart rate between 65–90 beats per minute. After 5 hours of surgery, estimated blood loss was minimal. A total of 1650 mL crystalloid and 500 mL colloid fluid were given. At closure of dura, 6 mg of morphine was administered for analgesia and consequently the patient was turned supine and all anesthetic agents discontinued.

During the following 30 minutes the patient failed to emerge from anesthesia. During this period only insufficient spontaneous breathing patterns and no response to painful stimuli were observed. Heart rate and blood pressure were within preoperative range. Core temperature was recorded as 36.2 °C despite intraoperative warming with forced heated air. The left pupil was 4 mm in diameter and minimally reactive to light, the right pupil was 2 mm in diameter and reacted briskly.

After checking for residual neuromuscular block and determining a normal train-of-four response an arterial blood gas sample was sent to the laboratory. Results returned within normal ranges except for a blood glucose of 180 mg/dL. A dose of 0.1 mg naloxone was given to antagonize opioid effects but no improvement in neurologic status was observed. An emergent computed tomography (CT) scan was obtained showing no hematoma, ischemia, pneumocephalus or brain-stem compression. A CT-angiogram was performed, which demonstrated an occluding mid-basilar artery clot. After consultation with radiologists, neurosurgeons, and family members a decision for intra-arterial local application of alteplase was made and partial recanalization achieved. The patient was transferred to the neurologic intensive care unit and kept on mechanical ventilation. One month postoperatively the patient was discharged to a nursing care facility with ataxia, and swallowing difficulties.

Discussion

In order to facilitate early detection of neurologic complications, anesthesiologists usually aim for an early emergence following intracranial surgery. However, some clinical conditions may require prolonged sedation. Hypothermia, hypertension, and coagulation disorders as well as prolonged surgery or intraoperative brain swelling might be reasons for delaying emergence.

Delayed awakening from anesthesia is defined as a failure to regain consciousness within 20–30 minutes after the end of surgery. The most common causes of delayed postoperative emergence include residual drug effects, respiratory failure, metabolic derangements, and neurologic complications (Table 8.1). Early recognition of these postoperative complications is extremely important since most of them require immediate surgical or medical attention.

Table 8.1. Common causes for delayed emergence after neurosurgery.

Systemic
   Residual drug effects
      Overdose, potentiation of drugs, prolonged neuromuscular
       blockade
   Central anticholinergic syndrome
   Respiratory failure
      Hypoxia, hypercapnia
   Metabolic and endocrine derangements
      Hypo-, hyperglycemia, electrolyte imbalance,
       hypothyroidism
   Hypothermia
   Hypotension

Neurologic
   Cerebral hypoxia
   Hemorrhage
   Thrombosis, embolism
   Seizure
   Cerebral swelling
   Pneumocephalus

Neuromuscular blockade is commonly used to better allow for ventilation and improved operating conditions. Residual neuromuscular blockade has been identified as a significant postoperative problem increasing morbidity and mortality [1]. Risk factors like advanced age and hepatic or renal dysfunction decrease clearance of muscle relaxants and thus prolong their effects. The duration of action and recovery time of muscle relaxants are significantly increased by hypothermia during anesthesia, mainly because of reduced elimination rate [2]. In this case hypothermia was identified as a possible risk factor and neuromuscular monitoring was used to exclude residual effects of muscle relaxant.

Opioids, in addition to analgesic action, can also have a strong sedative effect in susceptible patients. Remifentanil has an extremely short context-sensitive half life that allows for excellent analgesic control and rapid emergence. In order to avoid an analgesic gap at the end of surgery, postoperative pain therapy has to be initiated before discontinuation of remifentanil. The patient received morphine for translational analgesia, which might have contributed to sedation and delayed emergence. Naloxone was administered to rule out a possible opioid effect.

With conclusion of surgery the patient is weaned off controlled mechanical ventilation and transferred to a spontaneous breathing regimen before extubation. Ineffective spontaneous respiration results in hypoxia and hypercapnia. Arterial carbon dioxide levels exceeding 80 mmHg are associated with significantly impaired consciousness. This usually resolves without neurologic deficit as arterial $PaCO_2$ declines. In the present case arterial blood gas analysis revealed no abnormality.

Hypoglycemia, hyponatremia, and hypo-osmolality can cause delayed emergence from anesthesia. An underlying metabolic disorder, side effects of current medications or consequences of the surgical procedure may be responsible for these electrolyte derangements. In patients with type 2 diabetes mellitus frequent measurements of blood glucose levels are necessary to prevent potentially devastating complications of undetected hypoglycemia. Metformin, commonly used to treat diabetes mellitus, can cause lactic acidosis and hypothyroidism, both delaying recovery from anesthesia.

After excluding common systemic and anesthesia-related causes for prolonged awakening, a brief neurologic assessment should be performed to further differentiate cerebral complications.

Cerebral swelling can occur intraoperatively or preexist. In the context of posterior fossa surgery this is of particular concern. Extensive intraoperative manipulation close to the brainstem can lead to negative effects on the respiratory drive. Rapid emergence might increase risk and not be the optimal choice for these patients.

Pneumocephalus, the presence of air in the cerebral cavity, is a common complication of posterior fossa surgery and may occur in up to 78% of cases [3]. Surgical decompression, decreased brain volume following mannitol administration and hyperventilation are contributing factors. Positioning during surgery has been associated with increased incidences for sitting, park-bench, and prone positions. Tension pneumocephalus always represents a neurosurgical emergency requiring immediate surgical intervention.

Intracranial thrombotic events as well as hemorrhage can lead to rapid deterioration of the patient and cause failure to emerge after anesthesia. All of the abovementioned cerebral complications require radiologic imaging to diagnose and develop a treatment strategy. Due to the immediate nature of the complications and possibly fatal outcomes an emergent CT is considered the gold standard. The CT scan of the presented patient revealed none of the obvious complications of posterior fossa surgery. Computed tomography scans have a low sensitivity for early ischemia detection and interpretation is impaired by bony structures. Spiral CT–angiography, magnetic resonance imaging, or magnetic resonance angiography are more helpful in identifying occluded vessels.

A CT–angiogram led to the definite diagnosis in our patient. Basilar artery occlusion is a rare complication following neurosurgery and is associated with poor prognosis. The mechanisms are due to embolism or results of artherothrombosis. Abnormal level of consciousness and pupillary abnormalities were typical signs of basilar artery thrombosis demonstrated by our patient. Others would include hemi- or quadriparesis, coma, bulbar and pseudo-bulbar signs. These might be difficult to evaluate in the immediate perioperative setting.

A variety of treatment options are available, including anticoagulation with heparin, surgical thrombectomy, transluminal angioplasty and stenting, intra-arterial or systemic thrombolysis. The immediate postoperative period limited the therapeutic possibilities in our patient. In a multidisciplinary approach intra-arterial thrombolysis was considered the best balance between aggressive treatment to reverse the occlusion and the high risk of hemorrhage.

Conclusion

Early recovery after neurosurgical procedures is preferred in order to facilitate neurologic assessment and diagnosis of adverse outcomes. Multiple factors contribute to a delayed emergence from anesthesia and a systematic approach to rule out all possible causes is necessary.

References

1. **M. S. Arbous, A. E. Meursing, J. W. van Kleef** et al. Impact of anesthesia management characteristics on severe morbidity and mortality. *Anesthesiology* 2005; **102**: 257–68.

2. **T. Heier, J. Caldwell.** Impact of hypothermia on the response to neuromuscular blocking drugs. *Anesthesiology* 2006; **104**: 1070–80.

3. **T. J. K. Toung, R. W. McPherson, R. T. Donham** et al. Pneumocephalus: effects of patient position and the incidence and location of aerosol after posterior fossa and upper cervical cord surgery. *Anesth Analg* 1986; **65**: 65–70.

Craniotomy. Posterior fossa craniotomy

Trigeminal neuralgia

Basem Abdelmalak and Joseph Abdelmalak

Trigeminal neuralgia (also known as tic douloureux) is characterized by unilateral, severe, paroxysmal bursts of neuropathic facial pain, which causes severe disability and is limited to the distribution of one or more of the divisions of the trigeminal nerve. It is not homogeneous in presentation. It can be aching, throbbing, lancinating, or burning pain. Trigeminal neuralgia is multifactorial in etiology: it may be due to vascular compression, tumor, demyelination, or idiopathic causes. The treatment options are either medical (carbamazepine, oxacarbazepine, lamotrigine, neurontin, clonazepam, pregabalin, phenytoin, and baclofen) or surgical [1]. Surgical management includes microsurgical exploration/decompression [2], percutaneous procedures (rhizotomies) on the Gasserian ganglion (radiofrequency lesioning, glycerol injection, balloon compression), radiosurgery ("gamma knife" procedure), and neurectomy [1, 3]. General anesthesia is typically the technique of choice. Bradycardia and even asystole as a result of the trigeminocardiac reflex can complicate these procedures [4, 5].

Case description

The patient was an 88-year-old, right-handed female with a history of trigeminal neuralgia affecting the second division of the right trigeminal nerve (V2). She was treated with a gamma knife procedure, with very good results for 2 years. However, her pain recurred. It was severe, 9/10 on pain visual analog scale, and "electrical shock" in quality. She had some improvement with pregabalin to a pain score of 5/10. The patient was admitted for a percutaneous balloon compression procedure.

The patient's past medical history was also significant for essential hypertension, congestive heart failure, and coronary artery disease, status post single artery coronary artery bypass graft and aortic valve replacement 15 years ago, as well as abdominal aortic aneurysm repair around the same time. She had a 40 pack-year tobacco history but quit 6 years ago.

On physical examination, her blood pressure was 155/95 mmHg, pulse was 74. Her height and weight were 144.8 cm and 69 kg with a body mass index of 33. The patient's medication included: allopurinol, colchicine, furosemide, pregabalin, coumadin, tramadol, lisinopril, hydrochlorothiazide, and metoprolol.

After standard monitors were applied and two intravenous lines were inserted, general anesthesia was induced using propofol and fentanyl. Sevoflurane in air and oxygen was utilized for maintenance of anesthesia. The head was positioned for satisfactory stereotactic localization utilizing fluoroscopy. The cheek was sterilized and draped in the usual fashion. About 2.5 cm lateral to the labial crease, the skin was punctured. Through this puncture, a 20-gauge spinal needle was then advanced to the region of the foramen ovale using biplanar fluoroscopic guidance. The foramen was then punctured. A 14-gauge introducer needle was then advanced alongside this and it too punctured the foramen ovale. The 20-gauge needle was then removed and a 4-French Fogarty-type catheter was passed through the needle. The needle was withdrawn from the foramen, then the balloon inflated with 0.75 mL of contrast for 60 seconds, monitored by fluoroscopy. During inflation of the balloon, the patient became bradycardic and hypotensive. She was treated successfully with 0.6 mg glycopyrrolate given intravenously. The balloon was then deflated and the needle and catheter withdrawn. The case ended uneventfully.

Discussion

The etiology of trigeminal neuralgia is poorly understood, but common theories include vascular compression, tumor, demyelination, or idiopathic causes [3]. If the pain is refractory to medical treatment, the patient may try trigeminal nerve block or one of the following surgical procedures:

1. Microsurgical exploration/decompression. The surgery is done under general anesthesia, with an incision usually performed behind the ear. An opening is made in the skull about the size of a quarter. After opening the dura, the cerebellum is retracted and, using microsurgery, the trigeminal nerve inspected. If a vessel is found, it is dissected free of the trigeminal nerve and a Teflon sponge is placed to keep the vessel from recompressing the nerve. The wound is then closed.

2. Percutaneous procedures. These procedures include chemical, thermal, radiofrequency lesioning and the balloon compression procedure [1]. This is usually done under general anesthesia when the Gasserian ganglion is accessed percutaneously. General anesthesia is preferred as these procedures require a completely motionless patient often accomplished by adequate muscle relaxation, to facilitate the intervention and minimize injury to surrounding structures. This procedure is described above.

3. The gamma knife procedure. Topicalization is accomplished by injecting local anesthetics, at four sites on the scalp. A reference frame is then secured to the head at those sites. Some pressure is common for the first 5–10 minutes. Measurements are taken and then the patient is sent for magnetic resonance imaging and computed tomography scans. These are transferred to the planning computer to define the region to be treated. If there is a vessel compressing the nerve, the procedure may be aborted. A plan for focused radiation to the trigeminal nerve is created by the neurosurgeon. The radiation oncologist reviews the plan and assigns a dose of radiation. The patient lies down on the treatment couch. The head holder is used as a positioning device that will direct with great accuracy, up to 192 beams of radiation to converge at the point picked on the computer. The patient is usually monitored by 3 video cameras and 2 intercom systems. The patient then slides into the device up to their lower chest for about 25–30 minutes and then exits. When the treatment is completed, the patient is taken to the recovery room where the

Table 9.1. A summary of the trigeminocardiac reflex pathway, as well as the triggering events, clinical effects, possible predisposing factors, prevention, and treatment.

Afferent	Trigeminal nerve
Efferent	Vagus nerve
Triggers	1. Surgical manipulations of trigeminal nerve or its sensory branches (stimulation of the ophthalmic branch → oculocardiac reflex) 2. Surgical division of the dorsal sensory roots of the trigeminal nerve 3. Percutaneous microcompression of the trigeminal ganglion

Clinical effects	Lasts for as long as the trigger is applied, will cease on removing the trigger
	 Negative chronotropic and ionotropic responses:
	   Bradycardia
	   Hypotension
	   Asystole
	 Ventricular fibrillation
	 Apnea
	 Gastric hypermotility

Prevention and preparation	1. May consider local anesthetic infiltration in anticipation of the trigeminal nerve stimulation/manipulation 2. Gentle manipulation of the trigeminal nerve and its sensory branches 3. A noninvasive and temporary pacemaker may be prepared in advance for high-risk cardiac patients 4. May pretreat with glycopyrrolate in bradycardic patients 5. Tachycardia is not protective
Postulated predisposing factors	Hypercapnea Hypoxemia Light anesthesia Narcotics Preoperative beta-blockers Preoperative calcium channel blockers High resting vagal tone
Treatment	1. Stop the trigger 2. Spontaneous recovery 3. Mild bradycardia → glycopyrrolate ± ephedrine 4. Severe cases → atropine ± epinephrine

frame is removed and bandages applied. The patient is observed, typically between 30–120 minutes, then discharged.

In the above case, the patient had a gamma knife procedure in the past. Upon recurrence of symptoms, balloon compression procedure was considered. During inflation of the balloon, the anesthesiologist should be ready with atropine or glycopyrrolate to manage the bradycardia and/or asystole that is reported to occur frequently at this stage of surgery [5]. Sure enough we did encounter bradycardia and hypotension; it was of moderate degree and was treated successfully with 0.6 mg glycopyrrolate IV bolus. It should be noted that it is not recommended to give any more narcotics after induction as it may predispose the patient to a trigeminocardiac reflex (see Table 9.1) and can also hinder evaluating the success of surgery by observing postoperative pain relief.

The trigeminocardiac reflex is well described with such procedures and is described in the next case. The noxious stimulus on the trigeminal nerve during needle insertion and balloon inflation is thought to induce the reflex. This reflex can also be activated without surgery – the mere pain of trigeminal neuralgia has reportedly resulted in bradycardia that was severe enough to cause syncope and in other instances degenerated to complete cardiac arrest [4, 5]. Events such as these demonstrate the potentially debilitating nature of trigeminal neuralgias.

References

1. **S. Prasad, S. Galetta**. Trigeminal neuralgia: historical notes and current concepts. *Neurologist* 2009; **15**: 87–94.

2. **M. Sindou, J. M. Leston, C. Le guerinel** *et al.* Treatment of trigeminal neuralgia with microvascular decompression. *Neurochirurgie* 2009; **55**: 185–96.

3. **M. Obermann, Z. Katsarava**. Update on trigeminal neuralgia. *Expert Rev Neurother* 2009; **9**: 323–9.

4. **R. Campbell, D. Podrigo, L. Cheung**. Asystole and bradycardia during maxillofacial surgery. *Anesth Prog* 1994; **41**: 13–16.

5. **S. T. Cha, J. B. Eby, J. T. Katzen** *et al.* Trigeminocardiac reflex: a unique case of recurrent asystole during bilateral trigeminal sensory root rhizotomy. *J Craniomaxillofac Surg* 2002; **30**: 108–11.

10

Trigeminocardiac reflex

Heather Hervey-Jumper and Christopher R. Turner

Bradycardia and even asystole may occur suddenly during posterior fossa surgery and requires immediate evaluation and treatment in order to prevent potential ischemia and major neurologic complications. One important mechanism for this clinical presentation is the trigeminocardiac reflex (TCR).

Case description

A 53-year-old female with a history of progressive headaches and syncopal episodes was found to have a right-sided tentorial mass consistent with a falcine meningioma. She underwent a surgical resection of the mass via a right-sided occipitotemporal craniotomy in the left lateral decubitus position with her head rotated toward the floor. The pedicle of the meningioma was attached to the falx. During dissection of the mass from its pedicle, the patient experienced asystole that resolved upon cessation of falcine manipulation. Three subsequent individual and discrete mechanical stimulations of the falx reproduced similar but less severe hypotensive and bradycardic responses that resolved with cessation of stimulation. After administration of glycopyrrolate the bradycardia with falcine traction was no longer evident. The balance of the surgery and the patient's recovery were uneventful.

Discussion

Pathophysiology

The TCR is typically described as bradycardia and hypotension seen with mechanical stimulation of the distribution of the trigeminal nerve (cranial nerve (CN) V) [1]. The most common manifestation of the TCR is bradycardia, but other dysrhythmias including junctional rhythms, ventricular ectopy, AV blockade, asystole, and ventricular tachycardia can occur. This reflex is classically known as the "oculocardiac reflex" because of its prevalence in ophthalmologic surgery

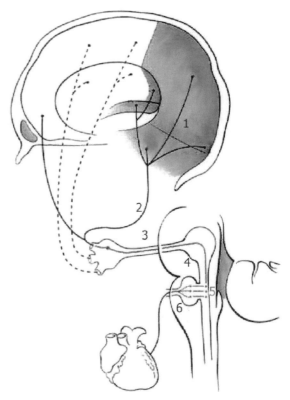

Figure 10.1. The diagram shows the pathway of a trigeminocardiac reflex originating from the posterior falx. Mechanical stimulation of the posterior falx causes activation of the nervus tentorii [1]. Signal travels through V1 [2] via the Gasserian ganglion and the trigeminal nerve [3] into the spinal trigeminal ganglion [4]. Short internuncial fibers [5] connect to the motor nucleus of the vagus [6]. Stimulation of this pathway results in reflex bradycardia.

[2]. The oculocardiac reflex is typically triggered by ocular or extraocular stimulation, which is transmitted via the ophthalmic branch (V1) of CN V to Gasserian (trigeminal) ganglion where V1 joins fibers from the maxillary (V2) and mandibular (V3) branches of CN V. From there the signal is transmitted to the trigeminal sensory nuclei located in the pons and medulla along the floor of the fourth ventricle (Figure 10.1).

The signal is then relayed via short internuncial nerve fibers in the reticular formation to the immediately adjacent vagal nuclei (in the medulla). The efferent limb is the vagus nerve, which when activated causes parasympathetic stimulation of the sinoatrial node resulting in bradycardia and subsequent hypotension. Most but not all of this pathway (from V1 to the sinoatrial node) appears to be cholinergically mediated.

While classically described as resulting from the pathway described above, in fact stimulation of any of the branches of CN V can result in the initiation of the TCR. The reflex has been documented with maxillary, mandibular, zygomatic, and petrosal bone manipulation, rhizolysis of the Gasserian ganglion, tumor resection in the cerebellopontine angle, irrigation of the temporomandibular joint, and endoscopic brow lift surgery.

Penfield and McNaughton [3] in the early twentieth century using silver nitrate preparations of human and rhesus monkey dura demonstrated extensive innervation of the meninges by all three divisions of CN V. As examples, branches of V1 form the ethmoid nerves that follow the small branches of the anterior meningeal artery. The meningeus medius nerve is a branch of V2 and runs with the anterior branch of the middle meningeal artery to innervate the middle fossa dura. The nervus spinosus, a branch of V3, follows the middle meningeal artery outside the cranium and through the foramen spinosum to innervate the middle fossa dura. The tentorial nerves arise from the intracranial portions of V1 and course into the dura of the parieto-occipital region and the posterior third of the falx, where there is a converging and bilaterally overlapping innervation at its midpoint. The posterior third of the falx seems to be the most sensitive region for the TCR. In the case described, it is likely the falcine distribution of V1 sensory fibers that resulted in the TCR [1].

The TCR has been reported to occur in 8–18% of cases involving surgical resection of lesions in the anterior and middle cranial base. In these cases however, none of the patients show postoperative neurologic deficits. Though the TCR does not appear to result in many major complications, there is evidence that an intraoperative TCR may be associated with a significantly worse postoperative hearing function after vestibular schwannoma surgery, and there is a higher occurrence of ipsilateral tinnitus postoperatively in patients that had intraoperative TCR than those that did not [4].

Treatment

When stimulation of the falx (or other structure) results in the TCR, cessation of the surgical manipulation in that area is the first step in correcting the hemodynamic instability. Often this alone terminates the reflex and allows restoration of hemodynamic stability [5]. If not, atropine or glycopyrrolate are both usually effective at blocking the cardiovascular effects of vagal stimulation [6]. Atropine has a faster onset and more pronounced heart rate effect and should be used if cessation of surgical stimulation does not immediately terminate the reflex. Advanced cardiac life-support measures should be instituted as conditions warrant, keeping in mind that patients in this scenario must usually be taken out of pins and returned to the supine position for effective CPR. This requires some time, but CPR must be instituted as rapidly as possible if the bradycardia is preventing effective circulation of the resuscitation medications or if hypotension lasts long enough to pose a risk of neurologic ischemia. External or internal cardiac pacing may be effective in particularly refractory cases of TCR.

While the TCR fatigues with repeated stimulation it nevertheless carries significant risk for recurrence if left untreated. Glycopyrrolate and atropine both block recurrence of the TCR by blocking the effects of vagal stimulation; glycopyrrolate may be advantageous if time permits in that the resulting tachycardia is less severe. Adequate depth of anesthesia (using volatile agents as opposed to opiates) serves to blunt the severity of the TCR as does correcting physiologic derangements such as hypoxia, hypercarbia and acidosis. In general, routine prophylactic anticholinergic use is not recommended as refractory tachydysrhythmias may develop.

Conclusion

In conclusion, TCR most commonly manifests as bradycardia and hypotension in response to mechanical stimulation of any of the branches of the trigeminal nerve. Trigeminocardiac reflex episodes that resolve do not appear to directly cause longstanding neurologic injury but some postoperative hearing deficits appear to correlate with its occurrence. Ultimately it is vigilant attention to the depth of anesthesia and the correction of physiologic derangements with continuous communication between the anesthesia and surgical teams during resection that are paramount in managing surgical procedures when TCR appears.

References

1. **D. F. Bauer, A. Youkilis, C. Schenck** *et al.* The falcine trigeminocardiac reflex: case report and review of the literature. *Surg Neurol* 2005; **63**: 143–8.

2. **M. Ostachowicz, J. Burau, A. Sadkiewicz.** The oculocardiac reflex during surgical correction of strabismus in local anesthesia. *Ophthalmologica* 1965; **150**: 259–62.

3. **W. Penfield, F. McNaughton.** Dural headache and innervation of the dura mater. *Arch Neurol Psychiatr* 1940; **44**: 43–75.

4. **B. Schaller, J. F. Cornelius, H. Prabhakar** *et al.* The trigemino-cardiac reflex: an update of the current knowledge. *J Neurosurg Anesthesiol* 2009; **21**: 187–95.

5. **A. Koerbel, A. Gharabaghi, A. Samii** *et al.* Trigeminocardiac reflex during skull base surgery: mechanism and management. *Acta Neurochir* 2005; **147**: 727–33.

6. **E. F. Meyers, S. A. Tomeldan.** Glycopyrrolate compared with atropine in prevention of the oculocardiac reflex during eye-muscle surgery. *Anesthesiology* 1979; **51**: 350–2.

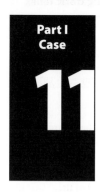

11

Sitting craniotomy

Michael D. Maile and George A. Mashour

Sitting craniotomies pose a unique set of problems for perioperative care of the neurosurgical patient. Although there are benefits to neurosurgery in this position, a number of potentially catastrophic complications may also result.

Case description

A 20-year-old morbidly obese male presented for resection of a pineocytoma via a supracerebellar approach in the sitting position. The patient had a long history of headaches that were recently increasing in severity; over the past year, he had also been experiencing visual loss with his headaches. The patient presented to the emergency department after having a seizure with loss of consciousness. A computed tomography scan demonstrated dilated third and lateral ventricles concerning for obstructive hydrocephalus. This finding was further investigated by magnetic resonance imaging, which showed a mass lesion in the pineal region. Subsequent open, stereotactic biopsy made the microscopic diagnosis of pineocytoma. The patient elected to proceed with resection of the tumor, for which the sitting position would be employed.

After induction of general anesthesia and placement of an endotracheal tube, a right-side internal jugular multi-orifice catheter and right radial arterial line were placed. The patient's head was secured in pins. Care was taken to pad all pressure points. Before the head was secured in place, a transesophageal echo (TEE) probe was inserted and an examination was performed that ruled out patent foramen ovale. After the patient was in his final position, a precordial Doppler monitor was secured to his chest. Precordial Doppler was monitored continuously and the TEE was used intermittently. Maintenance anesthesia consisted of isoflurane, fentanyl, and vecuronium. Somatosensory evoked potentials were monitored continuously throughout the case. The surgery was completed without complication, the patient emerged from anesthesia

quickly and the trachea was extubated in the operating room. Postoperative examination did not reveal any new deficits. The patient was then transferred to the neurosurgical intensive care unit for further recovery. He was discharged from the hospital on postoperative day 4.

Discussion

The sitting position for craniotomies offers several surgical advantages. Exposure to posterior cervical and posterior fossa structures is improved. Cerebral venous drainage and cerebrospinal fluid (CSF) drainage is enhanced by the effects of gravity, producing a less "tense" brain and allowing for better surgical exposure. Pooling of blood in the surgical field is minimized in the sitting position, potentially improving operating conditions and reducing blood loss. It has also been suggested that access to the airway and chest will allow easier patient resuscitation should their condition deteriorate [1].

The surgical advantages of the sitting position are offset by several issues for the surgical and anesthesia teams [2, 3]. The risk of venous air embolism (VAE) is increased because the surgical field is significantly higher than the level of the heart. Because of this risk, precordial Doppler and/or TEE are often used to monitor for VAE; a multi-orifice central line may be placed to aspirate a VAE should one occur.

Hemodynamic instability may complicate surgery in the sitting position. In addition to the usual vasodilatation and myocardial depression caused by many anesthetic agents, the sitting position leads to pooling in the lower extremities, which may further exacerbate intraoperative hypotension. The decrease in cerebral perfusion caused by placing the head above the heart may make hypotension more detrimental. In order to minimize intraoperative hypotension, the patient can be positioned slowly by incrementally elevating the back and head. Volume loading can decrease the effect of pooling of blood in the lower extremities. Vasopressors and inotropes should be available to maintain organ perfusion throughout the surgery.

The risk of pneumocephalus may be increased in the sitting position compared with other positions [4]. The drainage of CSF and venous blood out of the cranial vault by gravity provides more room for air to enter epidural or dural spaces. This can be compounded by other maneuvers that decrease CSF, blood, or brain volume such as CSF drainage, administration of diuretics, hyperventilation, or resection of a mass lesion. The use of nitrous oxide is generally avoided due to the risk of VAE and tension pneumocephalus.

Orthopedic, dermatologic, and peripheral nerve injuries have been reported in the sitting position and are likely due to pressures exerted on dependent regions of the body. Care should be taken when positioning the patient and liberal padding of all pressure points should be performed. Swelling of the tongue and oropharynx can occur during sitting craniotomies. This may be due to neck flexion obstructing venous and lymphatic drainage. Placement of a TEE probe may also contribute to this complication; smaller diameter probes may be utilized if available. If swelling is significant, extubation may have to be delayed after completion of the surgery. Common peroneal nerve injuries have been reported and are likely due to nerve compression and/or stretching of the nerve secondary to flexion of the thigh. Recurrent laryngeal nerve palsies have also been reported for sitting craniotomies and are likely also related to compression by the TEE probe and endotracheal tube.

A rare but catastrophic complication of the sitting position is quadriplegia [5]. Several factors have been postulated to contribute to this complication. Flexion of the neck may compress the cervical spine and result in ischemia. A decrease in intraoperative blood pressure will also decrease perfusion, especially with the head being elevated above the level of the heart. Monitoring evoked potentials may allow for early detection and intervention with spinal ischemia.

Conclusion

Overall, the benefits of the sitting position may outweigh the risk if patients are carefully selected and intraoperative management is conducted with care [6]. It has been suggested that a ventriculo-atrial shunt, pulmonary hypertension, a patent foramen ovale, and symptomatic cerebral ischemia may be absolute contraindications to this procedure. Performing surgery in the sitting position for patients with uncontrolled hypertension, significant chronic obstructive airway disease, or at the extremes of age should also be done with caution. However, there are few data to support appropriate patient selection.

References

1. **T. Gale, K. Leslie**. Anaesthesia for neurosurgery in the sitting position. *J Clin Neurosci* 2004; **11**: 693–6.

2. **J. Matjasko, P. Petrozza, M. Cohen** *et al*. Anesthesia and surgery in the seated position: analysis of 554 cases. *Neurosurgery* 1985; **17**: 695–702.

3. **M. Standefer, J. W. Bay, R. Trusso**. The sitting position in neurosurgery: a retrospective analysis of 488 cases. *Neurosurgery* 1984; **14**: 649–58.

4. **T. Sloan**. The incidence, volume, absorption, and timing of supratentorial pneumocephalus during posterior fossa neurosurgery conducted in the sitting position. *J Neurosurg Anesthesiol* 2010; **22**: 59–66.

5. **J. M. Porter, C. Pidgeon, A. J. Cunningham**. The sitting position in neurosurgery: a critical appraisal. *Br J Anaesth* 1999; **82**: 117–28.

6. **G. P. Rath, P. K. Bithal, A. Chaturvedi** *et al*. Complications related to positioning in posterior fossa craniectomy. *J Clin Neurosci* 2007; **14**: 520–5.

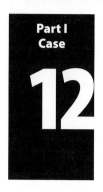

Craniotomy. Posterior fossa craniotomy

Cerebellar hemorrhage

Gene H. Barnett

Stroke can be either ischemic (due to an interruption of blood and oxygen to the brain) or hemorrhagic (due to bleeding into or around the brain). Here we explore the management issues surrounding a hemorrhagic stroke of the cerebellum – one of the most common sites for intracerebral hemorrhage, and one where proper management can have a profound impact on outcome.

Case description

The patient was a 75-year-old female with a history of hypertension and end-stage renal disease requiring dialysis. Shortly after breakfast, she developed a severe occipital headache. She gradually developed difficulty walking and called 911. By noon, she was transported to a nearby emergency department. Upon presentation she was awake, alert and appeared to be neurologically intact (although gait was not tested). She denied use of antiplatelet or anticoagulation agents. She was afebrile, but with a blood pressure of 190/110 mmHg, respiratory rate of 20 breaths per minute and pulse of 90 beats per minute. A computed tomography (CT) scan of the brain revealed a 2.5-cm, midline cerebellar hemorrhage, eccentric (to the left) without hydrocephalus. She was treated with labetalol and hydralazine to decrease systolic blood pressure to <160 mmHg. By 1:00 pm, a request for transfer to a tertiary care facility with neurosurgical service was made. While waiting for air transport, the attending physician noted that the patient was developing swallowing difficulty and respiratory distress. The patient was then sedated and pharmacologically paralyzed, and the trachea was intubated.

Upon arrival at our facility at 2:15 pm, she remained sedated and paralyzed with mechanical ventilatory support. Laboratory studies from the transferring hospital indicated normal prothrombin and activated partial thromboplastin times, as well as platelet

counts. A repeat CT scan showed enlargement of the clot to 3.5 cm in maximum dimension, yet without evidence of obstructive hydrocephalus (Figure 12.1). After telephone consultation with the family, the decision was made to take the patient to surgery on an emergent basis.

In the operating room she was positioned prone with the head flexed to optimize exposure to the posterior fossa. After clipping hair and allowing access for a Frazier burr hole (in the event that an emergency ventriculostomy was required), a midline incision was made from just above the inion to the mid-cervical area. The paraspinal muscles were split and dissected off the occiput and upper cervical spine. Then, a generous craniectomy was made, along with removal of the posterior arch of C1. By 3:15 pm the dura was opened with the cerebellum spontaneously delivering itself due to increased posterior fossa pressure. The cerebellar fissure was microsurgically split and it became apparent that the clot was in the left cerebellar hemisphere, herniating to the right, giving it a midline appearance on imaging. The hemisphere was entered and the clot evacuated. As is common with clot evacuation, multiple points of bleeding were identified. These were secured, the dura loosely patched with a dermal allograft material, and a titanium mesh cranioplasty made. After the wound was closed, she was returned to the intensive care unit, still intubated and sedated, and monitored with periodic reduction of sedation with neurologic examinations, as well as intermittent CT imaging.

Examination consistently revealed appropriate, symmetric limb movements and limited cranial nerve exams. Computed tomography scans showed satisfactory decompression of the posterior fossa and absence of hydrocephalus. The following day, sedation was withdrawn, she underwent dialysis, and was extubated (Figure 12.2). After several days each in the neurologic intensive care unit, step-down unit and regular

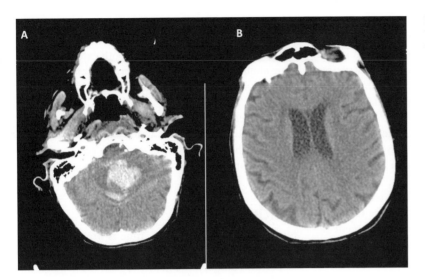

Figure 12.1. Preoperative computed tomography – (a) showing cerebellar clot and (b) absence of hydrocephalus.

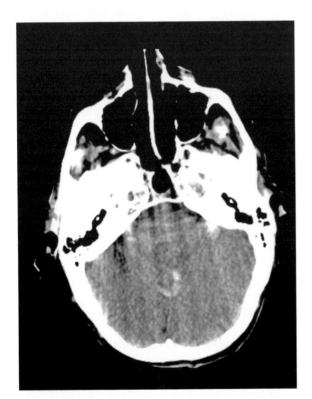

Figure 12.2. Postoperative computed tomography – showing resolution of cerebellar clot.

neurologic unit, she was transferred to a rehabilitation facility. At the time of hospital discharge she was neurologically intact, except for complaints of 'dizziness' and imbalance when trying to walk.

Discussion

Intracerebral hemorrhage is most commonly associated with chronic hypertension, amyloid angiopathy, anticoagulation, trauma or underlying pathology such as tumor or vascular malformation [1]. In this case, chronic hypertension was the suspected cause – preferentially affecting the deep hemispheric nuclei or cerebellum. When over-anticoagulation (usually related to coumadin) is the causative factor, then reversal with fresh frozen plasma, vitamin K, and/or factor VII is desirable before surgery (or to determine if it will thwart clot progression), although the time for such correction may lead to neurologic worsening.

The role of surgical intervention in supratentorial intracerebral hemorrhage is controversial, but most evidence suggests that patients with small (i.e., <40 mL) or large (>100 mL) clots have limited or no benefit from surgical intervention. The role, if any, of minimally invasive approaches to deep clots using thrombolysis remains undefined [2]. Many patients with deep clots may decompress their intraparenchymal clot with rupture into the ventricular system. This event may turn out to be a life-saving blessing, or result in a cascade of further problems related to obstructive or communicating hydrocephalus.

The posterior fossa has substantially less compartmental volume than the supratentorial space. Here, stable clots <2 cm in maximum cross-sectional dimension typically do not warrant surgical intervention, unless exhibiting radiographic progression, neurologic symptoms, signs of brainstem compression, or hydrocephalus. However, cerebellar clots ≥ 2.5 cm almost always require surgical intervention [3]. In cases where symptoms appear to be due to obstructive hydrocephalus, initial (or total) intervention may be placement of an external ventricular drainage device. In this case, however, the patient had evidence of brainstem dysfunction (swallowing and respiratory dysfunction) without overt hydrocephalus (along with enlarging clot >2.5 cm in size) so emergent surgery was warranted.

Although the midline posterior fossa can be accessed with the patient in either a sitting or prone position, the latter is usually preferred in urgent or emergent situations. As ventricular obstruction may occur when the patient is positioned, prepared or opened, allowing access for an emergency external ventricular drainage device is desirable in preparing and draping the patient [4]. Surgery itself is relatively straightforward. As noted above, often multiple sources of bleeding are encountered at the time of clot decompression making it difficult to determine a definitive source of the original hemorrhage. At times, an unexpected source of bleeding such as vascular malformation, aneurysm, or tumor may be encountered. The surgeon will need to use his or her experience to determine how to manage such findings when encountered. Appropriate blood products should, ideally, be available to deal with such unexpected findings, yet not unduly delay emergent surgery. Life-saving clot decompression and hemostasis generally take precedence over vascular anomaly correction or maximal tumor resection. Staging a second, definitive procedure under more controlled, studied conditions (i.e., with complete imaging, navigation, etc.) is perfectly appropriate under such circumstances. The primary goal of surgery is to save the patient's best-quality life, if possible.

Closure should consider whether some additional compartmental volume is desirable. In the supratentorial space, this extra capacity may be accomplished by partial lobectomy or hemicraniectomy. Infratentorially, leaving the dura open or a capacious dural graft and craniectomy are means to that end. Here, we placed a graft with excess capacity, and used a titanium mesh cranioplasty that provided both external protection, along with some extra intracranial capacity as this was an onlay, as opposed to a full thickness cranial repair.

In the end, an expeditious approach to treating this patient led to a good, but not great early recovery – however, this early result needs to be compared with the alternative of virtually certain severe disability or death.

Conclusion

Similar to ischemic stroke, "time is brain" for many hemorrhagic stroke patients [5]. In deciding if or when to perform surgery, the neurosurgeon must weigh the likelihood of the surgical benefit for a good recovery versus a futile intervention or sustaining a new, severely disabled life. In this case, many factors aligned to provide the optimal outcome for this patient.

Acknowledgments

The author wishes to thank the assistance of Ms. Christine Moore for her assistance with the preparation of this manuscript.

References

1. **A. I. Qureshi, S. Tuhrim, J. P. Broderick** *et al.* Spontaneous intracerebral hemorrhage. *N Engl J Med* 2001; **344**: 1450–60.

2. **D. W. Miller, G. H. Barnett, D. W. Kormos** *et al.* Stereotactically guided thrombolysis of deep cerebral hemorrhage: preliminary results. *Cleve Clin J Med* 1993; **60**: 321–4.

3. **S. Kobayashi, A. Sato, Y. Kageyama** *et al.* Treatment of hypertensive cerebellar hemorrhage – surgical or conservative management? *Neurosurgery* 1994; **34**: 246–50.

4. **E. S. Connolly, G. M. McKhann, J. Huang, T. F. Choudhri.** *Fundamentals of Operative Techniques in Neurosurgery.* New York: Thieme, 2002; 628.

5. **J. L. Saver.** Time is brain-quantified. *Stroke* 2006; **37**: 263–6.

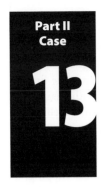
Vascular procedures. Aneurysm clipping

Preoperative evaluation

Milad Sharifpour and Paul S. Moor

Rupture of an intracranial aneurysm is the leading cause of nontraumatic subarachnoid hemorrhage (SAH) and accounts for 80% of the cases, with a high rate of death and complications [1]. Subarachnoid hemorrhage accounts for 2–5% of all new strokes and affects approximately 30 000 persons each year in the USA [2]. The most typical manifestation is sudden onset, severe headache that is described as "the worst headache of my life," with or without nausea, vomiting, and focal neurologic deficits.

Case description

The patient was a 45-year-old female who had presented to an outside hospital with a 1-month history of progressive right-sided facial and body numbness that had worsened acutely over the week prior to her admission. She was on home coumadin therapy for a history of upper extremity deep venous thrombosis. At the time of presentation she did not manifest any focal neurologic deficits and was awake, alert, and able to follow commands. Computed tomography (CT) scans with and without contrast demonstrated intraparenchymal hemorrhage centered in the midbrain in addition to periventricular white matter disease. Five days after the initial presentation, the patient became acutely somnolent. The trachea was intubated and she underwent a noncontrast CT scan of the head. In addition to the preexisting intraparenchymal hemorrhage, a new SAH with extensive cisternal blood and fourth ventricular compression was demonstrated. Based on the clinical exam this was classified as a Hunt–Hess grade III SAH (Table 13.1). A ventriculostomy catheter was placed and the patient's neurologic status improved subsequently. A radial artery catheter was replaced and large-bore intravenous access was obtained. At that time she was able to open her eyes spontaneously and answer yes and no appropriately to questions. She subsequently underwent a diagnostic angiogram that demonstrated a basi-

Table 13.1. Hunt–Hess classification.

Grade	Characteristics
I	Asymptomatic or minimal headache and slight nuchal rigidity
II	Moderate to severe headache, nuchal rigidity, no neurologic deficit other than cranial nerve palsy
III	Drowsiness, confusion, mild focal deficit
IV	Stupor, moderate to severe hemiparesis, possibly early decerebrate rigidity, vegetative disturbances
V	Deep coma, decerebrate rigidity, moribund

lar trunk aneurysm. The trachea remained intubated for airway protection during transfer under propofol sedation to our neurosurgical intensive care unit (ICU), for physiologic optimization before undergoing microvascular clipping. The patient's systolic blood pressure was maintained <140 mmHg and her mean arterial pressure was kept <80 mmHg in the context of an unsecured aneurysm. The external ventricular drain was set to drain at 20 cmH$_2$O above the level of the tragus. The patient was maintained normovolemic, using 0.9% normal saline. Cerebral vasospasm prophylaxis was initiated with nimodipine and magnesium sulfate. Levetiracetam was initiated for seizure prophylaxis. Sequential compressive devices were used for deep venous thrombosis prophylaxis as the patient was not suitable for anticoagulation. The patient underwent definitive correction of the aneurysm the following day.

Discussion

Aneurysmal SAH is a neurologic emergency, resulting from blood extravasation into the subarachnoid space normally filled with cerebrospinal fluid (CSF), that requires complex treatment and monitoring. Fifteen to 25% of patients die before reaching medical care and there is an approximately 50% mortality rate associated with SAH. Of those who survive, up to one third require life-long care and as many as 46% have residual cognitive deficits affecting their functional status and quality of life [3]. Subarachnoid hemorrhage is more common in women than in men (3:2 ratio) and it is 2× more common among African–Americans. It happens more frequently in persons >40 years old with peak rupture rates between 50 and 60 years. The main risk factors for SAH include hypertension, tobacco smoking, first-degree relatives with SAH, and heavy alcohol consumption. Furthermore, aneurysms are associated with heritable connective tissue disorders such as polycystic kidney disease, Ehlers–Danlos syndrome (type IV), Marfans syndrome, pseudoxanthoma elasticum, and fibromuscular dysplasia. Risk of rupture varies with size and location of the aneurysm. The most common sites of ruptured aneurysms are (1) anterior cerebral artery, (2) posterior communicating artery, and (3) middle cerebral artery. The most common manifestations include sudden onset of severe headache, with nausea, vomiting, neck pain, photophobia, loss of consciousness, and prolonged coma. Meningismus, focal neurologic deficits, third and sixth cranial nerve palsies, and altered level of consciousness can be present on physical examination.

The initial management of a patient with SAH should focus on (1) airway management depending on neurologic function, (2) avoiding hypertension that can lead to rupture of unsecured aneurysms or rebleeding, (3) maintenance of adequate cerebral perfusion pressure (CPP) to minimize the risk of cerebral ischemia in recently insulted brain with altered autoregulation, (4) determining the degree of neurologic severity, as well as serial assessment of neurologic function using the Hunt–Hess scale (Table 13.1), (5) detection of rebleeding or hydrocephalus, and (6) provision of seizure prophylaxis. Prevention, detection, and treatment of cerebral vasospasm are imperative in patients presenting between post-rupture day 4–14, the risk period for vasospasm and delayed ischemic neurologic deficit.

A noncontrast head CT scan should be the first diagnostic study performed in patients presenting with SAH symptoms as this detects more than 95% of SAHs if performed within the first 24 hours. The presence of xanthochromia on lumbar puncture helps diagnose SAH in patients with strong suspicion of SAH and negative or equivocal head CT. Meanwhile, cerebral angiography is the gold standard for detection of intracranial aneurysms and should be performed promptly once initial stabilization is achieved to facilitate early repair of the ruptured aneurysms.

Since rebleeding is associated with increased mortality and the risk of rebleeding is highest immediately after SAH, early intervention within the first 72 hours is recommended for patients with neurologic grades I–III. Definitive management of aneurysmal SAH includes endovascular coiling or microvascular clipping. According to the International Subarachnoid Aneurysm Trial, in patients who are equally suitable for endovascular coiling or surgical clipping, at one year, endovascular coiling is associated with significantly lower dependency or death compared with surgical clipping [4]. However, endovascular coiling is associated with a higher rate of late rebleeding. Other factors, including patient's age and other medical co-morbidities, aneurysmal properties such as size and neck, accessibility, and relationship to adjacent vessels should be considered while choosing the most appropriate treatment option.

In addition to a complete preoperative history and physical examination, evaluation of a patient with SAH should focus on assessing the presence and extent of the commonly associated physiologic derangements. Early complications, most often occurring within the first 72 hours, include (1) rebleeding, hydrocephalus, and elevated intracranial pressure (ICP), (2) elevated blood pressure in response to pain, anxiety, and sympathetic activation, (3) cardiac abnormalities including electrocardiographic changes, arrhythmias, myocardial injury, and stunned myocardium in response to SAH-associated catecholamine release, and (4) pulmonary complications including cardiogenic and neurogenic pulmonary edema, aspiration, and pneumonia. Late complications include (1) cerebral vasospasm, (2) intravascular volume contraction, (3) hyponatremia, and (4) shunt dependence. Hyperglycemia, anemia, fever, and hyperthermia are other complications that frequently occur in SAH patients and are associated with increased mortality and poor functional outcome (Table 13.2). In addition, systemic hypotension may occur in response to nimodipine therapy for vasospasm prophylaxis. Such derangements require thorough preoperative optimization, to help minimize their impact during anesthesia.

Patients with a ruptured aneurysm are at the highest risk of rebleeding within the first 24 hours following the initial rupture and this risk decreases over the next few days. Pain, anxiety, and SAH-associated catecholamine release can lead to elevated blood pressure, which increases the risk of rebleeding in

Table 13.2. Systematic approach to subarachnoid hemorrhage.

System	Comments
Nervous system	↑ ICP, hydrocephalus: can be managed w/ external ventricular drain Rebleeding; risk ↓ by early coiling or clipping. Blood pressure control with IV beta blockers for unsecured aneurysms Cerebral vasospasm: prophylaxis with nimodipine and magnesium sulfate. Tx: Permissive HTN and hypervolemia. Intra-arterial vasodilator injection and transluminal angioplasty for refractory cases Seizure: consider anticonvulsant therapy depending on degree of bleed
Cardiovascular	Electrocardiographic abnormalities: the majority are benign and require no treatment Arrhythmias: <5% are life threatening and require management according to advance cardiac life support guidelines Stunned myocardium: useful to evaluate ventricular function with transthoracic echocardiogram. May require inotropic/pressor support, diuresis
Respiratory	Cardiogenic or neurogenic edema, aspiration, pneumonia: Tx: ventilatory support, diuresis for pulmonary edema, antibiotics and infection management for pneumonia Airway compromise in patients with altered mental status: prompt intubation
Endocrine	Hyponatremia secondary to cerebral salt wasting or syndrome of inappropriate antidiuretic hormone; Tx: salt replacement with hypertonic saline Hypomagnesemia, hypokalemia, hypocalcemia Hyperglycemia is associated with worse outcomes; maintain normoglycemia with sliding scale insulin
Volume status	Volume contraction secondary to decreased intake and cerebral salt wasting; maintain normovolemia with 0.9% normal saline
Prophylaxis/prevention	Gastrointestinal: proton pump inhibitors Venous thrombosis: compression devices, as anticoagulation not deemed suitable for patients with a recent intracranial bleed and unsecured aneurysm Infectious disease: antibiotic prophylaxis for ventricular drain. Protocols for prevention of ventilator-associated pneumonia

ICP = intracranial pressure; Tx = therapy; HTN = hypertension.

unsecured aneurysms. Analgesics and antihypertensive infusions are frequently required to achieve adequate blood pressure control. Beta-blockers and labetalol are preferred since they do not induce cerebral vasodilation and do not further increase ICP.

Alternatively, nicardipine can be used to achieve blood pressure control. However, in the presence of hydrocephalus, aggressive management of blood pressure should be addressed only after hydrocephalus is treated. Twenty to 30% of the patients experience hydrocephalus within the first three days post-rupture; incidence is increased in higher grade SAH as a result of ventricular blood load, foraminal obstruction, increased CSF viscosity, and impaired CSF flow. Elevated ICP as a result of communicating hydrocephalus can be managed with an extraventricular drain.

Electrocardiographic abnormalities such as peaked T-waves, QT prolongation, and S-T segment elevation or depression are present in up to 70% of the SAH patients and these are often benign and do not require specific treatment. Rhythm disturbances are also common and up to 5% of the patients experience life-threatening arrhythmias, which should be managed according to advanced cardiac life-support guidelines. Stunned myocardium is the most severe cardiac complication associated with SAH. It can severely impair left ventricular function and decrease cardiac output and mean arterial pressure, resulting in decreased CPP and increased risk of ischemic cerebral insult as well as cardiogenic pulmonary edema. Management requires inotropic support, diuresis, and ventilatory support. Elevated cardiac enzymes and troponin are also frequently encountered laboratory values in SAH patients and may be associated with worse prognosis.

Patients with neurologic insults are at increased risk for pulmonary complications such as aspiration, pneumonia, and pulmonary edema, and may require mechanical ventilation. It is important to normalize and maintain PaO_2, $PaCO_2$, and pH in order to prevent increased ICP.

Patients are at risk for cerebral vasospasm from post-rupture days 4–14. About two-thirds of patients demonstrate angiographic evidence of vasospasm and up to 50% develop symptomatic vasospasm with clinical symptoms of cerebral ischemia, such as new onset focal neurologic deficits and altered mental status. The amount of blood in the subarachnoid space seen on the initial CT scan is the strongest predictor of vasospasm. Transcranial Doppler ultrasonography is the most frequently used noninvasive method to detect vasospasm while angiography remains the gold standard. Once clinical cerebral vasospasm is detected, medical therapy with induced hypertension, hypervolemia, and hemodilution ("triple-H" therapy) is often initiated. While induced hypertension and hypervolemia are effective and well established in the treatment of cerebral vasospasm, the utility of hemodilution remains controversial. Transluminal angioplasty and intra-arterial infusion of vasodilators should be reserved for patients whose vasospasm remains refractory to medical therapy.

Patients with SAH are at increased risk of intravascular volume contraction in the setting of cerebral salt wasting syndrome and decreased oral intake. Volume status should be frequently monitored and adequate volume replacement with 0.9% normal saline is required to prevent volume contraction.

Hyponatremia occurs in up to one-third of SAH patients and is secondary to syndrome of inappropriate antidiuretic hormone secretion, or cerebral salt wasting. Both syndrome of inappropriate antidiuretic hormone secretion and salt wasting can be managed with sodium and replacement with intravenous hypertonic saline. Fluid restriction is often avoided because of cerebral vasospasm risk. Other common electrolyte abnormalities that should be suspected and treated include hypokalemia and hypocalcemia.

While 10% of patients are at risk of seizures following SAH, the need for the routine administration of anticonvulsants remains unclear [2]. The cerebral metabolic rate increases in a seizing brain; seizure prophylaxis therefore helps prevent further ischemic injury in susceptible patients. Fever and hyperglycemia are also common in SAH patients and are associated with increased mortality and poor outcome, therefore therapy should be directed towards maintaining normothermia and normoglycemia [3].

Conclusion

In conclusion, SAH is a complex disease with high morbidity and mortality – management of patients with SAH requires a multisystem approach. Patients present for elective clipping of an unruptured aneurysm or emergent surgery following SAH. Prognosis depends on the severity of the initial bleed, prompt securing of the aneurysm, and the incidence and the extent of neurologic and systemic complications associated with SAH. Thorough assessment of the patient, effective organ support, and correction of pathophysiology are vital prior to leaving the ICU for what may be a challenging case in the operating room.

References

1. **J. I. Suarez, R. W. Tarr, W. R. Selman**. Aneurysmal subarachnoid hemorrhage. *N Engl J Med* 2006; **354**: 387–96.

2. **M. N. Diringer**. Management of aneurysmal subarachnoid hemorrhage. *Crit Care Med* 2009; **37**: 432–40.

3. **M. Smith**. Intensive care management of patients with subarachnoid haemorrhage. *Curr Opin Anaesthesiol* 2007; **20**: 400–7.

4. **A. Molyneux, R. Kerr, I. Stratton** *et al.* International Subarachnoid Aneurysm Trial (ISAT) of neurosurgical clipping versus endovascular coiling in 2143 patients with ruptured intracranial aneurysms: a randomised trial. *Lancet* 2002; **360**: 1267–74.

14

Intracranial aneurysm clipping with intraoperative rupture

Paul S. Moor

Cerebral aneurysm surgery is challenging for both surgeons and anesthesiologists, requiring close collaboration among all operating room team members. Although endovascular treatment for aneurysmal subarachnoid hemorrhage (SAH) has increased, operative management by clipping is likely to remain for the more distal, wide-necked aneurysms, or for those where coiling has failed. The process, however, has a risk of intraoperative rupture, which remains a potentially catastrophic event, adversely affecting outcome [1].

Case description

The patient was a 56-year-old African–American female smoker who presented with sudden onset of frontal headache, vomiting, and neck stiffness. Non-contrast head computed tomography (CT) revealed a right-sided SAH with minimal intraventricular blood and no obvious hydrocephalus. Her clinical condition represented a Hunt–Hess grade II SAH and she was admitted to the neurosurgical intensive care unit for observation. Cerebral angiography on day 1 demonstrated a large, wide-necked, anterior communicating artery aneurysm; craniotomy and clipping were arranged for later that day. Electrophysiologic monitoring with somatosensory evoked potentials and electroencephalography was arranged.

Anesthetic history and physical examination were obtained. Her past medical history was significant for controlled hypertension, treated with amlodipine, and obesity (body mass index = 35). Airway assessment was predictive of an easy intubation, the patient's cardiopulmonary status was normal and SAH induced sympathetic discharge did not appear to be significant. Nimodipine and magnesium vasospasm prophylaxis were commenced. Laboratory test values were all within normal limits, troponins were negative and cross-match for two units was performed.

The primary concerns of the anesthesiology team were (1) precise control of the aneurysmal transmural pressure gradient, (2) preservation of cerebral perfusion pressure (CPP) and oxygen delivery to the brain parenchyma to minimize risk of ischemia in recently insulted brain, (3) avoidance of large swings in intracranial pressure (ICP), (4) provision of optimal conditions for surgical exposure and minimal brain retraction, (5) anticipation and preparation for intraoperative aneurysm rupture and rapid blood loss, and (6) swift emergence from anesthesia to facilitate postoperative neurologic assessment.

A 14 g intravenous cannula was inserted in the preoperative holding area, prior to obtaining radial arterial access under midazolam anxiolysis. The patient was transferred to the operating room and further standard monitoring was applied. After preoperative verification, general anesthesia was induced carefully with lidocaine, fentanyl, and propofol. Paralysis was achieved with vecuronium. Direct laryngoscopy was performed after an esmolol bolus to ensure that systolic blood pressure remained <150 mmHg. The trachea was intubated and two further large-bore intravenous cannulae were placed. Further propofol was administered prior to application of the Mayfield skull clamp and end-tidal isoflurane was maintained at <1.0 minimum alveolar concentration, in addition to remifentanil and vecuronium infusions. Neurophysiologic monitoring was of satisfactory quality. Normovolemia was maintained with normal saline and albumin, with a systolic pressure variation between 6–8. On raising of the bone flap, the surgeons reported adequate brain relaxation as a result of moderate hyperventilation ($PaCO_2$ 30 mmHg) and 0.5 g/kg mannitol.

Anesthesia was unremarkable until the surgeons were preparing to place the temporary clip and microdissect the aneurysmal neck from the parent artery. Aneurysmal rupture and overwhelming hemorrhage occurred into the surgical site. Assistance was summoned and inspired oxygen increased to 100%.

Thiopental (3 mg/kg) was administered to induce burst suppression and lower blood pressure. A second suction device was utilized by the surgeons; systolic blood pressure of 60 mmHg and burst suppression was maintained with thiopental boluses. A bolus dose of adenosine induced transient circulatory arrest and allowed proximal artery identification and temporary clip placement.

Discussion

Anesthesia for patients with SAH is challenging. The maintenance of an adequate mean arterial blood pressure, and hence CPP, during the induction of anesthesia is key to prevent ischemic secondary injury. Aneurysmal rebleeding is possible if blood pressure surges from anesthetic and surgical stimuli that are not mitigated. The provision of an adequate CPP, while ensuring the transmural pressure gradient does not increase the risk of rebleeding, epitomizes the challenge.

Cerebral perfusion pressure and transmural pressure are essentially influenced by the same variables and are equal to the mean arterial pressure minus ICP [2]. The subtle difference between both values is that CPP represents the pressure driving cerebral blood flow and transmural pressure is the pressure acting across the aneurysmal wall, which is also influenced by local factors like clot organization, aneurysm size, and Laplace's law. The key is to keep CPP physiological while minimizing transmural pressure, as any increase in blood pressure or reduction in ICP increases the likelihood of aneurysmal rupture and rebleeding. Transmural pressure is at risk of increasing during direct laryngoscopy, application of Mayfield pins, incision and raising the bone flap.

Aneurysm rupture during laryngoscopy is an uncommon but life-threatening complication, which should be suspected if severe hypertension and bradycardia develop. Urgent CT and medical management of intracranial hypertension should commence, while future surgical options are being considered.

Historically, induced hypotension was advocated during aneurysm dissection due to the high risk of aneurysmal rupture. With the advent of temporary clipping, deliberate hypotension is now reserved for intraoperative rupture only. These cases require normotension as baseline. A mean arterial pressure of 60–80 mmHg is adequate.

Brain relaxation is essential to improve surgical access, reduce brain retraction, and assist in the clip application; it becomes more important in the high clinical grade SAH when intracranial compliance is reduced. This process demands a careful balance between the beneficial effect of brain volume reduction and the risk of brain ischemia. Methods to reduce the volume of intracranial contents such as hyperventilation, hyperosmolar agents and possible cerebrospinal drainage should be discussed with the surgeons as they may adversely affect transmural pressure. With mild hyperventilation to a $PaCO_2$ of 30 mmHg, use of mannitol osmotherapy 0.25–1 g/kg and/or furosemide, adequate relaxation can often be achieved.

Temperature control throughout aneurysm surgery has been controversial. Previously, hypothermia was induced to neuroprotect during surgery. The Intraoperative Hypothermia for Aneurysm Surgery Trial [3] found no benefit with induced hypothermia, although passive cooling is acceptable as long as it does not prevent an appropriate extubation. Hyperthermia should be avoided as it increases cerebral blood flow and oxygen requirements. As it is not uncommon for patients to be well insulated by surgical drapes, vigilance is required.

Temporary arterial occlusion of the aneurysm's parent vessel is now an integral part of cerebral aneurysm surgery, preventing aneurysmal rupture while aiding dissection, clipping, and vessel reconstruction [4]. The safe duration is considered to be in the range of 10–15 minutes. Although not supported by randomized controlled trials, many centers use neurophysiologic monitoring to assist in the detection of regional ischemia associated with clip placement. Pre-occlusion burst suppression can be achieved with a slow bolus of thiopental 3–4 mg/kg and subsequent infusion of 3–4 mg/kg/hour, titrating to effect throughout occlusion. Vasopressor infusion can also be administered during temporary clipping to offset barbiturate administration and to improve cerebral collateral blood flow.

Significant intraoperative aneurysmal rupture can be catastrophic as the brain receives approximately 15% of the cardiac output and accounts for approximately 20% of basal oxygen consumption. Intraoperative rupture can be defined as aneurysmal bleeding that interrupts the normal sequence of the aneurysm microsurgery [1] and is considered significant if the resultant hemorrhage is not cleared by a double

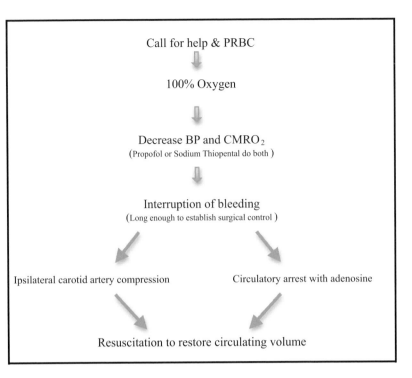

Call for help & PRBC

100% Oxygen

Decrease BP and CMRO$_2$
(Propofol or Sodium Thiopental do both)

Interruption of bleeding
(Long enough to establish surgical control)

Ipsilateral carotid artery compression   Circulatory arrest with adenosine

Resuscitation to restore circulating volume

Figure 14.1. Intraoperative rupture immediate action drill. BP, blood pressure; CMRO$_2$, cerebral metabolic rate; PRBC, packed red blood cells.

suction technique. The incidence of significant rupture is believed to be 3–4% [5], the majority occurring at time of aneurysm manipulation and dissection.

The immediate action drill for this potentially catastrophic event aims to allow surgical application of a temporary clip (Figure 14.1). The goals are to reduce cerebral metabolic rate, while decreasing the blood pressure to allow for proximal control of the aneurysm. The proximity and routine use of thiopental makes it a readily available agent for both purposes, but other drugs can be used. Associated hypotension is often sufficient to negate the requirement for a specific antihypertensive agent. Ipsilateral carotid compression and transient circulatory arrest with adenosine 12 mg may be utilized. On application of the clip, standard resuscitation of the intravascular compartment is essential.

Conclusion

In conclusion, intraoperative management of SAH is high-risk anesthesia with the potential for severe consequences. Constant vigilance regarding hemody-

namic control and preparedness for the possibility of intraoperative aneurysmal rupture are essential for good outcomes.

References

1. J. P. Chandler, C. C. Getch, H. H. Batjer. Intraoperative aneurysm rupture and complication avoidance. *Neurosurg Clin N Am* 1998; **9**: 861–8.

2. H. J. Priebe. Aneurysmal subarachnoid haemorrhage and the anaesthetist. *Br J Anaesth* 2007; **99**: 102–18.

3. M. M. Todd, B. J. Hindman, W. R. Clark *et al.* Mild intraoperative hypothermia during surgery for intracranial aneurysm. *N Engl J Med* 2005; **352**: 135–45.

4. C. L. Taylor, W. R. Selman, S. P. Kiefer *et al.* Temporary vessel occlusion during intracranial aneurysm repair. *Neurosurgery* 1996; **39**: 893–905; discussion 905–6.

5. T. J. Leipzig, J. Morgan, T. G. Horner *et al.* Analysis of intraoperative rupture in the surgical treatment of 1694 saccular aneurysms. *Neurosurgery* 2005; **56**: 455–68; discussion 455–68.

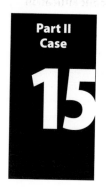

Vascular procedures. Aneurysm clipping

Awake fiberoptic intubation

Heather Hervey-Jumper and Christopher R. Turner

Patients who require fiberoptic-guided endotracheal intubation for the clipping or coiling of an intracranial aneurysm pose particular challenges for the safe completion of both procedures. The following case discussion highlights the considerations for awake endotracheal intubation in the patient with an unsecured aneurysm.

Case description

A 56-year-old female with a poorly documented history of "difficult intubation" presented for elective clipping of a middle cerebral artery aneurysm. Her past medical history was also significant for asthma and hypertension; prior treatment of her asthma with albuterol induced atrial fibrillation. Airway examination in the preoperative area revealed a Mallampati Class III oropharynx, mouth opening >3 cm, thyromental distance >6 cm, good mandibular subluxation, thick neck, slight limitation of the cervical spine and normal dentition. Given her further history of severe gastroesophageal reflux and hiatal hernia, the anesthesia team was concerned about the risk of aspiration with prolonged mask ventilation in the event that direct or indirect laryngoscopy proved difficult. A calm and clear discussion ensued with the patient, who subsequently agreed to an awake intubation. After placement of an intravenous and radial artery catheters, the patient was pretreated with glycopyrrolate as an antisialogogue, as well as ranitidine and sodium citrate. Twenty minutes later, nebulized lidocaine was started and the patient was then brought to the operating room. Standard monitors were applied and a low-dose remifentanil infusion (0.01 mcg/kg/min) was started. A "swish-and-swallow" technique of viscous lidocaine was performed, followed by atomized lidocaine sprayed in the posterior pharynx and directed at the vocal cords. Vigilance with respect to the blood pressure was maintained consistently. An oral airway was placed and

a flexible fiberoptic scope was passed into the posterior pharynx. The epiglottis then vocal cords were visualized – further lidocaine was sprayed onto the cords through an epidural catheter fed through the suction port of the scope. After a 30-second pause, the fiberoptic scope was inserted through the cords and into the trachea. Labetolol was administered for a systolic blood pressure of 165 mmHg, remifentanil was increased, and the endotracheal tube was passed after a pause and resolution of the hypertension. General anesthesia was then induced with propofol. After a brief period of bronchospasm that resolved with an increase of the inhalational anesthetic concentration, the case proceeded uneventfully and the aneurysm was secured. The patient was fully awake for tracheal extubation at the end of the case and recovered well.

Discussion

The indications for awake fiberoptic intubation (AFOI) in this case are essentially the same as for any difficult airway: concern for the ability to visualize the glottic opening via direct laryngoscopy combined with concern for the ability to mask ventilate. In a patient with an intracranial aneurysm, the additional concerns are ensuring pristine hemodynamic control in order to minimize the risk of aneurysmal rupture or re-rupture, which carries a significant risk of mortality or major morbidity [1], while maintaining sufficient blood pressure to ensure cerebral perfusion. Hemodynamic derangements may arise from two sources: the hemodynamic response of a poorly prepared patient to the stimulation of an awake intubation that is possibly premature, and the hemodynamic response to hypoxia and/or hypercarbia as a consequence of a failed or mismanaged awake intubation attempt. Hypertension is frequently a preexisting condition in patients with cerebral aneurysms, which is usually worsened with anxiety or the stimulation of an awake intubation. Thus, the ability to rapidly recognize and respond to changes in heart rate and blood pressure is critical to the safe completion of an awake intubation in a patient at risk for aneurysmal rupture. While an arterial catheter should be placed with the same concerns as apply to the intubation, i.e., hemodynamic control, it is easier to do so with minimal stimulation to the patient than it is to perform an AFOI.

Proper preparation of a patient for AFOI occurs in four overlapping steps. Psychological preparation and management of expectations should not be underestimated or underemphasized. It is critical that the patient understands the procedure about to occur, appreciates that they will be properly sedated and topicalized, and knows that they have the ability to pause the procedure if they are not tolerating it. Drying of the mucous membranes of the airway can be accomplished by the early administration of glycopyrrolate – again, the patient should be made aware of the consequent increase in heart rate and drying of the mouth. An antisialogogue serves both to increase the effectiveness of subsequent topical anesthetics and to decrease airway secretions that can obscure the fiberoptic view. Next comes the administration of topical anesthesia in order to anesthetize the glossopharyngeal innervation of the posterior pharynx, as well as the superior and recurrent laryngeal nerve branches of the vagus that provide sensory innervation to the superior and inferior aspects of the glottis, respectively. This can be done with a swish-and-swallow technique, staged administration of topical lidocaine via progressively deeper use of an atomizer, or administration of lidocaine via a hand-held nebulizer. Use of airway nerve blocks (glossopharyngeal, superior laryngeal, and transtracheal) is also a viable option, although they are more stimulating for the patient and probably should be reserved for situations where a need for rapid intubation is relatively more important than the desire for the least stimulating topicalization possible. While the airway is being topicalized, the patient should also be judiciously sedated. In general we have found that single-agent techniques are more effective than combining agents; in particular benzodiazepines augment amnesia but do little if anything to blunt the stimulation of an awake intubation. Combined agents also often act synergistically to suppress respiratory drive. With enough time, intravenous fentanyl can be effectively and safely titrated to an endpoint of a narcotized patient who is still breathing spontaneously and is oriented and cooperative. If time is short many providers find that using remifentanil has advantages over other agents in its rapid onset and recovery. This opioid may provide the ideal narcotization needed to facilitate intubation and the speedy recovery needed if airway compromise becomes an issue. Dexmedetomidine is an alpha-2 adrenergic agonist with significant sedative and analgesic properties. Dexmedetomidine, while slow in onset and more expensive than other agents, has the unique characteristics of providing sedation and analgesia while preserving respiratory drive and orientation. In the setting of an unsecured aneurysm, its sympatholytic effects are also beneficial. As further adjuncts, adrenergic blockade with esmolol or labetalol may also be useful to ensure blood pressure control without further respiratory depression, and one of these should be immediately available whenever an AFOI is attempted in a patient at risk for aneurysmal rupture. Supplemental oxygen via nasal cannula often increases the safety of the procedure but does little to lengthen the time to frank desaturation in the face of significant respiratory depression.

As the AFOI attempt is begun, one provider should be designated whose major responsibility is to monitor the patient's blood pressure. The blood pressure should not be allowed to rise above the preoperative baseline (or in our institution, a maximum systolic pressure of about 150 mmHg) and generally should be kept 20% below baseline in order to provide a margin of safety. If the patient is not tolerating the procedure by demonstrating a hypertensive response, it is necessary to pause to administer supplemental sedation and/or topicalization to prevent rapid or uncontrolled changes in blood pressure. Deep topicalization can often be supplemented via a catheter threaded through the suction port of the fiberoptic scope [2]. With this technique, local anesthetic can be directed at the tissue that is inadequately topicalized (often the glottic opening or the trachea itself), but it is necessary to remember that the onset of topical anesthesia requires at least 30–60 seconds. After the fiberoptic scope enters the trachea, the endotracheal tube should be advanced gently, again avoiding unnecessary reaction to the procedure by the patient. Stimulation of the carina by either the fiberoptic scope or the endotracheal tube should be assiduously avoided as the carina is commonly inadequately anesthetized and stimulation of the carina causes an intense reaction in the patient. Once the intubation is complete the patient should tolerate the presence of the endotracheal tube enough to permit an abbreviated postintubation neurologic examination.

If there is a high probability for successful mask ventilation, it is often better to intubate the trachea in a patient with a difficult airway after the induction of anesthesia. This may be particularly attractive in patients whose cooperation with an awake intubation is questionable, such as patients with mental status changes (Hunt–Hess Grade III or higher). There is a variety of techniques applicable to this scenario ranging from lightwands to rigid fiberoptics (e.g., Bullard, Glidescope, or C-Mac) to asleep flexible fiberoptic intubation. However, keep in mind that an asleep fiberoptic intubation is not necessarily less stimulating than asleep direct laryngoscopy. Fiberoptic intubation may affect the hemodynamic response or catecholamine levels as much as direct laryngoscopy when performed on an anesthetized patient [3]. Thus, even though a fiberoptic intubation may be performed after the induction of anesthesia, it does not obviate the need for vigilance with respect to hemodynamic control.

Intubation via an intubating laryngeal mask airway (e.g., Fastrach) or standard laryngeal mask airway and Aintree catheter assisted by a fiberoptic scope are also options, but should not be attempted if there is concern of not being able to mask ventilate the patient.

Conclusion

In conclusion, AFOI has the potential to trigger hypertension, tachycardia and, potentially, hypoxia or hypercarbia. These all pose an increased risk of rupture or re-rupture in aneursymal disease. Preventing the hemodynamic response to intubation in the awake patient should thus be with a multimodal approach of psychological preparation, suppression of the sympathetic reaction to instrumentation with opioids and topicalization, and the immediate availability of vasoactive medications to maintain a blood pressure within the target range to avoid rupture of the aneurysm. Hypercarbia or hypoxia during an awake fiberoptic intubation are frequently due to loss of respiratory efforts in a narcotized patient. Newer sedation regimens such as dexmedetomidine can provide sedation and analgesia while maintaining respiratory drive and reducing hypertension. In the presence of cerebrovascular disease where patient cooperation is questionable, asleep intubations utilizing an appropriate airway device may be the preferred option.

References

1. **L. Elijovich, R. T. Higashida, M. T. Lawton** *et al.* Predictors and outcomes of intraprocedural rupture in patients treated for ruptured intracranial aneurysms. *Stroke* 2008: **39**: 1501–6.

2. **F. S. Xue, H. P. Liu, N. He** *et al.* Spray-as-you-go airway topical anesthesia in patients with a difficult airway: a randomized, double-blind comparison of 2% and 4% lidocaine. *Anesth Analg* 2009: **108**: 536–43.

3. **M. Barak, A. Ziser, A. Greenberg** *et al.* Hemodynamic and catecholamine response to tracheal intubation: direct laryngoscopy compared to fiberoptic intubation. *J Clin Anesth* 2003: **15**: 132–6.

Vascular procedures. Aneurysm clipping

Patient with coronary artery stent

Richard Bowers and George A. Mashour

The increasing use of coronary artery angioplasty with deployment of stents for treatment of coronary artery disease poses several dilemmas for perioperative management. These conflicting requirements are manifested most acutely in the management of patients with neurovascular disease.

Case description

The patient was a 51-year-old female with a past medical history of ischemic heart disease, hypertension, and undifferentiated autoimmune disease with interstitial lung involvement. She presented with a 5-month history of episodic headache and retro-orbital pain with associated nausea and vomiting. Radiologic imaging revealed a saccular aneurysm of the posterior communicating artery. A decision was made for subsequent admission and aneurysm clipping on the basis of aneurysm morphology and the patient's age. A cardiac catheterization 7 months prior to the admission had revealed 80% stenosis of the right coronary artery. A paclitaxel-eluting stent was deployed to treat the lesion and the patient was taking regular aspirin and clopidogrel as advised by her cardiologist. These medications had been discontinued 7 days prior to surgery.

Anesthesia was uneventful and the patient was transferred to the neurologic intensive care unit postoperatively. Antiplatelet therapy was reintroduced at 24 hours post-surgery. No arrhythmia, troponin rise, or ECG changes were recorded.

Discussion

The presence of coronary stents in patients undergoing neurosurgical procedures warrants specific consideration prior to anesthesia. It is necessary to balance the risks of stent thrombosis, and the subsequent risk of myocardial infarction, arrhythmia, or cardiac arrest, against the risks of hemorrhage during or after a neu-

rosurgical procedure. There are several factors to be considered including:

1. Stent type.
2. Duration since cardiac intervention.
3. Antithrombotic regimen.
4. Urgency of neurosurgical procedure.

Other risk factors for stent thrombosis do exist, for instance diabetes mellitus, renal failure, and stent type, although the manipulation of these factors in the perioperative period to reduce the risk of stent thrombosis is limited [1].

There are two available stent types. Drug-eluting stents (DES) are now the commonest type used in coronary artery stenting and are estimated to represent more than 80% of stents deployed in the USA, although this rate has fallen somewhat over concerns for long-term risk of stent thrombosis [2]. Two subtypes of this stent type are available – sirolimus-eluting and paclitaxel-eluting. The goal of such agents is to prevent neointimal hyperplasia and occlusion. However, both of these agents also prevent neoendothelialization of the implanted stent over a variable period. Once all the drug is eluted from the stent, some degree of endothelialization may occur, although this has been reported as variable and incomplete [3]. The alternative is the bare metal stent (BMS). As the name suggests, this stent does not contain any antimitotic properties, so that, once implanted, it is covered by a layer of vascular endothelium.

Both stent varieties carry the risks of thrombosis and restenosis. Original coronary interventions using BMS carried an initial high risk of thrombosis, which ameliorated over the 6 weeks following stent deployment. This risk follows the natural progression of healing in the arterial wall and neoendothelialization of the stent. Thereafter the major risks encountered with BMS are restenosis, which may then require further treatment [1]. Drug-eluting stents (DES) were developed to avoid this late risk of restenosis.

Thrombosis risk continues until a stent is endothelialized. Consequently, antithrombotic strategies have been developed to reduce the risk of stent thrombosis. Current guidelines by the American College of Cardiology/American Heart Association (ACC/AHA) recommend the use of dual antiplatelet therapy. Aspirin is recommended at high doses for up to 6 months post-stent deployment, followed by lifelong aspirin therapy at a lower dose. Use of clopidogrel is recommended for a minimum of 1 month following BMS deployment [2]. Thrombotic risk is less than 1% if the appropriate regimen is adhered to [1]. There is a risk of late thrombosis due to the presence of antimitotic agents on the polymer coating of DES, particularly at times when antiplatelet therapy has been discontinued. The discontinuation of clopidogrel therapy within 6 months of the placement of a DES has been found to be the strongest independent risk factor for stent thrombosis within the subsequent 14 days [4]. The same study also found that the lack of clopidogrel therapy, though not necessarily acute discontinuation of therapy, beyond 6 months was also a risk factor for stent thrombosis. The ACC/AHA guidelines recommend 12 months clopidogrel therapy for all types of DES [2]. Mortality estimates for stent thrombosis range from 19 to 45% [5].

The risks of hemorrhage during or following intracranial neurosurgical procedures include excessive blood loss, neurologic deficits and disability, and risks related to blood transfusion. Small amounts of intracranial blood loss may result in significant changes of intracranial pressure and consequent neuronal insult. The use of antiplatelet agents may appreciably increase these risks. To date, no trial has been performed that demonstrates an excessive bleeding risk from maintenance of antiplatelet drugs during a neurosurgical procedure. There is evidence that aspirin and nonsteroidal anti-inflammatory drugs cause excessive hemorrhage in other surgical procedures, and while many of these studies measure different endpoints, the overall suggestion is that antiplatelet agents increase blood loss and hemorrhagic complications, and that combinations of drugs further increase these problems.

Standard practice in most centers is complete discontinuation of anticoagulation to remove any excess hemorrhage risk. This abrupt withdrawal results in a rebound phenomenon of increased platelet aggrega-

tion, which may compound the thrombotic risk posed from the surgical stress response.

Consequently, the clinician must balance the risks of major cardiac events on the one hand with neurologic sequelae on the other. The context in which the patient is seen will have a bearing on the approach taken to managing anticoagulation, and all options will need consideration among surgery, cardiology, and anesthesiology staff to minimize risks during the perioperative period. There are three scenarios that may arise:

1. The patient without a coronary stent but with concerning symptomatology.
2. The patient with coronary artery stents taking dual antiplatelet therapy.
3. The patient with coronary stents taking aspirin alone.

Scenario 1 – Patient with no coronary stents

A patient without previously documented coronary disease, but concerning cardiac symptoms, presenting for elective surgery should be referred for assessment by a cardiologist. The indications for preoperative coronary revascularization are limited, however, and an improvement in mortality from intervention has only been demonstrated for patients with significant left main stem disease treated prior to major vascular surgery [6]. This evidence may not be directly applicable to neurosurgical patients. *The ACC/AHA guidelines recommend avoiding noncardiac surgery following stent deployment for a minimum of 1 month in the case of BMS and 1 year if using a DES* [6]. This delay has been correlated with a reduction in major adverse cardiac events (MACE) [6]. In both cases, it is recommended that aspirin be continued throughout the perioperative period. It is unlikely that surgery for an intracranial aneurysm could be delayed for a year or aspirin continued in the perioperative period. It has been suggested that patients may instead have a BMS with the associated shortened period of anticoagulation cover, or a balloon angioplasty that may avoid the risks associated with use of a stent [1]. The choices would seem to be to (1) perform surgery before coronary intervention, (2) perform angioplasty without stenting and revisit the coronary artery disease postoperatively, or (3) perform angioplasty with a bare metal stent allowing at least 30 days, but preferably

90 days, before routine surgery on the basis of ACC/AHA guidelines [1, 3, 6].

Scenario 2 – Patient on dual antiplatelet therapy

This is a more frequent presentation: a patient presenting for surgery with coronary stents *in situ* and currently taking anticoagulation. Attention during the preoperative visit must be paid regarding the risk factors given earlier, although a decision as to when to proceed to surgery is usually based on the time elapsed since coronary stenting and the urgency of the neurosurgical procedure. The risks of coronary stent thrombosis do ameliorate with time as noted above, but the recommendations for antiplatelet therapy will still apply. Patients who prematurely discontinue clopidogrel are almost 60 times more likely to suffer a stent thrombosis [5]. The associated mortality rate was 45% [5]. Other studies corroborate this evidence, suggesting that discontinuation of thienopyridine therapy within the first 6 months after DES implantation was the strongest predictor for stent thrombosis with a hazard ratio of 13 [1, 3]. Aspirin withdrawal would also be necessary for intracranial surgery and this seems to compound the risks of stent thrombosis [3].

Scenario 3 – Patient on single antiplatelet therapy

The risk associated with discontinuation over 1 year from coronary stenting has not been defined in a large series; however, an observational study found that stent thrombosis at a mean duration of 15 months since deployment represented approximately 20% of all coronary events following aspirin withdrawal [3]. An odds ratio of 90 for the risk of myocardial infarction following acute aspirin withdrawal in patients with coronary stents has been reported [3, 5]. The average time from aspirin withdrawal to thrombotic event is 10 days [5]. There continue to be case reports of very late stent thrombosis during times of antiplatelet withdrawal and therefore the ACC/AHA guidelines state aspirin use should continue indefinitely [2].

Alternatives to complete anticoagulation discontinuation

Bridging therapies have been suggested, including withholding clopidogrel and covering the periopera-tive period with intravenous heparin or glycoprotein IIb/IIIa inhibitors, converting to short-acting cyclo-oxygenase inhibitors (such as flubiprofen) prior to surgery, or preoperative platelet transfusions [1, 3]. Most of these suggestions continue perioperative aspirin administration. There is unfortunately a lack of evidence and data to estimate the risks of continuing any form of antiplatelet therapy in the neurosurgical perioperative period. Studies in this area have examined major general, vascular, or cardiac surgery, and find an increase in blood loss with increased transfusion but which does not appear to affect mortality [1]. However, expert opinion unanimously agrees that antiplatelet therapy should be withheld in closed-space surgery [1, 3].

Conclusion

In conclusion, coronary artery stents present a challenging dilemma for the perioperative care of neurosurgical patients. There is currently an irresolvable conflict between the risks of withholding and continuing antiplatelet agents in the perioperative period. This conflict is most acute in closed-space surgeries such as intracranial procedures.

A delay of surgical intervention for as long as possible will allow coronary stent thrombosis risk to decrease, but not disappear entirely. Indeed, no period following coronary artery stenting appears to be able to be described as risk-free. Rapid percutaneous intervention is required in the event of stent thrombosis and access to coronary intervention laboratories is therefore a consideration. Attempts must be made to minimize the period of antiplatelet withdrawal and early reintroduction postoperatively should be considered. Please see Case 31 for further discussion.

References

1. **G. M. Howard-Alpe, J. de Bono, L. Hudsmith** *et al.* Coronary artery stents and non-cardiac surgery. *Br J Anaesth* 2007; **98**: 560–74.

2. **S. B. King, S. C. Smith, J. W. Hirshfeld** *et al.* 2007 focused update of the ACC/AHA/SCAI guideline update for percutaneous coronary intervention: a report of the American College of Cardiology/ American Heart Association Task Force on Practice guidelines. *J Am Coll Cardiol* 2008; **51**: 172–209.

3. **L. T. Newsome, R. S. Weller, J. C. Gerancher** *et al.* Coronary artery stents II: Perioperative considerations and management. *Anesth Analg* 2008; **107**: 570–90.

4. **J. W. van Werkum, A. A. Heestermans, A. C. Zomer** *et al.* Predictors of coronary stent thrombosis: the Dutch Stent Thrombosis Registry. *J Am Coll Cardiol* 2009; **53**: 1399–409.

5. **P. G. Chassot, A. Delabays, D. R. Spahn**. Perioperative antiplatelet therapy: the case for continuing therapy in patients at risk of myocardial infarction. *Br J Anaesth* 2007; **99**: 316–28.

6. **L. A. Fleisher**. Cardiac risk stratification for noncardiac surgery: update from the American College of Cardiology/American Heart Association 2007 guidelines. *Cleve Clin J Med* 2009; **76**: S9–15.

Vascular procedures. Aneurysm clipping

Deep hypothermic circulatory arrest for intracranial aneurysm clipping

Matt Giles and George A. Mashour

Over the last 15 years, advances in the fields of interventional neuroradiology and neurosurgical techniques have changed the way in which many intracranial aneurysms are managed. Many tertiary centers now rely on interventional neuroradiologists for coiling procedures of simple intracranial aneurysms, versus a more traditional and invasive neurosurgical approach. However, there still remains a subset of patients with large and/or complex intracranial aneurysms who are not candidates for neuroradiologic coiling procedures and for whom conventional neurosurgical approaches still carry exceptionally high risks of morbidity and mortality. The following is a case presentation and discussion of the application of deep hypothermic circulatory arrest (DHCA) for patients undergoing large and/or complex intracranial aneurysm clipping and repair.

Case description

A 62-year-old female presented to the operating room with a diagnosis of two large intracranial aneurysms. The first was a 17-mm aneurysm located at the junction of two temporal branches of the left posterior communicating artery (PCA), and the second was a 19-mm aneurysm located at the junction of the left posterior medial choroidal artery and the PCA. The patient was hemodynamically stable, awake, alert, and had presented to the emergency room earlier that day with vague complaints of severe headache, blurred vision, and difficulty with ambulation. Upon computed tomography-angiography (CTA) of the head, the neuroradiologist concluded that the two aneurysms were too large and complex in fusiform anatomy to allow for safe and effective coiling. Neurosurgery was consulted and concluded that an intracranial approach with clipping would likely prove successful. However, given the size and anatomy, circulatory arrest was necessary for adequate collapse of the aneurysms in order to facilitate surgical dissec-

tion and manipulation. After discussing the risks, benefits, and alternatives with the patient, and obtaining informed consent, a decision to perform the surgery under DHCA was made.

The patient was brought to the operating room, noninvasive monitors placed, and under local anesthesia a right radial arterial line was established. The patient was positioned supine, preoxygenated, and a titrated, mixed intravenous induction with midazolam, fentanyl, and propofol was conducted. The patient was easily bag/mask ventilated, and tracheal intubation was facilitated with rocuronium. Ventilation was adjusted to maintain an end-tidal CO_2 in the 32–36 mmHg range. Sevoflurane was titrated to adequately maintain anesthesia and hemodynamic stability. Two large-bore 16-gauge peripheral intravenous catheters were started, and a 9-French Cordis was placed in the patient's right subclavian vein for central access, through which a Swan–Ganz pulmonary artery catheter was placed. A Foley bladder catheter was inserted, and a transesophageal echocardiography (TEE) probe was gently placed. A brief TEE examination was performed. The patient was then positioned in the right lateral decubitus position with the lower torso gently turned to near-neutral supine position and supported with padding to facilitate surgical cannulation of the left femoral artery and vein for cardiopulmonary bypass (CPB). Temperature probes were placed in the nasopharynx, axilla, and bladder. Craniotomy with surgical dissection and isolation of the aneurysms commenced.

After common femoral artery and vein cannulation, positioning of the venous cannula for CPB was verified by TEE to be at the level of the right atrium. Upon near completion of aneurysm dissection, adequate CPB flow was initiated and hemodynamic stability was achieved. Systemic hypothermia commenced per CPB protocol until ventricular fibrillation occurred. At that point, potassium chloride was administered via the right atrial port of the pulmonary artery catheter to facilitate asystole. Systemic cooling continued to a core body and cortical temperature of 15 °C, at which point the CPB circulation was arrested, blood was drained via the venous cannula until vascular relaxation was reported by the neurosurgeon, and complete aneurysm reconstruction/clipping ensued. A total deep hypothermic circulatory arrest time of 32 minutes was documented. Upon clipping of both aneurysms, CPB was slowly reestablished and both extracorporeal flow and patient mean arterial pressure were brought to pre-CPB levels. Separation from CPB and surgical closure were uneventful.

Discussion

The rationale behind the technique of DHCA stems from the significant advantage the surgeon has once blood flow has stopped circulating to the aneurysm. In particular, by temporarily eliminating blood flow into an aneurysm, the vascular anomaly is converted from an otherwise hard, pulsating mass into a much more pliable, collapsed vascular sac [1].

The technique of DHCA is not without significant risk and should be considered an option of last resort for large or complex intracranial vascular anomalies. In general, aneurysms located in the anterior circulation are most often amenable to neurocoiling via interventional radiology, or more traditional neurosurgical clipping with a straightforward intracranial approach [1, 2]. Typically, larger aneurysms (10–25 mm) or complex aneurysms (fusiform, branching, etc.) predominantly occur within the posterior circulation, such as in the above case. Due in part to the size or complex nature of these aneurysms, conventional aneurysm coiling and even traditional neurosurgical clipping are both extremely difficult and with higher risk of rupture. Often these complex vascular anomalies cannot be collapsed easily intraoperatively because of the breadth of the neck, the irregularity/complexity of the network of arterial branches at the base, the presence of thrombus within the lumen, or extensive artheroma within the vessel walls [1, 2]. Cessation of the patient's blood flow allows for optimization of surgical exposure and provides an opportunity for clipping and reconstruction that would otherwise prove extremely difficult. When one or both proximal and distal arteries are inaccessible for complex aneurysm repair, DHCA may be the only safe and effective means of vascular control [1–4].

As discussed previously, there exists a subset of patients requiring extensive repair of large and/or complex intracranial vascular anomalies using DHCA. The circulatory arrest component of this technique affords the surgeon the advantage of a collapsed, bloodless aneurysm with which to work. However, the scientific rationale for the application of deep hypothermic temperatures during the cessation of circulation rests primarily upon the observed effect that a temperature-mediated reduction of metabolism occurs. Whole body and cerebral oxygen consumption during induced hypothermia decreases the metabolic rate for oxygen by a factor of 2 to 2.5 for every 10 °C reduction in temperature below normothermia (defined as 37 °C) [5–8]. These results are consistent in both in vivo and in vitro models, which suggest that the rate of cellular metabolism is directly proportional to temperature. The benefit of inducing hypothermia in the patient undergoing circulatory arrest, therefore, is observed as both a neuroprotective and systemic organ-protective effect. By decreasing the patient's temperature to 15–18 °C (common during DHCA), the systemic basal metabolic rates in all organs (including the brain) have decreased dramatically [5–8]. Hence by decreasing the basal metabolic rates for cellular substrates and oxygen utilization in all tissues, hypothermia helps exert a protective effect from ischemia while circulation is temporarily halted [9, 10]. Other studies have noted that the reduction in oxygen supply during deep hypothermic low-flow CPB is associated with preferential increases in vital organ perfusion (e.g., to the brain) and increased extraction of oxygen [8–10].

The protective effect of hypothermia during low-flow and no-flow circulatory states has also been demonstrated by studies looking at reductions in intracellular markers of ischemia. It has been well established that during episodes of brain ischemia, several excitatory amino acids (glutamate, aspartate, etc.) are released in relation to deprivation of cellular substrates (oxygen, glucose, etc.) indicating anaerobic metabolism and ischemia. However, hypothermia has been shown to significantly decrease the release of excitatory amino acids and other markers of focal and global ischemia [5–10].

Reducing a patient's temperature during surgery carries several risks, which have a wide range of implications on multiple organ systems. Moreover, the duration of the safe period of DHCA has not clearly been delineated. A number of studies aimed at determining a "safe DHCA time" have been conducted and suggest that an arrest period up to 40 minutes is tolerated without evidence of long-term neurologic sequalae [1–4]. But by no measure is neurologic ischemia and injury the only risk of DHCA. By inducing hypothermia, the patient is at increased risk for coagulation dysfunction and bleeding, which can be compounded in light of heparinization during (and separation from) cardiopulmonary bypass. Hypothermia also places the patient at increased risk of cardiac dysrhythmias, such as ventricular tachycardia and fibrillation. Recurrent ventricular tachycardia and fibrillation are commonly observed during rewarming and can persist into the postoperative period. Also associated with hypothermia is the increased risk of postoperative wound infection, which can significantly increase morbidity and mortality. Especially important to neurosurgical patients is the finding that cerebral autoregulation is lost during, and immediately after, extremes of temperature. In this setting, cerebral perfusion therefore becomes highly dependent upon the conduct of extracorporeal perfusion and post-bypass hemodynamic stability [1, 6–9].

In approaching the anesthetic management of a patient scheduled to undergo DHCA for aneurysm clipping, the goals of providing safe and effective anesthesia are no different than in any other patient undergoing general anesthesia, with the exception of a few added objectives. The additional goals of this particular anesthetic should include the prevention of cerebral injury, preserving overall hemodynamic stability before, during, and after CPB, and assisting the surgeon/CPB team in all efforts with special attention to blood loss/replacement, coagulation status/correction, and neurologic monitoring. With respect to the choice of monitors, all standard American Society of Anesthesiologists monitors should be employed, as well as an arterial catheter for blood pressure monitoring. Temperature probes in the bladder and nasopharynx, in addition to cerebral core temperature monitoring are critical to guiding systemic cooling efforts once CPB has been initiated. Multiple modalities for temperature monitoring are recommended for reliable measurements. The degree of induced hypothermia must be carefully controlled. In particular, slowly cooling the patient, maintaining a constant hypothermia, and finally slowly decooling the patient are key components to the success of DHCA [1–4].

As DHCA is becoming more widely employed as a technique for repairing complex aneurysms, the use of TEE for cardiac monitoring has proven very useful. Specifically, TEE allows for early intraoperative evaluation of overall cardiac function, including estimation of ejection fraction, assessment for wall motion abnormalities, valvular dysfunctions, as well as assessment of ventricular volume status and contractility. Transesophageal echocardiography is also very helpful with verifying the proper placement of the venous bypass cannulae into the right atrium while preparing for CPB [1]. Furthermore, assessing cardiac function immediately prior to separation of CPB, and after complete separation from CPB, can be invaluable at guiding the intraoperative management. In addition to TEE, a pulmonary artery catheter can be helpful in guiding the anesthetic management.

Conclusion

Overall, the application of DHCA has been successfully employed as a viable method of providing optimized surgical access to and control of large or complex intracranial aneurysms. However, DHCA is associated with unique risks and potentially devastating complications. The margin for error is small, and success depends upon an experienced and knowledgeable team. The safe practice and management of DHCA requires an extensive understanding of cardiac and neurosurgical anesthetic practice, CPB, as well as careful consideration and proper planning.

References

1. **W. L. Young, M. T. Lawton, D. K. Gupta** et al. Anesthetic management of deep hypothermic circulatory arrest for cerebral aneurysm clipping. *Anesthesiology* 2002; **96**: 497–503.

2. **W. L. Young**. Cerebral aneurysms: current anaesthetic management and future horizons. *Can J Anaesth* 1998; **45**: R17–31.

3. **A. Levati, C. Tommasino, M. P. Moretti** et al. Giant intracranial aneurysms treated with deep hypothermia and circulatory arrest. *J Neurosurg Anesthesiol* 2007; **19**: 25–30.

4. **M. G. Massad, F. T. Charbel, R. Chaer** et al. Closed chest hypothermic circulatory arrest for complex intracranial aneurysms. *Ann Thorac Surg* 2001; **71**: 1900–4.

5. **L. Berntman, F. A. Welsh, J. R. Harp**. Cerebral protective effect of low-grade hypothermia. *Anesthesiology* 1981; **55**: 495–8.

6. **J. Hartung, J. E. Cottrell**. Mild hypothermia and cerebral metabolism. *J Neurosurg Anesthesiol* 1994; **6**: 1–3.

7. **J. Hartung, J. E. Cottrell**. In response to: effects of hypothermia on cerebral metabolic rate for oxygen. *J Neurosurg Anesthesiol* 1994; **6**: 22.

8. **L. S. Fox, E. H. Blackstone, J. W. Kirklin** *et al.* Relationship of whole body oxygen consumption to perfusion flow rate during hypothermic cardiopulmonary bypass. *J Thorac Cardiovasc Surg* 1982; **83**: 239–48.

9. **L. S. Fox, E. H. Blackstone, J. W. Kirklin** *et al.* Relationship of brain blood flow and oxygen consumption to perfusion flow rate during profoundly hypothermic cardiopulmonary bypass. An experimental study. *J Thorac Cardiovasc Surg* 1984; **87**: 658–64.

10. **R. Busto, M. Y. Globus, W. D. Dietrich** *et al.* Effect of mild hypothermia on ischemia-induced release of neurotransmitters and free fatty acids in rat brain. *Stroke* 1989; **20**: 904–10.

Vascular procedures. Aneurysm clipping

18 Neuroprotection during surgical clip ligation of cerebral aneurysms

Neeraj Chaudhary, Joseph J. Gemmete, B. Gregory Thompson and Aditya S. Pandey

Subarachnoid hemorrhage (SAH) from a ruptured cerebral aneurysm is associated with significant morbidity and mortality. The endovascular treatment of ruptured cerebral aneurysms has become well established over the last decade as the preferred treatment modality [1]. However, there are no conclusive data yet regarding the best management of unruptured aneurysms. Not every aneurysm configuration and location is feasible for endovascular treatment due to technical limitations. Microsurgical clip ligation (MCL) is the treatment of choice for those aneurysms that cannot be safely treated from an endovascular approach. Here we discuss the different strategies of neuroprotection applied to prevent ischemic damage to the brain during clip ligation of cerebral aneurysms.

Case description

A 44-year-old male presented to our hospital with acute SAH; diagnostic cerebral angiogram was performed emergently that demonstrated an anterior communicating artery (ACOM) aneurysm. Two additional aneurysms were also identified at the origin of left superior hypophyseal artery and right posterior communicating artery. The ACOM artery aneurysm was deemed to be the cause of the SAH based on its morphology and the distribution of blood in the subarachnoid space. Endovascular embolization of the ACOM aneurysm was technically not feasible due to the complex shape and wide neck. Given these findings, MCL of the aneurysm via an open craniotomy was deemed the best option for the patient.

The patient was taken to the operating room, where general anesthesia was induced and endotracheal intubation established. The anesthesia was maintained by total intravenous anesthesia in order to minimize the use of inhalational anesthetic agents that can increase cerebral blood volume and intracranial pressure. The patient's blood pressure was tightly controlled to prevent any hypertensive surges during intubation

and pinning that could possibly cause rebleeding from the aneurysm. A right frontal craniotomy was performed followed by a meticulous durotomy and bone drilling of the sphenoid ridge to gain access to the ACOM aneurysm. Prophylactically, mannitol and furosemide were administered before the dural incision. The right and left A1 and A2 segments of the anterior cerebral artery and the ACOM complex were identified.

During further exposure of the aneurysm, as the right frontal lobe was retracted there was rupture of the aneurysm with hemorrhage from its contralateral aspect. The patient was put into "burst suppression" with a bolus dose of propofol, which also decreased the blood pressure. Temporary clips were applied to both A1 segments which controlled the hemorrhage to some extent; however, there was minimal retrograde bleeding from the A2 segments. The aneurysm was then decompressed. Subsequently, a permanent fenestrated clip was placed across the neck of the ACOM aneurysm, maintaining patency of the A2 division intimately related to the superior aspect of the aneurysm. This secured the aneurysm, which was confirmed upon removal of the temporary clips. Burst suppression was reversed after approximately 13 minutes of temporary clip occlusion.

The surgical field was then irrigated with saline antibiotic solution and the craniotomy closed with meticulous hemostasis. The patient was transferred to the neurosurgical intensive care unit in a stable condition. On the second postoperative day the trachea was extubated.

Discussion

An interdisciplinary approach to the management of cerebrovascular disease is necessary for optimal patient outcome. The role of the neuroanesthesiologist in supporting the cerebrovascular physiology to overcome the stress from SAH is crucial. Subarachnoid hemorrhage is a devastating disease that is accompanied by a marked stress response with increased plasma concentration of catecholamines. Electrolyte imbalances are also prominent, which have both cerebral and systemic effects. Hence, the American Society of Anesthesiologists class in this group of patients is often IV or V [2].

Currently, application of temporary clips to the parent vessel during MCL is increasingly utilized. This is used either to gain control over unforeseen rupture of the aneurysm before clip ligation or as part of a planned strategy to achieve optimal positioning of the definitive aneurysm clip. In either case anesthetic interventions can offer cerebral parenchymal protection during these periods of temporary cessation of blood supply. The interventions are based on the duration of occlusion of blood flow. If the temporary clip application is going to be for less than 60–120 seconds then no anesthetic intervention is necessary. However, if this duration of occlusion to blood flow is exceeded, the following anesthetic interventions can be undertaken:

- The inspiratory concentration of oxygen is increased to 100%.
- Propofol or barbiturates are administered intravenously to achieve "burst suppression" on electroencephalography. This offers cerebral protection by reducing cerebral metabolism to a minimum, which in turn reduces oxygen consumption.
- Additional doses of phenylephrine to increase arterial blood pressure to more than 20% of baseline may improve retrograde flow to the brain parenchyma temporarily deprived of blood flow but can prove potentially dangerous. It may induce bleeding in the surgical field and therefore make temporary clip removal more prolonged and difficult [3].
- In situations where the temporary clipping exceeds 10 minutes, the role of induced mild to moderate hypothermia has been questioned in the recent reports of the IHAST trial secondary data analysis [4].

Another method that has been reported to have some benefit in case of an unforeseen hemorrhage during clip ligation of a cerebral aneurysm is the use of adenosine to induce temporary cardiac arrest [5]. Nussbaum *et al.* in their series of 10 cases have demonstrated the use of 12 mg adenosine injected intravenously to induce cardiac arrest for approximately 10 seconds [5]. During this period of circulatory arrest, blood is suctioned off the surgical field and a temporary clip is applied to gain hemostasis as the normal rhythm returns. Although adenosine is not in itself neuroprotective, it can afford an opportunity to achieve rapid proximal control of a ruptured aneurysm.

There has been a recent explosion of interest in the mechanisms of cerebral ischemia, with over 1000 experimental papers and over 400 clinical articles appearing within the past 6 years. These studies, in turn, are the outcome of three decades of investigative work to define the multiple mechanisms and mediators of ischemic brain injury, which constitute potential targets of neuroprotection [6]. Apart from temporary clip occlusion there are other insults to the brain during MCL such as tissue retraction and intraoperative hemorrhage as discussed above. The IHAST trial was the first prospective multicenter study to assess patient outcome where hypothermia was applied as a neuroprotective adjunct [7]. The IHAST investigators concluded that there was no significant improvement in neurologic outcome in patients with good grade SAH who underwent a craniotomy. An inconclusive trend towards some benefit in the male population and in patients with craniotomy 8–14 days after SAH was shown on secondary analysis of the data. The result of this study is in complete discordance with the results of preclinical studies in the animal population [8]. Further analysis of the IHAST cohort revealed that there was no significant added protection offered not only by the induced hypothermia but also by the supplemental pharmacologic protective agents [4].

Another nonpharmacologic modulation that has demonstrated some benefit in animal studies is ischemic preconditioning. Feng *et al.* recently have demonstrated the neuroprotective effects of hypoxic preconditioning in neonatal rat brain [9]. They conclude that the underlying mechanism of neuroprotection is mediated during the period of reperfusion following hypoxic insult and is via an increase in expression of vascular endothelial growth factor A, which in turn decreases the apoptotic cascade. The upregulation of adenosine receptors in ischemic preconditioning in animal models again has been proposed as a potential neuroprotective agent [10]. Anesthetic preconditioning with volatile agents is also an area of active investigation.

There are several other pharmacologic agents that have been assessed for neuroprotective properties based on a growing understanding of the neuronal ischemic injury pathway. There is a clearer understanding from basic science research of the role of the N-methyl-D-aspartate (NMDA) glutamate receptor in this pathway. Hardingham, in his recent review on this receptor, opines that hypo- or hyper-NMDA stimulation can set off a neurodestructive cascade [11]. Although implicated in animal stroke models, NMDA receptor blockade has not shown any clinical benefit in acute ischemic stroke due to poor tolerance and efficacy [11]. Another study in an animal model has implicated downregulation and internalization of NMDA receptors in the regions remote and in fact contralateral to the area of infarct, which in turn causes cognitive impairment in ischemic stroke without actual cell death [12]. A detailed discussion of the relevant pathways is beyond the scope of this chapter. Competitive inhibition of the glycine site of the NMDA receptor by the general anesthetic gas xenon has been implicated in its neuroprotective role [13]. An in vivo model of rat hippocampus subjected to oxygen-glucose deprivation and then exposed to xenon showed significant neuronal protection for a period of 3–4 hours from the ischemic insult, which was also shown to be inhibited by increased glycine concentrations. A clinical trial to learn more about the neuroprotective role of xenon is being formulated. The NMDA receptor blocker nitrous oxide has also been implicated to potentially play a role in the ischemic pathway. However, the IHAST group has demonstrated no detrimental effect of the application of nitrous oxide in patients undergoing temporary clip occlusion during MCL [14]. They show that although the risk of delayed ischemic neurologic deficits is increased in this group, the overall neurologic outcome is not affected.

Erythropoietin (Epo) is another agent that is increasingly being studied for its neuroprotective properties. It is well established at a molecular level that Epo in general offers cytoprotection via decreased oxidative stress and lipid peroxidation. In the brain its potential mechanism of neuroprotection has been studied recently in an in vitro study [15]. The study demonstrated that the pathway of neuroprotection is mediated by an increase in concentration of glutathione (an antioxidant) that results from an upregulation of the cystine glutamate exchanger (system Xc).

Conclusion

Although there are promising revelations regarding neuroprotective pathways and how these can be modulated in cellular and animal models, there is currently no definite benefit shown in human subjects. The role and efficacy of the cerebral protective measures suggested to prevent ischemic brain damage from temporary clip occlusion during MCL are not clearly understood. Larger multicenter studies and more translational research are needed to demonstrate the efficacy of currently employed cerebral protective measures. The next decade will hopefully provide a clearer analysis of the pathways of ischemic neuronal cell death, which in turn will help to determine more effective neuroprotective options.

References

1. A. J. Molyneux, R. S. Kerr, J. Birks *et al.*; ISAT Collaborators. Risk of recurrent subarachnoid haemorrhage, death, or dependence and standardised mortality ratios after clipping or coiling of an intracranial aneurysm in the International Subarachnoid Aneurysm Trial (ISAT): long-term follow-up. *Lancet Neurol.* 2009; 8(5): 427–33. Epub 2009 Mar 28.

2. P. H. Manninen, A. W. Gelb. The anesthetic management of patients during posterior fossa aneurysm surgery. In C. G. Drake, S. J. Peerless, J. A. Hernesniemi (eds.), *Surgery of Vertebrobasilar Aneurysms. London, Ontario Experience on 1767 Patients.* Vienna: Springer-Verlag; 1996, pp. 280–4.

3. T. Randell, M. Niemelä, J. Kyttä *et al.* Principles of neuroanesthesia in aneurysmal subarachnoid hemorrhage: the Helsinki experience. *Surg Neurol* 2006; 66: 382–8.

4. B. J. Hindman, E. O. Bayman, W. K. Pfisterer *et al.* No association between intraoperative hypothermia and supplemental protective drug and neurologic outcomes in patients undergoing temporary clipping cerebral aneurysm surgery: findings from the Intra-operative Hypothermia for Aneurysm Surgery Trial. *Anesthesiology* 2010; 112: 86–101.

5. E. S. Nussbaum, L. A. Sebring, I. Ostanny *et al.* Transient cardiac standstill induced by adenosine in the management of intraoperative aneurysmal rupture: technical case report. *Neurosurgery* 2000; 47: 240–3.

6. A. Tuttolomondo, R. Di Sciacca, D. Di Raimondo *et al.* Neuron protection as a therapeutic target in acute ischemic stroke. *Curr Top Med Chem.* 2009; 9(14): 1317–34.

7. **M. M. Todd, B. J. Hindman, W. R. Clarke, J. C. Torner**. Mild intraoperative hypothermia during surgery for intracranial aneurysm. *N Engl J Med* 2005; **352**: 135–45.

8. **G. L. Clifton, J. Y. Jiang, B. G. Lyeth** et al. Marked protection by moderate hypothermia after experimental traumatic brain injury. *J Cereb Blood Flow Metab* 1991; **11**: 114–21.

9. **Y. Feng, P. G. Rhodes, A. Bhatt**. Hypoxic preconditioning provides neuroprotection and increases vascular endothelial growth factor A, preserves phosphorylation of Akt-Ser-473 and diminishes caspase-3 activity in neonatal rat hypoxic-ischemic model. *Brain Res* 2010; **1325**: 1–9.

10. **R. L. Williams-Karnesky, M. P. Stenzel-Poore**. Adenosine and stroke: Maximising the therapeutic potential of adenosine as a prophylactic and acute neuroprotectant. *Curr Neuropharmacol* 2009; **7**: 217–27.

11. **G. E. Hardingham**. Coupling of NMDA receptor to neuroprotective and neurodestructive events.

Colworth Medal Lecture. Biochem. Soc. Trans. 2009; **37**: 1147–60.

12. **J. Dhawan, H. Benveniste, M. Nawrocky, S. D. Smith**. Transient focal ischemia results in persistent and widespread neuroinflammation and loss of glutamate NMDA receptors. *Neuroimage* 2010; **51**: 599–605.

13. **P. Banks, N. P. Franks, R. Dickinson**. Competitive inhibition at the glycine site of the n-methyl-d-aspartate receptor mediates xenon neuroprotection against hypoxia–ischemia. *Anesthesiology* 2010; **112**: 614–22.

14. **J. J. Pasternak, D. G. McGregor, W. L. Lanier** et al. Effect of nitrous oxide use on long-term neurologic and neuropsychological outcome in patients who received temporary proximal artery occlusion during cerebral aneurysm clipping surgery. *Anesthesiology* 2009; **110**: 563–73.

15. **B. Sims, M. Clarke, W. Njah, E. S. Hopkins, H. Sonthiemer**. Erythropietin-induced neuroprotection requires cystine glutamate exchanger activity. *Brain Res* 2010; **1321**: 88–95.

Vascular procedures. Aneurysm clipping

Dexmedetomidine and nitrous oxide for cerebral aneurysm clipping

Michael J. Claybon and George A. Mashour

Dexmedetomidine and nitrous oxide are commonly used as adjuvants to volatile agents or other intravenous anesthetics – the following case describes these agents in combination with each other for anesthetic maintenance of a cerebral aneurysm clipping.

Case description

The patient was a 58-year-old female with multiple intact unsecured aneurysms, who presented for clipping of one paraclinoid aneurysm. She had a history of hypertension, obesity, and delayed emergence from general anesthesia. The anesthetic goals for this patient included (1) maintaining hemodynamic stability throughout the entire perioperative period, (2) maintaining the ability to monitor neurophysiologic signals, and (3) prompt emergence and neurologic evaluation.

General anesthesia was induced with propofol, fentanyl, and vecuronium. The patient was then maintained with dexmedetomidine at levels of 0.2–0.7 mcg/kg/min and nitrous oxide 60–70% in oxygen. Fentanyl boluses were given to total 500 mcg (7 mcg/kg) during and shortly after induction.

Hemodynamic stability was achieved both intraoperatively and postoperatively, preserving cerebral perfusion pressure and avoiding hypertension (Figure 19.1). Somatosensory evoked potentials were stable and without interference by anesthetics. The dexmedetomidine infusion was discontinued during surgical closure approximately 40 minutes prior to the reversal of muscle relaxant. The patient was transitioned to 100% oxygen after completion of surgery and removal of head pins. She was spontaneously ventilating and following commands within four minutes. Extubation was smooth and delayed emergence was avoided. Postoperatively the patient was hemodynamically stable, remained in the neurosurgical intensive care unit until postoperative day 1 and was discharged home on postoperative day 3. During her postoperative interview, she was specifically asked about intraoperative awareness and she reported no recall of surgical events.

Discussion

Since its public introduction by Horace Wells in 1845, nitrous oxide has been in continuous use. Clinicians continue to debate the use of nitrous oxide, perhaps most avidly within the field of neuroanesthesia. While a drug that offers analgesia, sedation, and rapid emergence seems optimal for neurologic surgery, some properties of nitrous oxide promote concern. These include increases in cerebral metabolic rate, cerebral blood flow, intracranial pressure, and ability to increase the volume of pneumocephalus. McGregor et al. published a study in which data from the Intraoperative Hypothermia for Aneurysm Surgery Trial were analyzed. Of the 1000 patients studied, 373 received nitrous oxide with no detrimental effect on long-term gross neurologic or neuropsychologic function [1]. This multicenter study had significant variability in the use of nitrous oxide, with some centers using it extensively and others seldom if at all. However, in light of the fact that much of the concern for nitrous oxide is based on in vitro data and animal studies, McGregor et al.'s analysis may be helpful in supporting those anesthesiologists who employ nitrous oxide for neurovascular surgery.

Dexmedetomidine was introduced far more recently. This selective alpha-2-receptor agonist was initially used in mechanically ventilated critically ill patients before it found use in the operating room. Dexmedetomidine is unique in its ability to produce sedation, anxiolysis and analgesia with little respiratory depression. It offers an interesting advantage in that patients may be sedated with dexmedetomidine but remain arousable and cooperative. The central action of dexmedetomidine at presynaptic neurons in the brainstem's locus ceruleus produces sedation,

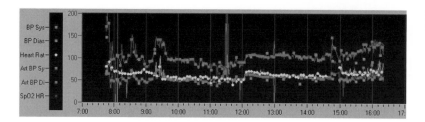

Figure 19.1. Intraoperative and recovery room vital signs.

while postsynaptic receptors in the spinal cord seem to be important in mediating analgesia. Additional benefits involving hemodynamics and "cooperative sedation" have been cited as advantages in using dexmedetomidine for monitored anesthesia care and as an adjunct in general anesthesia. Common use of dexmedetomidine involves a loading dose of 1 mcg/kg over 10 minutes followed by a continuous intravenous infusion between 0.2 and 0.7 mcg/kg/hour.

Dexmedetomidine decreases anesthetic requirements substantially with both opioid-sparing and minimum alveolar concentration (MAC)-sparing qualities. It is associated with reductions in MAC of inhaled anesthetics of 50–90% [2]; additionally, dexmedetomidine has been shown to reduce opioid requirements by 30–50% [3].

The benefits of dexmedetomidine as an anesthetic adjunct extend beyond sedation and analgesia. Sympatholytic effects blunt hypertension and tachycardia during surgery and anesthesia. Dexmedetomidine has been shown to reduce oxygen consumption perioperatively [2]. The hemodynamic stability associated with dexmedetomidine may also be cardioprotective. Alpha-2-agonists have been shown to decrease mortality after various types of surgical procedures; significant benefit has been noted in vascular surgery with a decrease in mortality and myocardial infarction [4].

It becomes especially important when discussing an anesthetic agent in neurosurgery to examine its neurophysiologic profile. Dexmedetomidine has been shown to decrease cerebral blood flow (CBF) in healthy human subjects [2]. Animal studies have similarly found a reduction in CBF, however, these studies did not find concomitant decreases in cerebral metabolic rate ($CMRO_2$) [3]. The concern for adequacy of cerebral oxygenation based on these animal studies was addressed in a human study of six healthy volunteers. In this study, both CBF and $CMRO_2$ were found to decrease in a dose-dependent man-

ner, and the $CBF/CMRO_2$ ratio was maintained [5]. This study correlates with data supporting dexmedetomidine having no detrimental effect on local brain tissue oxygenation in patients undergoing cerebrovascular surgery, even under conditions of cerebrovascular compromise and hyperventilation [3]. Animal studies have demonstrated decreases in intracranial pressure with dexmedetomidine; the limited human data available suggest that lumbar cerebral fluid pressures are unchanged intraoperatively [2]. An appropriate neuroanesthetic must also preserve neurophysiologic monitoring. Dexmedetomidine has been studied as an adjunct in spinal surgery and was not found to change either somatosensory evoked potentials or motor evoked potentials by any clinically significant amount [6].

Another favorable characteristic of dexmedetomidine is the potential for a neuroprotective effect. Cerebral ischemia is associated with increased brain catecholamine levels, and decreases in sympathetic tone have been shown to improve neurologic outcome [7]. Dexmedetomidine decreases norepinephrine levels in the brain and thus may be protective. Studies in animals have demonstrated that dexmedetomidine improves neuronal survival after transient global or focal cerebral ischemia [3, 7]. Additionally, animal and in vitro studies suggest that dexmedetomidine reduces glutamate release [3]. Reduction of this excitatory neurotransmitter is potentially neuroprotective.

Aside from neurovascular surgery, dexmedetomidine may be beneficial in other realms of neuroanesthesia. In various cases performed under monitored anesthesia care, the "cooperative sedation" availed by dexmedetomidine is especially valuable. Carotid endarterectomies, craniotomies, and implantation of deep brain stimulators have been performed successfully using dexmedetomidine as a sedative. In these cases, dexmedetomidine provides sympatholysis and facilitates detailed neurologic evaluation [3]. In a case series, Mack *et al.* reported that dexmedetomidine appeared to be a useful sedative for awake craniotomies when sophisticated neurologic testing was required [8]. Similar pharmacologic benefits may also be helpful in sedating neurocritical-care patients.

The most prominent side effects of dexmedetomidine involve hemodynamic changes including hypotension and bradycardia. Hypotension may predominate when central alpha-2a-receptor activity promotes vasodilation, an effect compounded by hypovolemia. Hypertension, however, has been attributed to peripheral alpha-2b-receptors, which may overwhelm the central effects after peak concentrations are reached initially. Blood pressure changes may have a temporal relationship to the use of a loading dose [2]. Bradycardia is most commonly found in younger patients with high levels of vagal tone; dexmedetomidine is not recommended for patients with heart block [3].

Nitrous oxide and dexmedetomidine are most commonly adjuncts to volatile or intravenous anesthetics. In this case, their combination provided a complete anesthetic while maintaining hemodynamic stability, enabling neurophysiologic monitoring, and facilitating a prompt emergence in a patient with a history of delayed recovery from general anesthesia. Although we do not recommend this combination for general use, it may be appropriate in certain clinical situations.

References

1. **D. G. McGregor, W. L. Lanier, J. J. Pasternak** *et al.* Effect of nitrous oxide on neurologic and neuropsychological function after intracranial aneurysm surgery. *Anesthesiology* 2008; **108**: 568–79.

2. **A. T. Gerlach, J. F. Dasta**. Dexmedetomidine: an updated review. *Ann Pharmacother* 2007; **41**: 245–52.

3. **A. Bekker, M. K. Sturaitis**. Dexmedetomidine for neurological surgery. *Neurosurgery* 2005; **57**: 1–10.

4. **D. N. Wijeysundera, J. S. Naik, W. S. Beattie**. Alpha-2 adrenergic agonists to prevent perioperative cardiovascular complications: a meta-analysis. *Am J Med* 2003; **114**: 742–52.

5. **J. C. Drummond, A. V. Dao, D. M. Roth** *et al.* Effect of dexmedetomidine on cerebral blood flow velocity, cerebral metabolic rate, and carbon dioxide response in normal humans. *Anesthesiology* 2008; **108**: 225–32.

6. **E. Bala, D. I. Sessler, D. R. Nair** *et al.* Motor and somatosensory evoked potentials are well maintained in patients given dexmedetomidine during spine surgery. *Anesthesiology* 2008; **109**: 417–25.

7. **J. Kuhmonen, J. Pokorny, R. Miettinen** *et al.* Neuroprotective effects of dexmedetomidine in the gerbil hippocampus after transient global ischemia. *Anesthesiology* 1997; **87**: 371–7.

8. **P. F. Mack, K. Perrine, E. Kobylarz** *et al.* Dexmedetomidine and neurocognitive testing in awake craniotomy. *J Neurosurg Anesthesiol* 2004; **16**: 20–5.

20 Anaphylaxis associated with indocyanine green administration for intraoperative fluorescence angiography

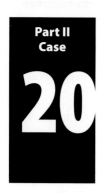

Marnie B. Welch and Laurel E. Moore

Indocyanine green (ICG; Cardio-green) is a tricarbocyanine organic dye that has diverse clinical uses including cardiac dye-dilution studies, liver function and blood flow determination, and ophthalmic angiography [1]. Fluorescence angiography with ICG dye is being increasingly utilized for the intraoperative visualization of the cerebral vasculature in patients undergoing neurosurgical procedures.

Case description

The patient was a 67-year-old American Society of Anesthesiologists Class III female scheduled to undergo elective left pterional craniotomy for clipping of intracranial aneurysms. In the course of evaluation for other issues, the patient was found to have three intracranial aneurysms: a complex middle cerebral artery (MCA) bifurcation aneurysm (10 mm × 11 mm), a small anterior communicating aneurysm, and a small distal MCA aneurysm. Her past medical history included extensive tobacco use, hyperlipidemia, well-controlled hypertension and known carotid atherosclerotic disease. A recent cardiac stress test was negative for ischemia. She had no known drug allergies.

General anesthesia was induced and maintained using a balanced technique. She remained hemodynamically stable throughout the case, but required small doses of ephedrine intermittently to keep her within 20% of her baseline mean arterial pressure of 65 mmHg. Four hours into the case, the large complex MCA aneurysm was successfully clipped and ICG angiography was performed to confirm patency of the parent and branch vessels, as well as the exclusion of the aneurysm from the cerebral circulation. Within 2 minutes of intravenous administration of ICG 12.5 mg (0.22 mg/kg), the patient's blood pressure dropped from 132/60 to 58/32 mmHg (Figure 20.1).

The patient's pulse, oxygen saturation, peak inspiratory pressures, and end-tidal CO_2 remained unchanged. This hypotension was poorly responsive to routine measures including crystalloid, ephedrine, and phenylephrine – anaphylaxis was presumed. Small doses of epinephrine (10 mcg) and diphenhydramine were administered with gradual return to a normal blood pressure. Hives became evident on her legs and arms, but no bronchospasm was observed. The neurosurgeons were informed of the reaction and the remaining two aneurysms were clipped promptly and without ICG angiography. The patient was neurologically intact upon emergence and proceeded to have an uneventful recovery. She had no awareness during the period of significant hypotension, despite the decrease in anesthetic concentration because of her cardiovascular status. Her family was informed of her reaction to ICG dye. Mast cell tryptase levels were drawn approximately 20 minutes after ICG administration and returned markedly elevated at 74.6 ng/ml (normal 0.0–11.4 ng/ml). Cardiac enzymes were negative.

Discussion

Indocyanine green is a water-soluble dye that contains iodine as a contaminant (<5%). It is stored as a powder and is dissolved in the accompanying aqueous solvent in preparation for intravenous injection. It has a peak spectral absorption at 800–810 nm when dissolved in blood. It is stable in blood and plasma, is not bound to plasma proteins, and is not metabolized [2]. It is excreted by the liver and secreted unchanged in the bile; potentially harmful effects on the kidneys are minimal. Because of these unique physical characteristics and its negligible renal, peripheral, lung, and cerebrospinal fluid uptake, ICG has multiple clinical uses, including cerebral angiography. Dosing varies depending on its indication. The manufacturer states that

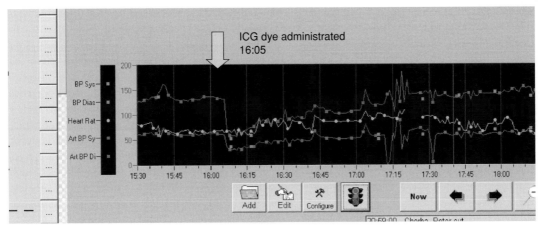

Figure 20.1. Intraoperative course from patient CC. Indocyanine green dye administered at 16:05 with subsequent immediate, severe hypotension, with eventual recovery. (Centricity CIS Copyright GE Medical Systems, 2002.)

dosing should not exceed 2 mg/kg. However, ICG dosing in adult case reports has ranged from 0.5 mg/kg to 5 mg/kg, or approximately 25–75 mg. Given its reported low incidence of serious adverse reactions and increasing indications in the neurosurgical literature, its clinical use is expected to expand.

Since its introduction in the 1950s, adverse reactions to ICG dye have been reported, although there are currently no reports in the neurosurgical or anesthesiology literature. Four adverse events involving the use of ICG were noted in the ophthalmology literature in or before 1978, with an estimated 240 000 procedures performed during that same time period [1]. A 1994 review of 1226 ophthalmology patients receiving ICG dye revealed one (0.05%) patient with a severe reaction [3]; a similar incidence was reported in Japan that same year in a review of 2820 ophthalmology patients [4]. Mild (0.15%) or moderate (0.2%) adverse reactions such as nausea, vomiting, sneezing, and itching were more common [3]. The manufacturer reports reactions to be one in every 42 000 doses [1]. In the cardiology literature, a higher incidence (4.3%; 4 out of 93 patients) developed reactions in cardiac output determination studies [5]; this was attributed to a higher dosage. In comparison, adverse reactions to radiocontrast media appear higher than with ICG dye [3].

Adverse reactions to ICG dye vary both in system involvement and severity. In one striking case report [1] the patient developed asphyxiation, tachycardia, and hypotension during a cardiac catheterization and could not be resuscitated. The cause of death at autopsy

was determined to be anaphylaxis, with multiple contributing patient factors including coronary occlusion and liver failure. A second fatal case report by Nanikawa et al. was attributed to laryngospasm [6]. In general, cardiopulmonary resuscitation is successful for ICG adverse reactions, but few data exist on the subject. Additional reactions documented in case reports include: urticaria, erythema, pruritis, hypotension, nausea, extreme dyspnea, pulmonary congestion, and laryngospasm. Our anesthetized patient experienced only two signs: severe hypotension and hives. Reactions to ICG dye usually develop quickly, as illustrated in our case. Patients have also received repeated doses of ICG over time, with worsening of symptoms with each administration [2]. To our knowledge, our patient had no prior exposure to ICG dye.

Treatment in case reports has included intravenous crystalloid and colloids, airway management if necessary, corticosteroids, epinephrine, diphenhydramine, beta-agonist nebulizers, and theophylline. The management of our patient followed established treatment of anaphylaxis; of note, epinephrine proved to be much more effective than other vasopressors.

Risk factors for developing adverse reactions to ICG dye are unknown. It was initially proposed that patients with iodine sensitivity were susceptible because of the solubilizing iodine component of the pharmaceutical product [1], but this has been refuted by a large case series [2]. The manufacturer does state, however, that a history of allergy to iodine is a contraindication to ICG administration, because the product itself contains iodine. Seventy-five percent of uremic patients were found to have adverse reactions in one evaluation [7]. Iseki noted that higher levels of eosinophils in chronic hemodialysis patients were found pre-ICG administration in patients both with and without reactions; the author then proposed this as the reason patients with end-stage renal disease seem to be at risk for adverse reactions to ICG [5]. It has been previously suggested that atopic individuals as well as a higher dose of ICG may predispose to adverse reactions, but a review of 17 cases by Benya do not support these as risk factors [2]. Our patient had none of these potential risk factors.

Both anaphylactoid and nonallergic reactions have been proposed as possible mechanisms for ICG dye reactions. Nonallergic (or anaphylactoid) reactions are triggered by mast cell degranulation and are not immune mediated. Drugs associated with nonallergic reactions include radiocontrast agents and opiates. As the reaction is non-immunologic, prior exposure to a drug is not necessary for the development of the reaction. Anaphylaxis, in contrast, is a true immunologic reaction involving IgE release defining it as a type I hypersensitivity reaction. The two different types of reactions are treated similarly; although true anaphylaxis is generally a more significant reaction. A case series with an unusually high incidence of ICG reactions occurred with higher doses of the medication [8]. These observations led the author to propose a dose-dependent mechanism that might support a nonallergic mechanism. But this proposed relationship was determined by a small number of cases and thus it is difficult to confidently ascertain a significant increase in incidence with a higher ICG dose. A case series by Michie et al. attempted to demonstrate that adverse reactions to ICG are nonallergic in nature [7]. The author states that the uremic patients in his case series have a decreased immunologic responsiveness and thus it is unlikely the high incidence of adverse reactions in this population could be due to anaphylaxis. However, patients do experience a prior sensitization to ICG dye with escalating symptoms, supporting anaphylaxis [2]. Patients, including ours, have had serious symptoms from ICG, but this does not conclusively support whether the reaction is nonallergic or anaphylactoid in nature.

Laboratory tests can assist in confirming the nature of hypotension under anesthesia. Our patient had a markedly elevated mast tryptase level. Tryptase is a neutral protease that is found almost exclusively in mast cells. When mast cells are activated during anaphylaxis, tryptase is released, along with other mediators such as histamine, for up to six hours after the reaction. Increased concentrations of mast cell tryptase are a highly sensitive indicator of anaphylactic reactions during anesthesia [9]. Their presence favors an IgE-mediated cause, based on a review of 416 specimens in anesthetic cases and confirmation with intradermal testing, radioimmunoassay, or both. However, an elevated mast cell tryptase does not always distinguish between an anaphylactic and nonallergic reaction. Tryptase elevation is usually less pronounced in nonallergic reactions, suggesting an immune-mediated reaction for our patient.

Conclusion

Awareness of adverse reactions associated with ICG dye is imperative given its increasing use in neurosurgery. Anesthesiologists need to understand the pharmacokinetics, incidence, and type of adverse reactions, as well as the relative and absolute contraindications to ICG usage. Administration of the dye to patients with a history of prior reaction to ICG, end-stage renal disease, and allergy to iodine (which the preparation of ICG contains) should be avoided. As with other radiocontrast agents, an appropriate resuscitative plan and equipment must be available.

References

1. **T. R. Carski, B. J. Staller, G. Hepner** et al. Adverse reactions after administration of indocyanine green. *J Am Med Assoc* 1978; **240**: 635.

2. **R. Benya, J. Quintana, B. Brundage**. Adverse reactions to indocyanine green: a case report and review of the literature. *Cathet Cardiovasc Diagn* 1989; **17**: 231–3.

3. **M. Hope-Ross, L. A. Yannuzzi, E. S. Gragoudas** et al. Adverse reactions due to indocyanine green. *Ophthalmology* 1994; **101**: 529–33.

4. **A. Obana, T. Miki, K. Hayashi** et al. Survey of complications of indocyanine green angiography in Japan. *Am J Ophthalmol* 1994; **118**: 749–53.

5. **K. Iseki, K. Onoyama, S. Fujimi** et al. Shock caused by indocyanine-green dye in chronic hemodialysis patients. *Clin Nephrol* 1980; **14**: 210.

6. **R. Nanikawa, T. Hayashi, Y. Hashimoto** et al. A case of fatal shock induced by indocyanine green (ICG) test. *Jpn J Legal Med* 1978; **32**: 209–14.

7. **D. D. Michie, D. G. Wombolt, R. F. Caretta** *et al.*
    Adverse reactions associated with the administration
    of a tricarbocyanine dye (Cardio-Green) to uremic
    patients. *J Allergy Clin Immunol* 1971; **48**: 235–9.

8. **R. Speich, B. Saesseli, U. Hoffmann** *et al.*
    Anaphylactoid reactions after indocyanine-green

    administration. *Ann Intern Med* 1988; **109**: 345–
    6.

9. **M. M. Fisher, B. A. Baldo**. Mast cell tryptase in
    anaesthetic anaphylactoid reations. *Br J Anaesth* 1998;
    80: 26–9.

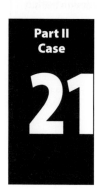

Vascular procedures. Aneurysm coiling

Subarachnoid hemorrhage during aneurysm coiling

Khoi D. Than, Anthony C. Wang, Neeraj Chaudhary, Joseph J. Gemmete, Aditya S. Pandey and B. Gregory Thompson

Intraprocedural rupture of an intracranial aneurysm is a potentially catastrophic complication, but can be even more devastating in a heparinized patient in an offsite interventional suite. Understanding how to respond to such an event is essential to good patient outcome.

Case description

A 67-year old woman with hypertension presented to the emergency department with the sudden onset of the worst headache of her life. Upon initial neurologic examination, she was drowsy but arousable, and was disoriented to place. The remainder of her examination was intact. A noncontrast head computed tomography scan was obtained, which showed expected diffuse subarachnoid hemorrhage (SAH) and a small hypo-attenuating spherical abnormality in the basilar artery tip. Small temporal horns were visible (an early sign of hydrocephalus) and the remainder of her ventricular system appeared slightly enlarged. After the scan's completion, the patient appeared increasingly lethargic, so a right frontal external ventricular drain was placed and set to drain at 20 cm above the tragus. The opening intracranial (ICP) pressure was 25 mm Hg.

Given the patient's presentation of a Hunt–Hess grade 3 SAH, a diagnostic cerebral angiogram was obtained, with the potential to perform endovascular coil embolization should an aneurysm be discovered. The patient was brought to the interventional neuroradiology suite, where an arterial line and further intravenous access was obtained and general anesthesia was induced. Neurophysiologic monitoring was performed throughout the case. An angiogram showed a 7 mm, wide-domed, small-necked saccular aneurysm at the basilar tip. It was decided to attempt coil embolization to treat the aneurysm.

While the last coil was being injected into the aneurysm, the patient acutely became hypertensive. The ICP measurement from the ventriculostomy precipitously increased to 40 mm Hg. An injection of contrast dye demonstrated extravasation from the aneurysm.

Discussion

The advent of endovascular coil embolization in the early 1990s represented a breakthrough in the care of patients with intracranial aneurysms. Particularly for aneurysms in locations difficult to access by conventional surgical approaches, many patients now have the option of endovascular treatment via a 2 mm incision in the groin. This technique is frequently employed as a primary modality for definitive treatment of both ruptured and unruptured aneurysms.

As with open clip ligation, aneurysm rupture during endovascular embolization is a dreaded complication [1–4]. The incidence of intraprocedural rupture is between 2–4%, with associated mortality as high as 40% (but generally 10–15%). Although the incidence of rupture is slightly lower than in open operative procedures, the associated mortality is higher given that, with coiling, the head is closed and direct access to the source of bleeding for proximal and distal control is unavailable.

The etiologies of intraprocedural rupture include elevation in blood pressure, increased aneurysmal intraluminal pressure secondary to contrast injection, mechanical perforation by the operator, and diversion of blood flow by inserted coils to the weak areas of the aneurysm wall. Intraprocedural rupture can occur both in elective procedures, as well as in the treatment of previously-ruptured aneurysms. Risk factors for intraprocedural rupture include (1) recent rupture, given that the aneurysm wall is already weakened,

(2) smaller aneurysms, given less room for error when manipulating guide-wires or coils, and (3) the presence of a "daughter" aneurysm (a smaller associated aneurysm).

To minimize morbidity and mortality, there are certain steps that need to be undertaken by the anesthesiologist in cases of intraprocedural aneurysm rupture. The following discussion assumes that the patient is already anesthetized and the trachea intubated. General anesthesia is beneficial, as this allows for perfect immobilization during coil injection and stent placement, and significantly decreases the risk of microvascular perforation once the small intracerebral vasculature is catheterized. In addition, seizure often occurs as a result of intraprocedural aneurysm rupture and thus airway control could potentially be compromised.

With "airway" and "breathing" already controlled and the FiO_2 increased to 100%, the next step in a case of intraprocedural rupture relates to "circulation" or management of blood pressure. Aneurysmal rupture is typically accompanied by a rise in blood pressure, which can be a cause of the rupture as well as an effect mediated by the Cushing reflex. Reduction in blood pressure minimizes the amount and severity of resultant subarachnoid hemorrhage, decreases the likelihood of further re-rupture, and aids the interventionalist in obtaining control. Blood pressure control will also assist in the management of intracranial pressure. In general, a mean arterial pressure (MAP) between 60 and 80 mm Hg will help to accomplish these goals. Agents such as esmolol, labetolol, nitroglycerin, nitroprusside, and nifedipine can be used. Adenosine may also be used to induce a transient cessation of pulsatile blood flow to the aneurysm. Another priority at this time is to lower the cerebral metabolic rate and thus minimize the brain's need for blood flow. This can be achieved with the use of thiopental or propofol, which will both decrease systemic blood pressure, as well.

Endovascular procedures always involve periodic injections of heparin to prevent thromboembolic events during the procedure. Clearly, this anticoagulation will prove problematic in the event of intraprocedural aneurysm rupture, as any bleeding will be more difficult to control. Immediately after obtaining an ideal blood pressure, attention should be turned to reversing anticoagulation. Reversal of heparin using protamine sulfate should be performed immediately, administered at a dose of 1 mg for every 100 units of heparin given. Given that patients often either present with, or are prescribed pre-procedural platelet inhibition with aspirin and/or clopidogrel, consideration should be given to platelet transfusion. In many institutions, platelets are kept in the interventional suite throughout the procedure in case of such an event.

After maximizing oxygen delivery, reducing blood pressure, decreasing cerebral metabolic rate and reversing both anticoagulation and platelet inhibition, the team's next focus should be management of increased ICP. Immediate hyperventilation to a goal $PaCO_2$ around 30 mmHg is a physiologic mechanism to acutely reduce ICP. The first-line pharmaceutical agent in these situations is typically mannitol, an osmotic diuretic administered at a dose of 0.25-1g/kg. Management of external ventricular drainage is a direct means by which ICP can be controlled. However, when adjusting the rate of ventricular drainage, one must take care not to decompress the brain too rapidly, as this can result in aneurysmal re-rupture (recall that transmural pressure gradient = MAP – ICP, so lowering the ICP increases the pressure across the wall). With unsecured ruptured aneurysms, a ventriculostomy catheter should not drain at a level lower than 15–20 cm H_2O above the tragus.

When subarachnoid hemorrhage occurs, seizures must also be prevented. Thiopental can be administered for neuroprotection and anti-seizure prophylaxis. Phenytoin (dose = 20 mg/kg) is perhaps the most common anticonvulsant agent, however, this must be infused at a rate no faster than 1 mg/kg/min (slower for older patients and those with cardiac disease). Rapid infusion of phenytoin (and its accompanying solvent, polyethylene glycol) can result in severe hypotension and even cardiovascular collapse. For this reason, the water soluble fosphenytoin is preferred in cases of intraprocedural rupture, as it can be infused more rapidly. Levetiracetam is a newer agent growing in popularity due to its ease of administration and more benign side-effect profile.

While the anesthesiologist is stabilizing the patient's respiratory, cardiovascular, sedative, and neurophysiologic issues, as well as managing intracranial hypertension, the attention of the neurosurgeon and/or interventional neuroradiologist is typically focused on securing the aneurysm, as this is the definitive measure to control further SAH. As a salvage measure, liquid embolization administered to seal the vascular defect can be employed.

Inevitably, some cases that begin in the interventional neuroradiology suite will be unsuccessful in protecting the aneurysm. Such cases complicated by rupture will commonly need to be brought emergently to an operating room for open clipping of the aneurysm. The anesthesiology team must therefore always be prepared for expeditious transport to the operating room in the event that an endovascular procedure fails. They must also be ready to rapidly lighten anesthesia if an accurate neurologic examination is required.

By following the steps outlined above – control of blood pressure, reduction of cerebral metabolism, reversal of anticoagulation and platelet inhibition, control of ICP, prevention of seizures, and timely transport, if necessary – the neuroanesthesiologist can be prepared for such cases of intraprocedural aneurysm rupture and greatly improve the chances for a good patient outcome.

References

1. A. Doerfler, I. Wanke, T. Egelhof *et al.* Aneurysmal rupture during embolization with Guglielmi detachable coils: causes, management, and outcome. *AJNR Am J Neuroradiol* 2001; **22**: 1825–32.

2. E. Levy, C. J. Koebbe, M. B. Horowitz *et al.* Rupture of intracranial aneurysms during endovascular coiling: management and outcomes. *Neurosurgery* 2001; **49**: 807–13.

3. H. J. Priebe. Aneurysmal subarachnoid hemorrhage and the anaesthetist. *Br J Anaesth* 2007; **99**: 102–18.

4. M. K. Varma, K. Price, V. Jayakrishnan *et al.* Anaesthetic considerations for interventional neuroradiology. *Br J Anaesth* 2007; **99**: 75–85.

Vascular procedures. Aneurysm coiling

Cardiac abnormalities after subarachnoid hemorrhage

William R. Stetler, Jr. and George A. Mashour

The intimate connection between the brain and heart has long been speculated to affect neurologic disease. This relationship is perhaps most clearly demonstrated in the significant cardiac dysfunction that may occur following subarachnoid hemorrhage (SAH). Common cardiac abnormalities include arrhythmias, diastolic and systolic dysfunction, and subendocardial infarction. Understanding the neurocardiac axis is essential to the clinician managing the patient with cardiac dysfunction following SAH.

Case description

The patient was a 54-year-old male with no significant past medical history who suddenly developed a "thunderclap headache" while playing basketball and then collapsed onto the court. Emergency Medical Service was alerted, the trachea was intubated, and he was taken directly to the emergency department where computed tomography (CT) of the head revealed significant SAH. Neurosurgery was consulted and a ventriculostomy catheter was placed emergently. A CT angiography of the brain revealed a 15-mm anterior communicating artery aneurysm and the patient was subsequently taken to the angiography suite where the aneurysm was occluded by coil embolization. The patient was taken postoperatively to the neurosurgical intensive care unit (ICU), intubated and on a norepinephrine infusion, where he was noted to exhibit flexor posturing.

On admission the patient's cardiac troponin I (cTnI) was <0.10 ng/mL (normal <0.20 ng/mL), but after the procedure it was noted to be 0.96 ng/mL and an electrocardiogram (ECG) was performed showing significant S-T segment changes (Figure 22.1). Overnight the patient had increasing oxygen requirements and chest radiograph revealed diffuse pulmonary edema bilaterally. An uptrend of the cTnI continued to a peak value of 7.5 ng/mL on postoperative day 3. Falling blood pressures requiring

increasing vasopressor requirements and difficulty with oxygenation secondary to worsening pulmonary edema continued during this time. A transthoracic echocardiogram (TTE) was performed that showed an estimated left ventricular ejection fraction (LVEF) of 22% with significant anterior wall motion abnormality.

On postoperative day 12 a repeat TTE was obtained, this time revealing an estimated LVEF of 47% with only minimal anterior wall motion abnormality. He underwent an uneventful ventriculoperitoneal shunt placement and after 2 more weeks in the neurosurgical ICU was transferred to the general care ward, following commands in all four extremities.

Discussion

Anatomically, the heart is innervated through the intermediolateral gray column in the spinal cord and the parasympathetic ganglia from the vagus nerve. These are in turn served by many nuclei within the medulla that are connected to cortex on many levels. Likewise, afferent fibers from the heart ascend to the nucleus tractus solitarius (NTS) and the dorsal vagal nucleus, which indirectly send fibers back to the ventrolateral medulla [1].

However, the connection between brain and heart was theorized long before the anatomy was understood. The idea of sudden unexplained death and death from fright, has been thought to arise from a connection between brain and heart in which a neural insult causes the heart to stop. Examples include death during grief, natural catastrophes, alcohol withdrawal, and many other periods of significant emotional stress. It is thought that the emotional or neurologic insult is so severe that the heart ceases to function, possibly as a result of a neurally induced arrhythmia. In fact there are well described ECG changes noted with neurologic disease, most notably arrhythmias and repolarization changes (S-T and T wave changes), as

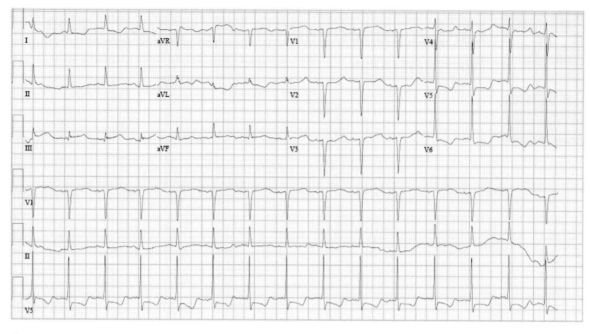

Figure 22.1. Electrocardiogram of a patient with subarachnoid hemorrhage and no history of coronary artery disease. Note the S-T segment depressions in lead V5.

were seen in our case. Our patient developed S-T changes that mimicked coronary ischemia as well as repolarization changes seen in the many T-wave inversions. These changes can often leave the heart vulnerable to the development of ventricular tachycardia/fibrillation [1–3]. These ECG abnormalities often improve with time [2] and after any circumstance that disconnects the heart from the brain, including heart transplantation or brain death, offering further evidence towards the direct connection between heart and brain [3].

Although any neurologic insult may affect the heart, SAH is perhaps the prototype and has been recognized to cause considerable cardiac dysfunction, including ECG changes and elevation of serum cardiac enzymes indicative of myocardial cell death. The effect on the heart following SAH significantly increases both morbidity and mortality, as seen in our case above with both increasing vasopressor and oxygen requirements following left ventricular dysfunction. Increased levels of cTnI following neurologic insults were found to result in higher in-hospital, all-cause mortality. With respect to SAH in particular, in-hospital mortality is nearly four times as high and patients have more severe disability at discharge with a significant elevation of cTnI [4].

It has further been shown that the degree of neurologic injury as based on the Hunt–Hess grading system following SAH correlates with the elevation of cTnI. Mild elevations of cTnI may be related to signs of diastolic dysfunction such as pulmonary congestion seen on chest radiograph. As cTnI increases it is more likely that the patient will develop signs of left ventricular systolic dysfunction and a decline in LVEF observed on echocardiogram. In our patient with a high grade hemorrhage, the cTnI rose rapidly and correlated with his significant ventricular failure. Fortunately, cardiac dysfunction following SAH is usually transient in nature. Repeat echocardiogram at 5–10 days post-bleed improves in nearly 75% of patients who initially demonstrated wall motion abnormalities following SAH [5], as was seen in our patient on his repeat preoperative echocardiogram several days following the bleed.

Frequently hypothesized mechanisms of neurogenic cardiac dysfunction include a systemic elevation of circulating catecholamines, elevated levels of serum steroids in the setting of stress, and a direct nervous system stimulation of the heart. Experimental infusion of catecholamines has been shown to produce ECG changes and histopathologic changes consistent with neurocardiac disease. Similar pathology is seen in animal models after infusion of steroids and exposure to environmental stressors and in humans following significant emotional stress producing what resembles an acute Takotsubo cardiomyopathy. Finally, direct stimulation of the hypothalami has been shown to cause distinctive pathologic changes in cardiac muscles less than 2–4 micrometers away from nerve fiber endings, implicating a direct neural insult to the heart [3].

The unifying link to the above proposed mechanisms of neurogenic cardiac disease is sympathetic nervous system overactivity. It is proposed that following a neurologic insult like SAH, the brain causes a "sympathetic storm" in which there is a local increase in neurally released catecholamines, systemic elevation of catecholamines from adrenal production, and an endogenous increase in the production of steroids [3]. The rise in catecholamines causes a depletion of adenosine triphosphate, which contributes to the failure of cardiac calcium channels. This results in an influx of calcium that produces microscopic contraction bands and causes failure of mitochondrial permeability, which leads to cell death [2].

The histopathology of neurogenic cardiac lesions is distinct from the coagulation necrosis observed following myocardial infarction. Lesions following neurologic disease (such as SAH) are characterized by contraction band necrosis in which myocytes die in a contracted state following calcium influx. This lesion is totally separate from the coagulation necrosis seen following traditional infarction [3], pointing towards an entirely different mechanism of injury following a neurologic insult than those following local cardiac disease. In fact, patients who have undergone cardiac catheterization during the period of elevated cardiac enzymes following SAH have been shown to have no coronary artery disease, redirecting the cause of cardiac dysfunction to a nonischemic etiology such as increased sympathetic tone [2].

Although it was originally believed that cardiac muscle was controlled predominantly by the sympathetic nervous system, it is increasingly accepted that there is a large influence of parasympathetic innervation to myocardium via the vagus nerve [1, 2]. Thus, even as sympathetic activity is implicated as the likely culprit surrounding neurocardiogenic pathology following SAH, more attention has recently been directed towards parasympathetic dysfunction as an important contributor to cardiac injury [2, 6]. Independently of neurologic disease, higher parasym-

pathetic tone has been shown to be an independent positive predictor for reduced all-cause mortality. Furthermore, stimulation of the parasympathetic nervous system has been shown to cause reduced inflammation. This parasympathetic mediated anti-inflammatory response is directed through cholinergic receptors on macrophages making the response immediate, as opposed to the systemic anti-inflammatory response mitigated by cytokines and glucocorticoids. Following the sympathetic stimulation caused by SAH, macrophages release inflammatory cytokines, which activate afferent vagus fibers via the NTS. Efferent vagus fibers then reflexively stimulate the cholinergic receptors on macrophages to decrease release of inflammatory cytokines while at the same time fibers from NTS to hypothalamus cause release of adrenocorticotropin hormone to increase glucocorticoid production [6]. Dysfunction in this system following SAH results in unregulated inflammatory changes, and is thought to contribute to cardiac pathology.

Thus, it seems that the most likely mechanism of cardiac abnormalities following SAH is both a catecholamine release after brain injury as well as parasympathetic dysfunction. Catecholamine release depletes adenosine triphosphate, causes increases in permeability of calcium that leads to a calcium influx, and eventually leads to myocardial necrosis. At the same time, parasympathetic dysfunction leads to unchecked inflammation that worsens adenosine triphosphate depletion and further contributes to myocardial cell death. Additionally, both sympathetic overactivity and parasympathetic dysfunction result in a pro-arrhythmogenic state as well that worsens ECG changes associated with myocardial necrosis [2].

Conclusion

In conclusion, there are significant cardiac abnormalities observed following SAH that vary depending upon the grade of SAH, but correlate with the degree of elevation of cTnI. These effects are likely mitigated through sympathetic and parasympathetic dysfunction that results from global cerebral dysfunction following SAH.

References

1. **A. M. Davis and B. H. Natelson**. Brain-heart interactions: The neurocardiology of arrhythmia and

sudden cardiac death. *Tex Heart Inst J* 1993; **20**: 158–69.

2. **H. A. Mashaly and J. J. Provencio**. Inflammation as a link between brain injury and heart damage: the model of subarachnoid hemorrhage. *Cleve Clin J Med* 2008; **75**: S26–30.

3. **M. A. Samuels**. The brain-heart connection. *Circulation* 2007; **116**: 77–84.

4. **R. Sandhu, W. S. Aronow, A. Rajdev** *et al.* Relation of cardiac troponin I levels with in-hospital mortality in patients with ischemic stroke, intracerebral

hemorrhage, and subarachnoid hemorrhage. *Am J Cardiol* 2008; **102**: 632–4.

5. **M. Tanabe, E. A. Crago, M. S. Suffoletto** *et al.* Relation of elevation in cardiac troponin I to clinical severity, cardiac dysfunction, and pulmonary congestion in patients with subarachnoid hemorrhage. *Am J Cardiol* 2008; **102**: 1545–50.

6. **M. H. Shishehbor, C. Alves, V. Rajagopal**. Inflammation: implications for understanding the heart-brain connection. *Cleve Clin J Med* 2007; **74**: S37–41.

23 Postoperative retroperitoneal bleed

Stacy Ritzman

Retroperitoneal hematomas are more commonly described after patients have had procedures within the retroperitoneum (kidney or lumbar spine) or may even arise spontaneously in an anticoagulated patient. Iatrogenic injuries leading to retroperitoneal hematomas are becoming more common due to the increasing popularity of interventional procedures.

Case description

This case is a 71-year-old male with a past medical history of anterior communicating artery (ACOM) aneurysm status post coiling 5 years previously who presented to the emergency room with new onset headache, stiff neck, and slight confusion. A head computed tomography (CT) showed a left frontal lobar intracranial hemorrhage. His past medical history was also significant for left bundle branch block, coronary artery disease status post percutaneous transluminal coronary angioplasty and bare metal stent to left anterior descending artery two years previously, and hypertension. His blood pressure was 184/96 and heart rate was 88 upon arrival.

He was taken to the interventional radiology suite where a pre-induction arterial line was placed; anesthesia was induced and the trachea intubated uneventfully. The systolic blood pressure was closely controlled with nitroglycerin and labetalol to maintain values <120 mmHg. After access was gained through the left common femoral artery, a cerebral angiogram showed a 2 mm × 3 mm recurrence of a previously coiled ACOM aneurysm at its neck. A stent was deployed across the ACOM and the aneurysm was successfully coiled. The patient was loaded with 600 mg of clopidogrel and the groin access site was closed with the StarClose device (a clip that closes the femoral artery access site in a purse-string fashion). The patient did sustain a 20-second bout of supraventricular tachycardia intraoperatively, which resolved with intravenous esmolol but the remainder of his intraoperative course was uneventful. The trachea was extubated at the end of the procedure and he was neurologically intact. He was then transported to the neurocritical care unit.

Shortly after arrival at the intensive care unit (ICU), the patient became hypotensive (systolic pressure in 80s) and tachycardic (heart rate 110) and complained of nausea. He was beta-blocked with metoprolol due to his cardiac history to treat his tachycardia. While treating his blood pressure with crystalloids and phenylephrine, baseline laboratory values and cardiac enzymes were sent. Concomitantly, a stat bedside 2-D echocardiogram was done to rule out a cardiac etiology for the hypotension. It was essentially normal without wall motion abnormalities. The patient then began to complain of abdominal pain and it was noted on exam that his left abdomen was swollen and tense. He was taken emergently to the radiology suite where an abdominal CT revealed a large left-sided retroperitoneal hematoma (Figure 23.1). The patient was transfused three units of packed red blood cells (PRBC) to treat a hematocrit of 21. He was closely monitored in the ICU with serial hematocrits but required six additional units of PRBC. He continued to be hypotensive, requiring a norepinephrine infusion. The decision was then made to take him emergently to the operating room to repair the iliac artery and evacuate the hematoma. Anesthetic concerns at this time were: (1) inducing anesthesia in an acutely hypovolemic patient, (2) the potential hemodynamic collapse once the tamponade effect on the retroperitoneal space was relieved, and (3) the potential for massive blood loss and transfusion.

A central line was placed pre-induction since he had poor peripheral access. He was transfused two units of PRBC and then was induced with etomidate. He became profoundly hypotensive during induction requiring small boluses of epinephrine. He was maintained on isoflurane and resuscitation was

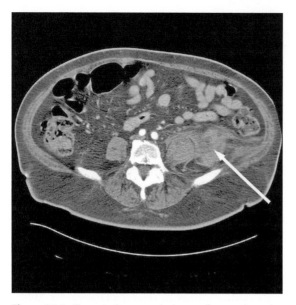

Figure 23.1. Computed tomography image of retroperitoneal hematoma. Arrow pointing to hematoma.

continued with administration of blood and crystalloid. After incision, his BP dropped again requiring boluses of epinephrine but the surgeon was able to quickly gain proximal control of the bleeding vessel. The posterior wall of the iliac artery had been lacerated and the source of the bleeding was localized and controlled. The hematocrit stabilized, but he continued to require norepinephrine to maintain his blood pressure. He was further resuscitated and monitored and was extubated the following day. He was discharged to home a week later.

Discussion

Retroperitoneal hematoma is a rare clinical entity but is becoming increasingly more common due to the higher number of interventional procedures being done. It may develop after a femoral artery puncture regardless of whether a device was used to close the vessel at the end of the procedure. It is caused by the puncture of the posterior wall of the femoral or iliac artery during cannulation. This complication may be more likely to occur in female patients (smaller vessel size), a higher femoral artery puncture site (unable to compress above the inguinal ligament), and uncontrolled hypertension [1].

The clinical manifestations of retroperitoneal hematoma are vague and thus the clinician must have a high index of suspicion to make the diag-

nosis. Initially patients may have very subtle signs such as relative hypotension and mild tachycardia that resolves transiently with fluid administration. They may complain of back, lower abdominal or groin pain and may develop swelling of the groin or abdomen. Eventually they will manifest a drop in hematocrit. Our patient's symptoms and signs were initially attributed to a cardiac etiology due to his past medical history and the inability to assess S-T segment changes with his coexisting left bundle branch block. There was also concern that the intraoperative run of supraventricular tachycardia may have been due to cardiac ischemia. The correct diagnosis was not made however until his retroperitoneal hematoma had expanded, causing abdominal pain and swelling.

Sometimes if the hematoma develops near or within the iliopsoas muscle, patients will present with a femoral neuropathy. This will manifest as severe pain in the affected groin or hip with radiation to the anterior thigh and may eventually progress to paresthesia in the antero-medial thigh and leg paresis [1, 2]. If iliopsoas muscle spasm occurs due to the hematoma, the hip will be maintained in a flexed and externally rotated position and any attempt to straighten the hip will cause pain.

Cutaneous signs such as Grey–Turner (ecchymosis in the flank region) or Cullen (ecchymosis in the periumbilical region) signs are characteristically associated with retroperitoneal hematoma. These, however, are late findings and will not aid in making the initial diagnosis.

Abdominal compartment syndrome may also develop with resultant impaired respiratory, cardiovascular (impaired venous return and increased systemic vascular resistance leading to decreased cardiac output), and renal function (increased renal vascular resistance and compression of renal veins and ureters). This may necessitate abdominal decompression through a laparotomy [2].

Diagnosis of retroperitoneal hematoma is made either via CT or angiography. Ultrasound of the abdomen and pelvis is usually not sensitive enough to diagnose retroperitoneal hematoma as blood in the retroperitoneum will often pass into the abdominal or pelvic cavity, confusing the diagnosis [1]. Computed tomography, however, is highly sensitive in diagnosis and visualization of extravasating contrast will locate the source of bleeding.

Management of retroperitoneal hematoma depends on the clinical status of the patient. All patients should be monitored in an ICU with fluid resuscitation, blood transfusion, and correction of coagulopathy if it exists. If the patient is hemodynamically stable, without evidence of ongoing bleeding, conservative management should be tried with the above measures. However, if the patient is unstable or has ongoing bleeding, endovascular therapy with stent-grafting across the injured vessel is a treatment option if interventional radiology is available. If not, surgery can be undertaken realizing that it may release the effect of the tamponade and initially make matters worse. This occurred transiently in our patient but was promptly treated with epinephrine and proximal control of the bleeding vessel by the surgeon. Surgery may also be indicated to decompress the retroperitoneal space if nerve or ureteral compression exists [3].

Conclusion

Retroperitoneal hematoma is an uncommon clinical entity that may be encountered more frequently as iatrogenic injuries occur during interventional procedures. Since signs and symptoms are initially non-specific, it requires a high index of suspicion on the part of the clinician for prompt diagnosis and treatment.

References

1. **Y. C. Chan, J. P. Morales, J. F. Reidy, P. R. Taylor.** Management of spontaneous and iatrogenic retroperitoneal haemorrhage: conservative management, endovascular intervention or open surgery? *Int J Clin Pract* 2008; **62**: 1604–13.

2. **C. Gonzalez, S. Penado, L. Liata** *et al.* The clinical spectrum of retroperitoneal hematoma in anticoagulated patients. *Medicine* 2003; **82**(4): 257–62.

3. **S.I. Daliakopoulos, A. Bairaktaris, D. Papadimitriou** *et al.* Gigantic retroperitoneal hematoma as a complication of anticoagulation therapy with heparin in therapeutic doses: a case report. *J Med Case Reports* 2008; **2**: 162.

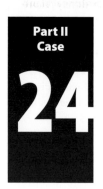

Vascular procedures. Aneurysm coiling

Angiography in the patient with kidney failure

Jerome O'Hara and Mauricio Perilla

Introduction

Contrast-induced nephropathy (CIN) from iodine contrast media during radiologic procedures is one of the most common causes of acute kidney injury. This risk increases in patients with chronic renal insufficiency. Balancing efforts to control blood pressure and prevent further worsening of renal function during cerebral artery coiling after subarachnoid hemorrhage can be challenging.

Case description

A 65-year-old, 88-kg female presented for cerebral angiography and planned coiling of a large middle cerebral artery aneurysm. During the physical examination in the emergency department, the patient was lethargic and complained of a headache. Blood pressure was 205/95 mmHg and oxygen saturation was 98% on supplemental nasal cannula oxygen. Initial management included a noncontrast computed tomography (CT) scan, which diagnosed extensive subarachnoid hemorrhage suggestive of aneurysmal rupture. The patient was admitted to the neurosurgical intensive care unit for observation and invasive arterial blood pressure monitoring. The patient's medical history included chronic renal insufficiency (admission serum creatinine = 1.8 mg/dL) secondary to non-insulin dependent diabetes and uncontrolled hypertension. On the day of the planned coiling serum creatinine was 2.3 mg/dL, serum glucose was 91 mg/dL, and arterial pressure was 130/70 mmHg.

In preparation for the procedure the patient was maintained on a normal saline intravenous infusion supplemented with a sodium bicarbonate solution infusion during and after the procedure. This was initiated in an attempt to prevent further decline in renal function when additional contrast dye exposure was administered during angiography. General anesthesia with endotracheal intubation, central venous pressure

monitoring, and careful blood pressure control was planned for the aneurysm coiling procedure.

Discussion

Anesthetic concerns included (1) aggressive arterial blood pressure management to prevent further intracranial hemorrhage prior to completing aneurysm coiling, (2) maintenance of euglycemia, and (3) managing intravascular volume within the balance of providing adequate renal blood flow without risking volume overload. With this patient having chronic renal insufficiency and uncontrolled hypertension prior to the procedure, renal autoregulatory mechanisms to maintain optimal renal perfusion likely required higher systemic blood pressure. This poses a great challenge to balance adequate renal perfusion yet maintain lower blood pressure to avoid an extension of cerebral hemorrhage until coiling is completed. Central venous pressure and urine output can only act as a guide in assessing renal perfusion, but less so if diuretics have been administered.

Contrast-induced nephropathy from the administration of iodinated contrast media remains a potentially serious complication associated with angiographic procedures. The many therapeutic efforts studied to ameliorate CIN have met little success over the last two decades and the incidence remains at ~12% [1]. In patients without risk factors for CIN, the incidence is lower (<5%), but as high as 50% in patients with multiple risk factors. It has been well established that patients who develop CIN have an increased risk of morbidity, prolonged hospitalization, and mortality [2].

Risk factors for CIN include chronic renal insufficiency, diabetes mellitus, advanced age, congestive heart failure, nephrotoxic drug use, metabolic syndrome, hyperuricemia, hypovolemia, and large volumes of contrast media exposure [1, 2]. The most important risk factor for CIN remains chronic renal insufficiency.

With more angiographic procedures being performed in the setting of cerebral aneurysm coiling, cerebral and coronary artery angioplasty/stenting, anti-arrhythmic cardiac ablations, and major vascular stenting, the ability to minimize the incidence of CIN carries a major impact on both patient outcomes and medical costs. This realization has led to many clinical studies in an attempt to determine if there is a "best practice" standard in the setting of angiography to prevent CIN.

Etiology and diagnosis of contrast-induced nephropathy

The pathophysiology of CIN is suspected to be related to contrast media-triggered vasoconstriction and development of oxidative stress leading to accumulation of reactive oxygen species [3]. Contrast-induced nephropathy is defined as an absolute increase in baseline serum creatinine concentration of at least 0.5 mg/dL or with a relative increase of 25% in the setting of chronic renal insufficiency. There must be no alternate etiology and the event must occur within 48–72 hours after contrast exposure [4].

Potential therapeutic interventions

In the setting of potential exposure to contrast dye during angiography, the focus should be the identification of patients at risk and subsequent prevention of CIN rather than treatment after exposure has already occurred. Consensus exists that proper intravascular hydration is the most important first-line therapy for prevention of CIN. The electrolyte solution of choice is 0.9% (vs 0.45%) saline [5]. The choice of the iodinated contrast dye is very important and should either be an iso-osmolar or low-osmolar contrast media.

Systemically administered vasodilators, such as dopamine agonists (dopamine and fenoldopam), adenosine antagonists, prostaglandins, and endothelin antagonists have presented disappointing conclusions when studied in an attempt to lessen the incidence of CIN [6]. It remains inconclusive if theophylline, ascorbic acid, or simvastatin provide any advantage in this clinical setting [1]. Furosemide has been reported to increase the risk of developing CIN [7]. Multiple studies evaluating N-acetylcysteine and bicarbonate to prevent CIN have concluded these therapies "appear" to lessen the incidence of CIN, but are not conclusive.

Numerous prophylactic strategies have been studied, which have allowed several meta-analyses to be published on different single therapies in CIN. The conclusion of many of the meta-analyses reflect on the heterogeneous nature of the studies, publication bias, inability to absolutely recommend a therapy, and suggest that further adequately powered studies are needed even if it appeared a benefit was derived.

Alkalinization of renal tubular fluid with bicarbonate may prevent the development of CIN. Renal injury may be reduced by slowing the free radical production in the renal medulla [2]. In a meta-analysis, Meier et al. [3] reported that the use of sodium bicarbonate reduced the incidence of CIN, but revealed no difference in the need for renal replacement therapy or mortality. Two recently published randomized controlled studies suggest hydration with normal saline was as efficacious as using sodium bicarbonate for the prevention of CIN [8, 9]. Hemodialysis has been reported to reduce the degree of CIN in patients with chronic renal insufficiency after angiographic procedures [10]. This invasive therapeutic modality reflects additional medical costs and potential morbidity, but may be of benefit in this specific patient population to lessen further renal injury.

Conclusion

We presented a case that necessitated continued perioperative assessment of renal function during cerebral aneurysm coiling in a patient with chronic renal insufficiency. The co-morbidities of this patient placed her at high risk for CIN, which could lead to further impaired renal function and a negative outcome. The best plan for preventing acute renal failure secondary to CIN includes hydration with normal saline, intravenous sodium bicarbonate infusion prior to the procedure, minimization of dye exposure, and consideration of postprocedure hemodialysis.

References

1. **D. Reddan, M. Laville, V. D. Garovic**. Contrast-induced nephropathy and its prevention: what do we really know from evidence-based findings? *J Nephrol* 2009; **22**: 333–51.

2. **M. Kanbay, A. Covic, S. G. Coca** et al. Sodium bicarbonate for the prevention of contrast-induced

nephropathy: a meta-analysis of 17 randomized trials. *Int Urol Nephrol* 2009; **41**: 617–27.

3. **P. Meier, D. T. Ko, A. Tamura** *et al.* Sodium bicarbonate-based hydration prevents contrast-induced nephropathy: a meta-analysis. *BMC Med* 2009; **7**: 23.

4. **S. K. Morcos, H. S. Thomsen, J. A. Webb**. Contrast-media-induced nephrotoxicity: a consensus report. Contrast Media Safety Committee, European Society of Urogenital Radiology (ESUR). *Eur Radiol* 1999; **9**: 1602–13.

5. **H. S. Trivedi, H. Moore, S. Nasr** *et al.* A randomized prospective trial to assess the role of saline hydration on the development of contrast nephrotoxicity. *Nephron* 2003; **93**: C29–34.

6. **A. M. Kelly, B. Dwamena, P. Cronin** *et al.* Meta-analysis: effectiveness of drugs for preventing contrast-induced nephropathy. *Ann Intern Med* 2008; **148**: 284–94.

7. **M. Rudnick, H. Feldman**. Contrast-induced nephropathy: what are the true clinical consequences? *Clin J Am Soc Nephrol* 2008; **3**: 263–72.

8. **A. M. From, B. J. Bartholmai, A. W. Williams** *et al.* Sodium bicarbonate is associated with an increased incidence of contrast nephropathy: a retrospective cohort study of 7977 patients at Mayo clinic. *Clin J Am Soc Nephrol* 2008; **3**: 10–18.

9. **P. Schmidt, D. Pang, D. Nykamp** *et al.* N-acetylcysteine and sodium bicarbonate versus N-acetylcysteine and standard hydration for the prevention of radiocontrast-induced nephropathy following coronary angiography. *Ann Pharmacother* 2007; **41**: 46–50.

10. **P. T. Lee, K. J. Chou, C. P Liu** *et al.* Renal protection for coronary angiography in advanced renal failure patients by prophylactic hemodialysis. A randomized controlled trial. *J Am Coll Cardiol* 2007; **50**: 1015–20.

25

Postoperative normal perfusion pressure breakthrough

Juan P. Cata and Andrea Kurz

Altered flow dynamics after the surgical correction of vascular malformations create the risk for perfusion abnormalities in the postoperative period. Vigilance for edema or hemorrhage due to this complication is imperative in the postoperative setting.

Case description

A 37-year-old female with a 2-month history of generalized tonic-clonic seizures underwent a successful left craniotomy for clipping and resection of a 4 cm (in maximum diameter) arteriovenous malformation (AVM) located in the left parieto-occipital lobe. Six hours after surgery the patient presented with sudden and progressive right-sided motor weakness and rapid deterioration in mental status. She subsequently required emergent tracheal re-intubation due to hypercapnic respiratory failure and inability to protect her airway. Emergent computed tomography (CT) scan of the brain showed massive cerebral edema, as well as enlarged vascular enhancement suggesting hyperperfusion and a small intracerebral hemorrhage. A single photon emission computed tomography (SPECT) and cerebral angiography showed marked hyperperfusion with a regional cerebral blood flow of 73 mL/100 g/min and left posterior cerebral artery dilatation, respectively. Once admitted to the intensive care unit the patient was placed in a barbiturate coma, started on fluid restriction and aggressive systemic blood pressure control. Four days after surgery, a CT brain scan showed significant reduction in brain swelling and no signs of cerebral hyperperfusion. On postoperative day five, the barbiturate coma was stopped, the patient was successfully extubated and her neurologic status gradually improved. One month after surgery, examination demonstrated no neurologic deficit and a cerebral angiography showed normalization of flows and diameter of the left posterior cerebral artery.

Discussion

Normal perfusion pressure breakthrough (NPPB) is a major cause of morbidity and mortality following AVM surgery. It can also be present in the postoperative period of carotid endarterectomies and Galen vein malformations. The actual incidence of this vascular phenomenon is not well known, but Young et al. found an incidence of 2.6% [1]. Risk factors for NPPB include a large-sized AVM, large-diameter feeders and an AVM located in a border zone. The NPPB etiology is unclear. The brain tissue surrounding the AVM is supplied by blood vessels showing impaired autoregulation, consequently a rapid resumption of "normal" blood flow after AVM occlusion leads to hyperemia and vascular leak. Also, prolonged hypoperfusion results in the development of new blood vessels in the brain tissue surrounding the AVM. The sudden occlusion of the AVM after clamping or embolization resulting in an abrupt increase in perfusion through the newly formed blood vessels may be responsible for capillary leak and brain edema (Figure 25.1). Another hypothesis suggests that NPPB might be associated with impaired autonomic perivascular innervation in vascular beds proximal and distant (contralateral) to the AVM, which can explain the fact that global CBF may be increased after resection of the AVM [1]. "Occlusive hyperemia" [2] has also been suggested as a hypothesis in which postoperative flow restriction and spontaneous thrombosis of the venous system associated with the AVM causes occlusive hyperemia, which in turn is responsible for capillary dysfunction and rupture of the blood–brain barrier [3]. Abnormal vasomotor reactivity has also been demonstrated in peri-AVM areas of the brain [4].

The clinical manifestation of NPPB ranges from vague symptoms such as nausea, vomiting, and headache to more severe problems such as aphasia, hemiparesis, rapid deterioration of mental status, or seizures. Postoperative neuroimaging studies (CT scan, SPECT, and magnetic resonance imaging)

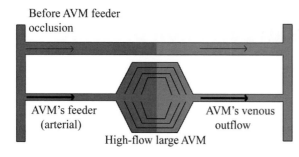

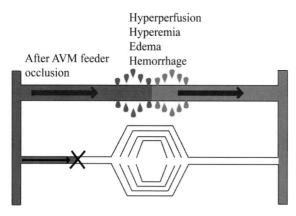

Figure 25.1. The picture depicts the vascular changes before (upper panel) and after (lower panel) arteriovenous malformation (AVM) feeder occlusion. It can be noticed that after occlusion, the blood flow in collateral circulation to the AVM increases and as a consequence hyperperfusion, tissue edema, and bleeding occur.

may demonstrate localized or generalized brain edema, hyperemia, and focal or multifocal intracranial hemorrhage. Transcranial cerebral Doppler may show vasomotor paralysis represented by decreased flow velocities in cerebral arteries without response to the administration of acetazolamide or during carbon dioxide challenge. Cerebral angiography may show stagnation in the feeders of the resected AVM and delayed circulation. Preoperative measures such as staged feeders and nidus embolization of large-size, high-grade AVM have been proposed to prevent NPPB.

Aggressive intraoperative control of systemic blood pressure and intracranial pressure, as well as meticulous hemostasis of feeders >1 mm, is recommended. It is unknown if the use of volatile anesthetic agents or total intravenous agents have an effect on the occurrence of NPPB. More aggressive measures such as carotid artery clamping and hypothermia have been proposed to prevent NPPB. It is noteworthy that none of the proposed preventive modalities are based on well-conducted clinical studies.

In the postoperative period, the use of low to normal systemic blood pressure, reduced fluid intake, anticonvulsants and diuretics are indicated in the management of patients at risk for or with mild forms of NPPB. Barbiturate coma, hyperventilation, and invasive intracranial pressure monitoring may be used in those patients with generalized brain edema and increased intracranial pressure [5]. Again, none of these therapeutic measures is supported by randomized controlled trials.

Vasomotor paralysis may last for several days to weeks after surgery. Thus, neuroimaging evidence of normal pattern of cerebral vasoreactivity along with neurologic status improvement may warrant barbiturate withdrawal and careful liberalization of the blood pressure control.

Conclusion

Normal perfusion pressure breakthrough is a potentially catastrophic event after AVM surgery. Anesthesia providers should strive for tight perioperative blood pressure control and should be vigilant for signs of postoperative neurologic deterioration.

References

1. **W. L. Young, A. Kader, E. Ornstein** et al. Cerebral hyperemia after arteriovenous malformation resection is related to "breakthrough" complications but not to feeding artery pressure. The Columbia University Arteriovenous Malformation Study Project. Neurosurgery 1996; **38**: 1085–93.

2. **N. R. al-Rodhan, T. M. Sundt Jr, D. G. Piepgras** et al. Occlusive hyperemia: a theory for the hemodynamic complications following resection of intracerebral arteriovenous malformations. J Neurosurg 1993; **78**: 167–75.

3. **J. Hai, Q. Lin, S. T. Li** et al. Chronic cerebral hypoperfusion and reperfusion injury of restoration of normal perfusion pressure contributes to the neuropathological changes in rat brain. Brain Res Mol Brain Res 2004; **126**: 137–45.

4. **H. H. Batjer, M. D. Devous Sr.** The use of acetazolamide-enhanced regional cerebral blood flow measurement to predict risk to arteriovenous malformation patients. Neurosurgery 1992; **31**: 213–17.

5. **D. Chyatte.** Normal pressure perfusion breakthrough after resection of arteriovenous malformation. J Stroke Cerebrovasc Dis 1997; **6**: 130–6.

Vascular procedures. Carotid endarterectomy

Preoperative evaluation

Maged Argalious

Stroke remains the third leading cause of death overall, and the second leading cause of death for women in the USA [1]. It has been estimated that 103 000 carotid endarterectomies (CEA) were done in the USA in 2005 [1]. Among patients undergoing CEA, the incidence of coronary artery disease is around 35% [2], and 25% of patients undergoing CEA have concomitant diabetes mellitus [2], highlighting the importance of preoperative evaluation and optimization in this patient population.

Case description

A 76-year-old male was scheduled for a right CEA under general anesthesia after an episode of transient monocular blindness (amaurosis fugax) prompted a duplex ultrasound of the carotid vessels. This showed a >90% occlusion of the right internal carotid artery as well as a 50–79% stenosis of the left internal carotid artery [3]. His medical history included hypertension, coronary artery disease with a documented non S-T segment elevation myocardial infarction (NSTEMI) 15 months prior, which required a percutaneous coronary intervention (PCI) with a cypher drug-eluting stent to the right coronary artery. He was able to walk around the house until a year ago when osteoarthritis of his knees markedly reduced his activities of daily living. His medications included metoprolol, amlodipine, atorvastatin, aspirin, and clopidogrel.

At the time of his NSTEMI, a 2-D echocardiogram revealed basal and mid-inferior and inferoseptal hypokinesis with a left ventricular ejection fraction of 42%. Preoperative laboratory work-up was significant for a hematocrit of 33 and a serum creatinine of 1.6 mg/dL. The vascular surgeon consulted the anesthesia team for preoperative evaluation.

Discussion

Carotid endarterectomy is considered an intermediate risk surgery. The classification of cardiac risk in noncardiac surgery is based on the incidence of cardiac death and nonfatal myocardial infarction (1–5% in intermediate risk surgeries).

The goal of preoperative preparation for noncardiac surgery is to:

1. Assess the need for emergent or urgent surgery that cannot be postponed even if the risk of coronary artery disease is high.
2. Exclude active cardiac conditions that require preoperative evaluation and treatment before noncardiac surgery (see Table 26.1).
3. Assess functional capacity since asymptomatic patients with good functional capacity (four or more metabolic equivalents) can proceed with their planned surgery and rarely require further noninvasive testing since their management will unlikely be changed based on the results of testing.
4. Assess the presence of clinical risk factors according to the Lee's revised cardiac risk index (see Table 26.2) in patients with low or unknown functional capacity to determine the need for further cardiac testing especially in patients with three or more clinical risk factors and those undergoing vascular surgery (high incidence of underlying coronary artery disease). The consensus is to only perform further cardiac testing (noninvasive: i.e., functional stress test; invasive: i.e., cardiac catheterizations) if the results of those tests are likely to change management.

While the American College of Cardiology/American Heart Association (ACC/AHA) offers an algorithm for evaluating cardiovascular risk [4], there are some clinical scenarios with inconclusive data to determine "best strategy" and more than one plausible option can be followed. This patient had no active cardiac conditions, had an unknown functional capacity and had three clinical risk factors (history of heart disease, cerebrovascular disease, and renal insufficiency) and was undergoing an intermediate risk vascular surgery. The

Table 26.1. Active cardiac conditions for which the patient should undergo evaluation and treatment before noncardiac surgery (Class I, Level of Evidence: B).

Condition	Examples
Unstable coronary syndromes	Unstable or severe angina* (CCS class III or IV)[†] Recent MI[‡]
Decompensated HF (NYHA functional class IV; worsening or new-onset HF) Significant arrhythmias	High-grade atrioventricular block Mobitz II atrioventricular block Third-degree atrioventricular heart block Symptomatic ventricular arrhythmias Supraventricular arrhythmias (including atrial fibrillation) with uncontrolled ventricular rate (HR greater than 100 beats per minute at rest) Symptomatic bradycardia Newly recognized ventricular tachycardia
Severe valvular disease	Severe aortic stenosis (mean pressure gradient >40 mmHg, aortic valve area less than 1.0 cm^2, or symptomatic) Symptomatic mitral stenosis (progressive dyspnea on exertion, exertional presyncope, or HF)

* According to L. Campeau [8].
[†] May include "stable" angina in patients who are unusually sedentary.
[‡] The American College of Cardiology National Database Library defines recent MI as more than 7 days but less than or equal to 1 month (within 30 days).
CCS indicates Canadian Cardiovascular Society; HF, heart failure; HR, heart rate, MI, myocardial infarction; NYHA, New York Heart Association.
Reprinted with permission from L. A. Fleisher, J. A. Beckman, K. A. Brown *et al.* ACC/AHA 2007 [1].

Table 26.2. Clinical risk factors [7].

History of heart disease
History of compensated or prior heart failure
History of cerebrovascular disease
Diabetes mellitus
Renal insufficiency

first option is to proceed with the planned surgery with heart rate control and no further testing. This would be based on the following rationale:

- This patient had an episode of amaurosis fugax and the right CEA could be considered urgent and not totally elective.
- Even if functional noninvasive stress testing showed reversibly ischemic myocardium, PCI with balloon angioplasty would require postponement of the CEA for 2–4 weeks to allow

healing of the vessel injury, while PCI with a bare metal stent (BMS) or a drug eluting stent (DES) may require postponing surgery for 4 weeks and 12 months respectively especially if the surgeon does not want to operate while patients are receiving dual antiplatelet therapy (aspirin and clopidogrel) [5]. The surgeon's rationale for stopping clopidogrel preoperatively was that any postoperative bleeding into a closed space (neck) could result in catastrophic airway compromise.

The second option was to proceed with noninvasive cardiac testing with the following rationale:

- Patients undergoing vascular surgery have a high incidence of concomitant coronary artery disease and cardiac causes are the most common causes of morbidity and mortality after CEA.
- Studies document the beneficial effects of clopidogrel combined with aspirin in reducing cerebral emboli in patients undergoing CEA [6]. Therefore, even if this patient required a PCI with a BMS or DES, surgery should proceed with dual antiplatelet therapy.

Conclusion

The role of the anesthesiologist as a perioperative consultant requires a thorough knowledge of current guidelines, a deep understanding of perioperative risk associated with various noncardiac surgeries in order to follow an evidence-based approach to perioperative management.

References

1. **W. Rosamond, K. Flegal, K. Furie** *et al.* Heart disease and stroke statistics – 2008 update: a report from the American Heart Association Statistics Committee and Stroke Statistics Subcommittee. *Circulation* 2008; **117**: e25–146.

2. **GALA** Trial Collaborative Group, **S. C. Lewis, C. P. Warlow**. General anesthesia versus local anesthesia for carotid surgery (GALA): a multicentre, randomized controlled trial. *Lancet* 2008; **372**: 2132–42.

3. **W. S. Moore, H. J. Barnett, H. G. Beebe** *et al.* Guidelines for carotid endarterectomy. A multidisciplinary consensus statement for the Ad Hoc Committee, American Heart Association. *Circulation* 1995; **91**: 566–79.

4. **L. A. Fleisher, J. A. Beckman, K. A. Brown**. ACC/AHA 2007 Guidelines on Perioperative Cardiovascular Evaluation and Care for Noncardiac Surgery. Executive Summary: A Report of the

American College of Cardiology/American Heart Association Task Force on Practice Guidelines (Writing Committee to Revise the 2002 Guidelines on Perioperative Cardiovascular Evaluation for Noncardiac Surgery): Developed in Collaboration With the American Society of Echocardiography, American Society of Nuclear Cardiology, Heart Rhythm Society, Society of Cardiovascular Anesthesiologists, Society for Cardiovascular Angiography and Interventions, Society for Vascular Medicine and Biology, and Society for Vascular Surgery. *Circulation* 2007; **116**: 1971–96.

5. **American Society of Anesthesiologists Committee on Standards and Practice Parameters.** Practice alert for the perioperative management of patients with coronary artery stents. A report by the American Society of Anesthesiologists Committee on Standards and Practice Parameters. *Anesthesiology* 2009; **110**: 22–3.

6. **D. A. Payne, C. I. Jones, P. D. Hayes.** Beneficial effects of clopidogrel combined with aspirin in reducing cerebral emboli in patients undergoing carotid endarterectomy. *Circulation* 2004; **109**: 1476–81.

7. **T. H. Lee, E. R. Marcantonio, C. M. Mangione** *et al.* Derivation and prospective validation of a simple index for prediction of cardiac risk of major noncardiac surgery. *Circulation* 1999; **100**: 1043–9.

8. **L. Campeau.** (Letter): Grading of angina pectoris. *Circulation* 1976; **54**: 522–3.

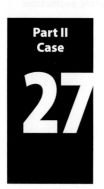
Monitoring modalities

Todd Nelson and Paul Picton

Carotid endarterectomy (CEA) has been proven to reduce the incidence of embolic stroke in symptomatic patients with >70% internal carotid artery stenosis [1]. The perioperative risk of stroke is significant [2], the pathogenesis of which include emboli, hemorrhage, and hypoperfusion. Intraoperative neurologic monitoring has been the subject of intense research for many years, the goal being to accurately identify intraoperative cerebral ischemia, and predict which patients may benefit from intraoperative shunting.

Case description

The patient was a 73-year-old male scheduled for a right CEA under general anesthesia. He presented with recurrent transient right-sided visual loss and had a past medical history significant for well-controlled hypertension, ischemic heart disease, and obesity. Carotid Doppler revealed 79% stenosis of his right internal carotid artery and 30% stenosis of his left.

He was premedicated with midazolam and a 20-gauge catheter was placed in his left radial artery for blood pressure monitoring. Following preoxygenation, anesthesia was induced with fentanyl and propofol; muscle relaxation was achieved with vecuronium. Anesthesia was maintained with isoflourane, oxygen, air, and remifentanil. Phenylephrine was titrated by infusion to maintain a stable arterial blood pressure that was increased by no more than 25% above baseline during cross-clamping. The mean stump pressure was 64 mmHg; shunting was not used. The carotid cross-clamp time was 35 minutes. Following cerebral reperfusion, an intraoperative angiogram was performed and was unremarkable.

The patient experienced delayed emergence and displayed signs of a left hemiparesis. Once fully awake he was safely extubated and was sent immediately for imaging. A diffusion-weighted magnetic resonance imaging confirmed the presence of a right-sided ischemic stroke in the middle cerebral artery (MCA) territory.

Discussion

Awake neurologic monitoring is considered the gold standard for evaluation of intraoperative neurologic status during CEA. The development of new neurologic symptoms is an indication of ischemia and necessitates shunt placement. For patients undergoing CEA under general anesthesia a number of monitoring modalities exist (Table 27.1): monitors of cerebral hemodynamics, monitors of cerebral oxygenation and metabolism, and monitors of electrophysiologic parameters [3].

Monitors of cerebral hemodynamics

Transcranial Doppler sonography can measure blood flow in the MCA, but can be difficult to localize in a significant proportion of patients. It demonstrates perioperative embolic showers and decrements in blood flow during cross-clamping. Carotid artery stump pressure provides an indication of the degree of perfusion from the contralateral circulation via the circle of Willis. The pressure in the carotid stump is measured immediately following placement of the carotid cross-clamp. Although invasive, it is technically easy. A mean pressure of >50 mmHg is commonly regarded as an indication of sufficient collateral flow, though a proven cutoff value remains under investigation.

Monitors of cerebral oxygenation and metabolism

Regional cerebral oximetry measured using near-infrared spectroscopy is convenient and noninvasive. Variability in pad placement can lead to unreliable regional oximetry readings. High inter- and

Table 27.1. Comparison of cerebral monitoring modalities for CEA under general anesthesia.

Cerebral monitor	Advantages	Limitations
Cerebral hemodynamics		
Transcranial Doppler	Allows direct evaluation of blood flow in MCA	MCA sometimes difficult to localize
	Possible to visualize embolic showers	Only provides information regarding MCA territory
		High likelihood of intraoperative probe dislocation
Stump pressure	Simple, inexpensive	No consensus on appropriate threshold value for ischemia
	No additional equipment or personnel needed	One time measurement
Cerebral oxygenation and metabolism		
Regional cerebral oximetry	Noninvasive	High inter- and intrasubject variability
	Easy, rapid to apply	Unclear contribution of non-brain blood sources
	Continuous measure of cerebral oxygenation	Absolute values less helpful than trends
Jugular bulb monitoring	Can give information regarding cerebral O_2 demand versus supply	Provides only a global value of oxygenation, nonspecific
		Invasive, requires some skill
Electrophysiologic monitors		
EEG	Direct measure of brain electrical activity	Expensive
		Requires constant presence of a trained technician
		Overly sensitive
SSEP	Ability to identify lesions in the sensory pathways	Expensive
	Requires fewer electrodes than EEG	Requires constant presence of a trained technician
		Extra-cerebral lesions in sensory pathway can influence readings

MCA, middle cerebral artery; EEG, electroencephalography; SSEP, somatosensory evoked potentials.

intra-individual variability exists. Trends are probably of greater value than absolute readings.

Jugular bulb monitoring provides a global measure of oxygenation in the ipsilateral hemisphere during cross-clamping: a rostrally placed oximeter is used to continuously measure jugular venous oxygen saturation. Alternatively, a jugular venous catheter is placed and periodic samples are drawn simultaneously with arterial line samples to compare pertinent values. It is an invasive technique that cannot identify specific areas of ischemia.

Electrophysiologic monitors

Electroencephalography (EEG) directly detects electrical potentials within the brain, providing a measure of brain activity. Cerebral blood flow is closely related to cerebral electrical activity and EEG thereby provides an indication of blood flow. It is very sensitive for ischemia in the brain and has a better ability to localize ischemic areas. Electroencephalography has been used for many years worldwide and, therefore, most clinicians are familiar with it as a monitoring tech-

nique for CEA. Unfortunately, EEG can be overly sensitive for ischemia. It is costly, cumbersome, and the presence of a trained technician is required throughout surgery.

With somatosensory evoked potentials, peripheral nerves (i.e., median and posterior tibial) are stimulated and the evoked potentials monitored via electrodes placed on the scalp. Lesions are diagnosed within sensory pathways. Like EEG, somatosensory evoked potentials are expensive and require the presence of a trained technician.

The GALA trial, a multicenter, randomized controlled trial which enrolled over 3000 patients, evaluated the difference in outcomes between general anesthesia and regional anesthesia for CEA [4]. This study showed no significant difference in stroke rates or 30-day mortality between CEA performed under general anesthesia versus those performed using local anesthesia alone. Multiple studies have been performed to attempt to determine the effectiveness of each modality used perioperatively in conjunction with general anesthesia. Despite extensive research, no single method has been proven to be more effective than any other in identifying ischemia, nor has any been proven to reduce the risk of stroke [5].

The challenge for all monitoring modalities is to identify thresholds for ischemia and stroke. As values are chosen that provide increased sensitivity to brain ischemia, the results become less specific. This leads to the placement of unnecessary shunts, which exposes the patient to the risk of stroke associated with shunt placement. The converse is also true. No value has been identified for any monitoring device that is both highly sensitive and highly specific.

Conclusion

In conclusion, a frequent basic neurologic examination on an awake patient remains the gold standard for neurologic monitoring during CEA. However, no difference in outcomes between general anesthesia and regional anesthesia has been proven. None of the monitoring modalities commonly used for CEA under general anesthesia have been shown to either reliably identify or prevent cerebral ischemia or stroke, nor predict which patients may benefit from shunt placement.

References

1. **North American Symptomatic Carotid Endarterectomy Trial Collaborators**. Beneficial effect of carotid endarterectomy in symptomatic patients with high-grade carotid stenosis. *N Engl J Med* 1991; **325**: 445–53.

2. **J. M. Findlay, B. E. Marchak, D. M. Pelz** *et al.* Carotid endarterectomy: a review. *Can J Neurol Sci* 2004; **31**: 22–36.

3. **S. Moritz, P. Kasprzak, M. Arlt** *et al.* Accuracy of cerebral monitoring in detecting cerebral ischemia during carotid endarterectomy: a comparison of transcranial Doppler sonography, near-infrared spectroscopy, stump pressure, and somatosensory evoked potentials. *Anesthesiology* 2007; **107**: 563–9.

4. **GALA Trial Collaborative Group**. General anaesthesia versus local anaesthesia for carotid surgery (GALA): a multicentre, randomized controlled trial. *Lancet* 2008; **372**: 2132–42.

5. **R. Bond, K. Rerkasem, C. Counsell** *et al.* Routine or selective carotid artery shunting for carotid endarterectomy (and different methods of monitoring in selective shunting). *Cochrane Database Syst Rev* 2002; **2**: CD000190.

Vascular procedures. Carotid endarterectomy

Neurologic decline after carotid surgery

Phil Gillen

Carotid endarterectomy (CEA) is a surgical procedure that typically involves the removal of atheromatous plaque and tunica intima from the lumen of a stenosed extracranial segment of the internal carotid artery (ICA), via an open approach. Due to the marked changes in cerebral perfusion, there is a spectrum of neurologic sequelae directly attributable to this procedure, ranging from intraoperative stroke and death to more subtle perioperative neurocognitive deterioration. This decline is becoming increasingly recognized as a consequence of CEA.

Case description

The patient was a 68-year-old male with demonstrated occlusive cerebrovascular disease (>70% stenosis of right carotid artery) with a history of a right-ICA territory transient ischemic attack (TIA) 3 months previously. He was scheduled for a right CEA under general anesthesia. His past medical history also included a myocardial infarction 5 years prior, along with mild peripheral vascular disease.

The primary anesthetic goals were maintenance of the patient's normal blood pressure, prevention of tachycardia and subsequent myocardial ischemia, analgesia, and prevention of coughing on emergence. A right radial arterial catheter was inserted preoperatively. Premedication involved a small bolus of benzodiazepine and the patient was carefully induced with small boluses of propofol and a concurrent infusion of remifentanil; neuromuscular blockade was achieved with vecuronium. Care was taken to blunt the sympathetic response to laryngoscopy and endotracheal intubation was achieved. The patient's anesthesia was maintained with isoflurane, oxygen and air, along with remifentanil. The procedure proceeded uneventfully with good control of blood pressure (within 20% of baseline) and smooth emergence was achieved with low-dose remifentanil. Prior to removal of the endotracheal tube, gross neurologic function was examined along with observation of the patient's pupils.

On arrival at the recovery ward, the patient – while able to demonstrate gross neurologic movement – was persistently disorientated in time, place, and person. Blood gas analysis including blood sugar and electrolyte levels were normal with adequate gas exchange. The patient's blood pressure was maintained at slightly elevated than normal throughout.

Following careful observation and after ruling out physiologic and pharmacologic causes, a computed tomography scan of the patient's head was performed, which proved unremarkable. He was admitted to the intensive care unit for further management and observation. The patient's cognition gradually improved over the following 3–4 days and he was discharged to the floor and eventually home. Follow-up at 6 weeks revealed normal gross neurologic function but the patient still complained of slight but persistent deficits in concentration.

Discussion

The recognized indications for CEA are numerous, but usually involve the presence of 70% or greater stenosis and/or the presence of ipsilateral TIA or stroke. During the dissection of the narrowed vessel, the carotid artery is clamped to facilitate dissection and reduce blood loss. This clamping significantly reduces the ipsilateral hemisphere's blood flow and has the potential to cause further cerebral hypoperfusion. Upon clamp release there is a demonstrable hyperperfusion on the affected side. The proposed mechanisms for neurologic damage are the hypo/hyperperfusion states, as well as cerebral ischemia combined with microembolic phenomena in patients who are likely to already have a compromised cerebral blood flow.

Carotid endarterectomy may be associated with both gross and subtle neurologic damage. While this case demonstrated no gross neurologic deficit and normal postoperative neuroimaging findings, there was a clear decline in postoperative neurocognition.

However, a comprehensive preoperative neurocognitive assessement was not performed.

Predicting neurologic decline

Postoperative cognitive dysfunction is a well recognized phenomenon following many surgical procedures performed under general anesthesia. Its presence is associated with preexisting cognitive deficit along with cardiopulmonary and pharmacologic factors. However, there is evidence that CEA itself is a risk factor for intraoperative neurologic damage. There is demonstrable neurocognitive decline in approximately 25% of CEA patients following postoperative day one neuropsychometric tests as compared with a paired cohort undergoing a similar anesthetic regimen including the use of benzodiazepines. Unfortunately, there has also been some debate and little consensus as to which psychometric tests are most appropriate. A recent review article [1] highlighted the many confounding variables in postoperative cognitive testing, which may explain why this area of research continues to be contentious.

Examining the risk factors for intraoperative CEA neurologic decline, one study found increased age to predict neurocognitive dysfunction. Of note, the authors found that other risk factors (including those associated with cerebrovascular disease such as smoking, diabetes, hypertension) and surgical parameters (including previous contralateral CEA, operative side, duration of surgery, cross-clamp time, and the need for shunt placement) did not appear to correlate with postoperative day 1 cognitive deterioration [2].

Preventing neurologic decline

A number of interventions have been examined to determine their efficacy in the early demonstration and subsequent prevention of neurologic damage.

Blood pressure: Blood pressure control has long been recognized as crucial during and after CEA to prevent critical hypo- or hyperperfusion states. It is for this reason that intra-arterial blood pressure is routinely measured and controlled perioperatively, including the careful administration of balanced anesthesia, analgesia, and vasoactive drugs.

Surgery under local anesthesia: The performance of CEA under local anesthesia has the potential to demonstrate immediate neurologic decline. However, the gross neurologic tests performed on awake patients during a CEA may be unable to detect anything more

than a large neurocognitive deficit. Recent studies have found there to be no significant difference in risk of stroke or death, hospital stay, or postoperative quality of life between local or general anesthetic techniques. However, further subgroup analysis demonstrated an improved neurologic outcome in surgery performed under local anesthesia [3].

Shunt placement: One method to reduce ipsilateral hypoperfusion is the use of a shunt, inserted proximal to the clamp, to allow for improved blood flow. As above [2], this bore no correlation to postoperative day 1 cognitive decline. Shunt placement is not universal in CEA surgery. Indeed its use may even be predictive of poor neurologic outcome as shunt usage is more likely in patients with more pronounced cerebrovascular disease.

Electrophysiologic analysis: The efficacy of a number of electrophysiologic parameters in the prediction of neurologic deficit has been assessed. These have included transcranial Doppler sonography (TCD), near-infrared spectroscopy (NIRS), stump pressure (SP) measurement, and somatosensory evoked potentials (SSEP).

Transcranial Doppler sonography analysis of arterial blood flow (usually the ipsilateral middle cerebral artery) has demonstrated that high numbers of microembolic signals, along with indicators of inappropriate intraoperative hypo/hyperperfusion correlate with postoperative ischemic events. Upon findings indicative of intraoperative cerebral ischemia, the administration of agents including platelet glycoprotein IIB/IIIA receptor antagonists or Dextran-40 in the immediate postoperative phase has shown an improved mortality. However, the efficacy of this modality in the *prevention* of embolic events has been questioned along with its ability to predict postoperative cognitive dysfunction. Its routine use in CEA remains contentious.

Near-infrared spectroscopy cerebral oximetry has been shown to be efficacious in those patients in whom TCD analysis is technically more difficult to perform in the perioperative course, due to the lack of a temporal bone window. Its values have also been shown to correlate to EEG changes indicative of ischemia.

One study found these parameters (TCD, NIRS, SP) to be equally efficacious in determining ischemia, but with SSEP being less accurate [4]. Analysis of electrophysiologic parameters has shown electroencephalography to be comparable with SSEP analysis in determining cerebral ischemia although its use is associated with a high false positive rate. Investigation into the use of Bispectral index monitoring has not been shown to be efficacious in determining neurologic decline in awake patients undergoing CEA.

Enzyme markers of neurologic damage: The presence and quantity of intracellular neuronal enzymes has been predicted to correspond to the degree of neuronal damage. For example, elevated levels of S100beta protein (S100B) have been shown to be a prognostic indicator of stroke size and outcome when measured 2–3 days post-event whereas immediate rises may not be associated with neurologic decline. In patients undergoing cardiopulmonary bypass, elevated S100B correlated with significant impaired cognition only later than 5 hours postoperatively.

Elevated serum S100B in CEA, but not neuron-specific enolase, has been associated with a subclinical neurologic decline. However, this has been questioned by further investigators [5]. Furthermore, the use of quantitative enzyme analysis via a jugular-venous bulb failed to link enzyme rise with neurocognitive decline. There is much debate as to the impact of the time of measurement of these enzymes. For example, S100B has a half life of only 2 hours.

Conclusion

In conclusion, the perioperative management of patients undergoing CEA, along with attempts to pre-vent its associated neurologic decline, continues to be a challenge to clinicians. Further investigation is warranted to ensure the best neurologic outcomes in patients undergoing this common procedure.

References

1. **P. De Rango, V. Caso, D. Leys** et al. The role of carotid artery stenting and carotid endarterectomy in cognitive performance: a systematic review. *Stroke* 2008; **39**: 3116–27.

2. **J. Mocco, D. A. Wilson, R. J. Komotar** et al. Predictors of neurocognitive decline after carotid endarterectomy. *Neurosurgery* 2006; **58**: 844–50.

3. **C. F. Weber, H. Friedl, M. Hueppe** et al. Impact of general versus local anesthesia on early postoperative cognitive dysfunction following carotid endarterectomy: GALA Study Subgroup Analysis. *World J Surg* 2009; **33**: 1526–32.

4. **S. Moritz, P. Kasprzak, M. Arlt** et al. Accuracy of cerebral monitoring in detecting cerebral ischemia during carotid endarterectomy: a comparison of transcranial Doppler sonography, near-infrared spectroscopy, stump pressure, and somatosensory evoked potentials. *Anesthesiology* 2007; **107**: 563–9.

5. **L. S. Rasmussen, M. Christiansen, J. Johnsen** et al. Subtle brain damage cannot be detected by measuring neuron-specific enolase and S-100beta protein after carotid endarterectomy. *J Cardiothorac Vasc Anesth* **14**: 166–70.

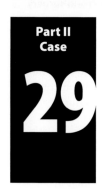

Vascular procedures. Carotid endarterectomy

Postoperative hematoma and airway compromise after carotid endarterectomy

Maged Argalious

In the North American Symptomatic Carotid Endarterectomy Trial (NASCET), the incidence of postoperative wound hematoma was 5.5% [1]. While the majority of cases is the result of venous oozing and only require temporary external compression while reversal of anticoagulation takes effect, prompt recognition and management of an expanding neck hematoma reduces the risk of progression to airway compromise, a potentially fatal complication.

Case description

A 76-year-old female arrived in the postanesthesia care unit (PACU) after an uneventful left carotid endarterectomy (CEA) for a severe left internal carotid artery stenosis (99%). Her medical history included stable coronary artery disease, chronic atrial fibrillation, hypertension and chronic obstructive pulmonary disease (COPD) with an 80 pack-year smoking history. Her surgical history included a remote cholecystectomy and cervical spine fusion. Her medications included aspirin, atorvastatin, amlodipine, metoprolol, hydrochlorothiazide as well as supplemental potassium. She had been taking coumadin (for atrial fibrillation), which was switched to an intravenous infusion of heparin on admission to the hospital. Her lab work showed a prothrombin time/International Normalized Ratio (PT/INR) of 13.2 seconds and 1.2 respectively. Her partial thromboplastin time (PTT) was maintained at 40–60 seconds. Apart from a serum potassium of 3.3 mEq/L, her laboratory values were within normal limits.

On emergence from anesthesia, she developed severe hypertension (190/115) requiring intravenous nitroglycerin boluses as well as intravenous labetalol. Her blood pressure on arrival to the PACU was 150/80 mmHg. Thirty minutes after, the PACU nurse noticed some swelling at the incision site. Immediately thereafter, the patient started to complain of shortness of breath despite increased supplemental oxygen. The

staff surgeon and anesthesiologist were called to the bedside.

Discussion

Airway management is often challenging in the PACU or critical care unit. Factors including surgery near the airway, intraoperative airway instrumentation or manipulation, previous neck dissection or radiation [2], large volumes of intraoperative fluids, and residual anesthetic effects contribute to these difficulties [3]. Postoperative bleeding after CEA is particularly hazardous because bleeding into a closed space can quickly result in an expanding neck hematoma that can cause impingement on laryngeal structures and airway compromise. Even patients considered as having an "easy airway" in the operating room can pose airway challenges in the PACU or critical care unit [4]. In patients recovering from neck surgery who develop respiratory insufficiency, the possibility of an expanding neck hematoma must be considered. Other possible causes of dyspnea in this patient are outlined in Table 29.1.

If the neck hematoma is visible but is not causing respiratory distress, pressure should be applied to the surgical site to avoid further expansion. In addition to notification of the surgeon, control of postoperative hypertension by infusions of short-acting medications (nitroglycerin, esmolol) is important in reducing the bleeding at the site of the fresh vascular anastomosis. In addition, confirmation of reversal of anticoagulation is important. If these measures are successful and the neck hematoma is small in size, close observation of the patient in a critical care environment as well as marking of the boundaries of the hematoma to ensure early identification of further expansion is important.

In cases of progressive expansion of the neck hematoma, even in the absence of airway compromise, awake intubation (possibly fiberoptic-guided

Table 29.1. Common causes of dyspnea after carotid endarterectomy (CEA) not related to expanding hematomas.

1. **Cardiac**
   Myocardial ischemia
   Acute postoperative hypertension with resultant
       pulmonary edema
   Atrial arrhythmia with rapid ventricular response

2. **Pulmonary**
   Right to left shunting most commonly due to atelectasis
   Exacerbation of COPD

3. **Nerve**
   Recurrent laryngeal nerve injury (especially in the setting of
       prior contralateral CEA or neck surgery with bilateral
       recurrent laryngeal paralysis)
   Phrenic nerve paresis after cervical plexus block (especially
       in patients with severe COPD)
   Carotid body denervation (more common after bilateral
       CEA)

COPD, chronic obstructive pulmonary disease.

Table 29.2. Management of postoperative neck hematoma.

Apply pressure to bleeding site

Notify surgery and anesthesia team (call for help)

Consider reversal of residual anticoagulation

Tight blood pressure control

Outcome:
No further hematoma expansion
   Communication with surgical team
   Mark the boundaries of the hematoma for early identification
       of further expansion
   Close observation and extended monitoring (8–12 hours) in
       a critical care environment

**Continuous expansion of hematoma with no airway
compromise**
   Awake (fiberoptic) intubation either in the PACU or after
       immediate transfer to the operating room after
       topical anesthesia to the airway followed by general
       anesthesia for exploration of wound and drainage of neck
       hematoma
   Assess neurologic status at the end of the case
   Consider maintaining endotracheal intubation
       postoperatively until resolution of reactionary airway
       edema

**Expansion of neck hematoma with rapidly progressive
airway compromise (dyspnea, stridor, airway
obstruction)**
   Emergent intubation (ASA algorithm)
   Cannot intubate/*can* ventilate: using face mask, oral or nasal
       airways, laryngeal mask airway:
   Consider immediate surgical drainage of the neck
       hematoma followed by further attempts to secure the
       airway
   Cannot intubate/*cannot* ventilate:
   Surgical airway (emergent cricothyroidotomy, percutaneous
       or surgical tracheostomy)
   Evacuation of hematoma and wound exploration,
       neurologic assessment
   Maintain airway secured postoperatively

PACU, postanesthesia care unit.

according to the American Society of Anesthesiologists difficult airway algorithm) [5] may be prudent, followed by surgical exploration of the wound and drainage of the hematoma. In some cases, airway edema persists despite drainage of the hematoma; it is advisable to maintain endotracheal intubation and postoperative sedation after confirming the absence of neurologic deficits.

In most instances of progressively expanding neck hematomas, airway obstruction ensues quickly as a result of encroachment and distortion of airway anatomy. If emergent intubation attempts are unsuccessful, the decision to proceed with a surgical airway (emergency cricothyroidotomy or tracheostomy) depends on the ability (vs inability) to ventilate the patient with a face mask or laryngeal mask airway. If ventilation is unsuccessful or becomes inadequate despite drainage of the neck hematoma, invasive airway access should proceed. Table 29.2 summarizes the management steps in cases of expanding neck hematoma.

References

1. Beneficial effect of carotid endarterectomy in symptomatic patients with high grade carotid stenosis. North American Symptomatic Carotid Endarterectomy Trial Collaborators. *N Engl J Med* 1991; **325**: 445–53.

2. **C. M. Burkle, M. T. Walsh, S. G. Pryor** *et al.* Severe postextubation laryngeal obstruction: The role of prior neck dissection and radiation. *Anesth Analg* 2006; **102**: 322–5.

3. **G. S. Murphy, J. W. Szokol, J. H. Marymont** *et al.* Residual neuromuscular blockade and critical respiratory events in the postanesthesia care unit. *Anesth Analg* 2008; **107**: 130–7.

4. **M. Argalious.** PACU Emergencies ASA Refresher Courses in Anesthesiology 2009. **37**; 1–12.

5. **American Society of Anesthesiologists Task Force on Management of the Difficult Airway**. Practice guidelines for management of the difficult airway: An updated report by the American Society of Anesthesiologists Task Force on Management of the Difficult Airway. *Anesthesiology* 2003; **98**: 1269–77.

Vascular procedures. Carotid endarterectomy

30 Postoperative stroke after carotid endarterectomy

J. Javier Provencio

Perioperative stroke can be a devastating complication of surgery and has a particularly high incidence in association with vascular procedures such as carotid endarterectomy (CEA).

Case description

The patient was a 75-year-old right-handed male with a history of a previous stroke 1 month before admission, which manifested as left upper extremity weakness that steadily improved over about a week. His initial evaluation at the hospital revealed a 60–79% stenosis of the right internal carotid artery. He returned to the hospital for an elective CEA. He was a >100 pack year smoker of cigarettes but had recently "cut down" to 10 cigarettes per day since his original stroke. In addition, he had a history of hypertension, hypothyroidism, and dyslipidemia. His medication regimen consisted of aspirin, clopidogrel, levothyroxine, an HMG-CoA reductase inhibitor, and three antihypertensive medications (a beta-blocker, a calcium channel blocker, and a peripherally acting alpha-blocker). In addition, he was taking hydrocodone-acetaminophen for low back pain. Interestingly, he was allergic to lobster, which had prompted physicians to administer diphenhydramine prior to dye-containing radiology tests.

On physical exam, the patient was a well-appearing man with no obvious signs of stroke. His blood pressure was high at 186/90 mmHg and he was tachycardic at 92 beats per minute. He had bilateral carotid bruits on auscultation and mild weakness of his left lower extremity but was able to hold the leg up against gravity for 10 seconds. He had no facial droop or weakness in the arm on the left side. He was noted to have visual field deficit in the left visual field. The rest of his examination was unremarkable.

Upon emergence from anesthesia, the patient was noted to be hemiplegic on the left side with a prominent facial droop. His National Institutes of Health Stroke Scale score was noted as 17 putting him in a high-risk group for poor outcome. Computed tomography (CT) scan showed no evidence of intracerebral hemorrhage but a CT angiogram suggested a deficit of perfusion in the right hemisphere suggesting an occluded artery. It was felt by the surgeon and the stroke physician that intravenous tissue plasminogen activator (tPa) was too risky due to the recent surgery. The patient was taken for arterial thrombolysis with a mechanical clot retrieval device. Postprocedure, he was awake with slightly improved arm and leg strength on the left side. He continued to improve through his hospital stay but ultimately had multiple strokes in the right hemisphere (Figure 30.1).

Discussion

The risk of stroke in patients with symptomatic or asymptomatic carotid stenosis is quite high. A number of studies have shown that the risk of subsequent stroke is decreased in correctly selected patients who have CEA. Despite this, stroke is a common perioperative complication, ranging from 0 to 8.4% [1–3]. Treatment of patients postoperatively after CEA who experience stroke can be a challenging situation for the clinician. On the one hand, they are in the hospital and usually come to the attention of medical staff very early (which is the most important goal of stroke therapy). On the other hand, the fact that they have had a recent surgery limits the interventions that can be offered to a patient with an acute stroke.

There are three causes of acute lateralized deficits after CEA: one is a physiologic abnormality and two are ischemic consequences. Hyperperfusion syndrome is loss of autoregulation of the intracerebral carotid system on the side of the surgery, which leads to loss of control of blood flow. When the arterial blood flow overwhelms venous return, blood pools in the capillary beds resulting in ischemia and hemorrhage. The

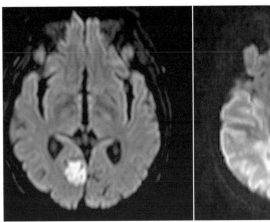
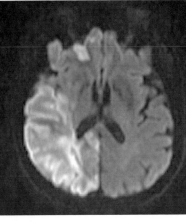

Figure 30.1. Diffusion weighted magnetic resonance images. The left image shows an area of stroke noticed after emergence from anesthesia. The area is relatively small considering the symptoms included complete hemiparesis. The right image shows the massive stroke the patient had after recovery from his original episode.

treatment is unclear but systemic hypotension to control the blood flow is currently the accepted standard [4].

The two common causes of ischemic stroke after CEA are acute occlusion of the carotid artery at the surgical site and embolization of clot to the distal cerebral vasculature [5]. The standard treatment of acute occlusion of the carotid artery includes emergent surgical revascularization of the carotid followed by intravenous anticoagulant administration to prevent clot reformation at the surgical site [6]. In patients with significant areas of infarcted brain, there is a risk of reperfusion cerebral edema, venous congestion and hemorrhage. In addition, anticoagulation in patients with large stroke volumes may increase the risk of hemorrhagic conversion of a bland stroke. Obviously, surgery is not indicated for patients who have distal emboli.

There are very few prospective data on acute intervention for stroke in patients who have distal embolism after CEA. There are a few reports at scientific meetings of systemic administration of recombinant tPa for patients after carotid endarterectomy with mixed results. It is unclear from these reports whether this is an effective or safe intervention.

More recently, intravascular interventional techniques to revascularize occluded intracerebral arteries has become a tempting option to open acute distal embolic strokes. Interventional procedures include a number of devices and drugs (including anticoagulants, antiplatelets, and lytic agents) used individually or in combination [7]. The use of more devices and drugs in combination increases the risk of bleeding but also increases the probability of successful recanalization. There are no prospective trials to support using

this paradigm but it is unlikely that there will ever be a trial with sufficient power to answer the question of efficacy. Anecdotal evidence suggests some patients benefit from this approach. There is no good evidence to inform the risk of bleeding.

In addition to strategies to revascularize the blood vessel, there are a number of interventions aimed at preventing subsequent stroke. They include aspirin, clopidogrel, the combination of extended-release dipyridimole and aspirin. In addition, there is evidence that HMG-CoA reductase inhibitors (statins) improve outcome after stroke. Fortunately, most patients with carotid endarterectomy take aspirin and statins as part of the treatment of their carotid stenosis.

Conclusion

Finally, there is an argument to be made for urgent neurologic consultation after stroke from CEA. Neurologists can quickly stratify patients for eligibility for acute intervention. In addition, improvement in stroke outcome has been shown to correlate with early and aggressive physical therapy and rehabilitation. This is an important and potentially overlooked aspect of care in patients with stroke after any surgery. A neurologic consultation may make aggressive evaluation and rehabilitation more likely.

References

1. **M. R. Mayberg, S. E. Wilson, F. Yatsu** *et al.* Carotid endarterectomy and prevention of cerebral ischemia in symptomatic carotid stenosis. Veterans Affairs Cooperative Studies Program 309 Trialist Group. *J Am Med Assoc* 1991; **266**: 3289–94.

2. L. G. Ludington, G. I. Kafrouni, M. H. Peterson *et al.* Clinical review of 106 consecutive carotid endarterectomies. *Int Surg* 1976; **61**: 155–9.

3. Endarterectomy for asymptomatic carotid artery stenosis. Executive Committee for the Asymptomatic Carotid Atherosclerosis Study. *J Am Med Assoc* 1995; **273**: 1421–8.

4. T. Karapanayiotides, R. Meuli, G. Devuyst *et al.* Postcarotid endarterectomy hyperperfusion or reperfusion syndrome. *Stroke* 2005; **36**: 21–6.

5. J. B Towne, V. M. Bernhard. Neurologic deficit following carotid endarterectomy. *Surg Gynecol Obstet* 1982; **154**: 849–52.

6. J. P. Berthet, C. H. Marty-Ané, E. Picard *et al.* Acute carotid artery thrombosis: description of 12 surgically treated cases. *Ann Vasc Surg* 2005; **19**: 11–18.

7. S. H. Kim, A. I. Qureshi, E. I. Levy *et al.* Emergency stent placement for symptomatic acute carotid artery occlusion after endarterectomy. Case report. *J Neurosurg* 2004; **101**: 151–3.

Part II
Case

31

Postoperative myocardial infarction

Maged Argalious

Patients with atherosclerotic carotid disease have a high incidence of concomitant coronary artery disease [1]. In the GALA study, a multicenter randomized controlled trial to evaluate general anesthesia (GA) versus local anesthesia (LA) for carotid surgery, the primary outcome of stroke, myocardial infarction, and death occurred in 4.7% of cases [2]. Since the risk of major adverse cardiac effects after carotid endarterectomy (CEA) is between 1 and 5%, CEA is considered an intermediate risk surgery [3].

Table 31.1. Medical management of patients with S-T segment elevation myocardial infarction (STEMI).

Oxygen
Aspirin
Statin drugs
Nitrates
Beta blockers
Narcotic analgesics (morphine)
ACE inhibitors/angiotensin receptor blockers
Management of hyperglycemia (insulin)

Case description

A 59-year-old male presented for a right CEA under regional anesthesia (superficial cervical plexus block). He had a history of hypertension, hyperlipidemia, and peripheral vascular disease. He was a current smoker and refused to quit smoking. He had a transient ischemic attack 5 weeks earlier and underwent a preoperative cardiac evaluation prior to his carotid surgery, including a dobutamine stress echocardiography for evaluation of orthopnea. This showed a reduced left ventricular function of 40% and regional wall motion abnormalities in the anterolateral wall of the left ventricle (LV). A cardiac catheterization was followed by percutaneous coronary intervention with two bare metal stents to the left anterior descending and obtuse marginal vessels. The patient was instructed to hold his clopidogrel 5 days prior to his scheduled carotid surgery and to continue his aspirin perioperatively [4]. The rest of the patient's medications included lisinopril, carvedilol, and rosuvastatin. After a stable intraoperative course, the patient was transferred to the recovery room in a stable condition.

One hour later, however, he developed crushing substernal chest pain followed by acute hemodynamic decompensation (hypotension, bradycardia). His electrocardiogram showed marked S-T segment elevation in the anterior chest leads.

Discussion

Patients with S-T segment elevation myocardial infarction (STEMI) of sufficient size have a reduction in LV function resulting in a reduced stroke volume, reduced systemic blood pressure, and a consequent reduction in coronary perfusion pressure. The reduction in stroke volume results in an increase in LV filling pressures, causing LV dilation and increasing LV end diastolic pressures. This leads to worsening coronary perfusion pressure, ultimately resulting in cardiogenic shock unless this vicious circle is reversed by reperfusion (fibrinolytic therapy or invasive percutaneous intervention) [5]. In STEMI of smaller size, the unaffected portion of the ventricle becomes hyperkinetic in order to sustain overall ventricular function.

Surgical patients with postoperative STEMI are poor candidates for fibrinolytic therapy [6]. Initial medical management options (Table 31.1) are usually limited in patients with STEMI in the setting of cardiogenic shock, because many of the recommended medications in STEMI are contraindicated for fear of worsening the hypoperfusion state (e.g., beta blockers, nitrates, ace inhibitors). In this patient, Advanced Cardiac Life Support guidelines (including the use of inotropes) should be followed to restore hemodynamic stability. In STEMI secondary to stent thrombosis as in this case, the definitive treatment is percutaneous

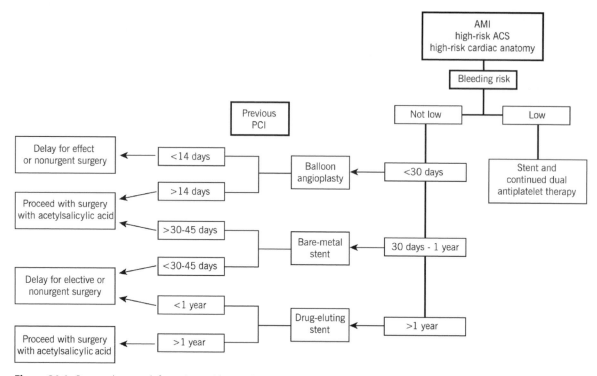

Figure 31.1. Proposed approach for patients with a previous percutaneous coronary intervention (PCI) who need subsequent surgery (left panel of the figure) and for patients who require nonsurgical revascularization before noncardiac surgery. ACS, acute coronary syndrome; AMI, acute myocardial infarction. Reprinted with permission from S. G. DeHert. Preoperative cardiovascular assessment in noncardiac surgery: an update. *European Journal of Anaesthesiology* 2009; 26(6): 449–57.

coronary intervention to re-establish blood flow to the thrombosed stent [6]. Surgical procedures in patients with prior percutaneous coronary intervention (PCI) should therefore be performed in institutions where 24-hour interventional cardiology is available.

In patients undergoing preoperative cardiac evaluation prior to noncardiac surgery, the decision to proceed with PCI has to be discussed among the management team (surgeon, anesthesiologist, and cardiologist) [5]. Patients with a recent transient ischemic attack have a higher incidence of subsequent stroke within the first year and CEA should not be considered totally elective. Therefore, if noncardiac surgery cannot be postponed until the minimum period of dual antiplatelet therapy after PCI is achieved (Figure 31.1), alternative management options should be considered including performing the CEA on dual antiplatelet therapy, bridging therapy with GIIb/IIIa receptor antagonists (e.g., tirofiban or eptifibatide), maximizing medical management before CEA followed by postoperative management of coronary artery disease, or pursuing a combined approach (CEA

and coronary artery bypass grafting) [7]. Premature discontinuation of antiplatelet therapy has been shown to markedly increase the incidence of stent thrombosis and should not be done for elective surgery [8].

Regardless of the revascularization technique, aspirin should be a lifelong therapy since its abrupt discontinuation results in a rebound increase in inflammatory prothrombotic state, adding to the prothrombotic state caused by surgical intervention [6].

References

1. **N. R. Hertzer, J. R. Young, E. G. Beven** *et al.* Coronary angiography in 506 patients with extracranial cerebrovascular disease. *Arch Intern Med* 1985; **145**: 849–52.

2. **GALA Trial Collaborative Group, S. C. Lewis, C. P. Warlow** *et al.* General anesthesia versus local anesthesia for carotid surgery (GALA): a multicentre, randomized controlled trial. *Lancet* 2008; **372**: 2132–42.

3. **L. A. Fleisher, J. A. Beckman, K. A. Brown** *et al.* 2009 ACCF/AHA Focused Update on Perioperative Beta

Blockade Incorporated Into the ACC/AHA 2007 Guidelines on Perioperative Cardiovascular Evaluation and Care for Noncardiac Surgery. A Report of the American College of Cardiology Foundation/ American Heart Association Task Force on Practice Guidelines. *Circulation* 2009; **120**: e169–276.

4. **C. L. Grines, R. O. Bonow, D. E. Casey, Jr** *et al.* AHA/ACC/SCAI/ACS/ADA Science Advisory. Prevention of premature discontinuation of dual antiplatelet therapy in patients with coronary artery stents. A science advisory from the American Heart Association, American College of Cardiology, Society for Cardiovascular Angiography and Interventions, American College of Surgeons, and American Dental Association, with representation from the American College of Physicians. *Circulation* 2007; **115**: 813–18.

5. **F. G. Kushner, M. Hand, S. C. Smith, Jr** *et al.* Focused Updates: ACC/AHA Guidelines for the Management of Patients with ST-Elevation Myocardial Infarction and Guidelines on Percutaneous Coronary Intervention. A Report of the American College of Cardiology Foundation /American Heart Association Task Force on Practice Guidelines. *Circulation* 2009; **120**; 2271–306.

6. **L. T. Newsome, R. S. Weller, J. C. Gerancher** *et al.* Coronary artery stents. II. Perioperative considerations and management. *Anesth Analg* 2008; **107**: 570–90.

7. **E. S. Brilakis, S. Banerjee, P. B. Berger**. The risk of drug-eluting stent thrombosis with noncardiac surgery. *Curr Cardiol Rep* 2007; **9**: 406–11.

8. **American Society of Anesthesiologists Committee on Standards and Practice Parameters**. Practice alert for the perioperative management of patients with coronary artery stents. A Report by the American Society of Anesthesiologists Committee on Standards and Practice Parameters. *Anesthesiology* 2009; **110**: 22–3.

Functional neurosurgery

Preoperative evaluation for deep brain stimulator surgery

Milind Deogaonkar

Deep brain stimulation (DBS) is now a routine therapeutic option for patients with Parkinson's disease, essential tremors (ET), and dystonia. The success of DBS surgery depends on proper patient selection, proper placement of the DBS electrode in the intended nucleus and proper programming. In view of this, the preoperative evaluation of the DBS patient assumes added importance.

Case description

A 65-year-old male was seen in our outpatient clinic to be evaluated for DBS surgery. He had symptoms of Parkinson's disease for 15 years, primarily motor fluctuation, tremors, and dyskinesia. The patient had an improvement of 60% on his motor unified Parkinson's disease rating scale when compared in the off and on state. The symptoms improved significantly with levodopa though the improvement was short-lasting. In addition, he had long-standing but stable coronary artery disease for which he was taking aspirin. He also had cervical spine fusion in the past and was asymptomatic except for a reduced range of motion. He had significant anxiety on his neuropsychological testing but no significant cognitive decline. The patient was deemed to be a good candidate for staged bilateral subthalamic nucleus DBS surgery. He was told to stop his aspirin 10 days in advance. An anxiety counselor was arranged in the operating room. Preoperative cervical magnetic resonance imaging was done to rule out any residual cervical stenosis or compression. The patient underwent a unilateral DBS followed by the second side DBS 3 weeks later. He then underwent bilateral implantable pulse generators 2 weeks after the second side. An awake intubation was performed and intraoperative electrophysiologic monitoring was employed during the surgery. The surgeries were uneventful and he had good therapeutic benefits.

Discussion

This case highlights the following important preoperative evaluation issues in DBS patients:

1. General surgical patient evaluation.
2. Disease-specific evaluation.
3. Neuropsychological evaluation.
4. Evaluation of associated medical conditions.
5. Airway evaluation.

General surgical patient evaluation

In general, patients must be able to tolerate the various components of surgery and have the social support structure to comply with the demands of surgery and postoperative care. For those undergoing DBS surgery, both the patient and family members need to have a detailed understanding of reasonable outcomes, potential complications, and the multiple steps involved in the preoperative assessments, surgery, perioperative management, and follow-up care. The patient needs to be cooperative with follow-up programming and adjustment of medications in the outpatient setting. Additionally, the patient and family need to have realistic expectations about surgical outcome.

Disease-specific evaluation

Parkinson's disease

In general, surgery is most likely to benefit symptoms affecting the extremities versus axial symptoms such as posture, balance, gait, and speech. Surgical candidates typically have severe tremors; "Off" medication-related rigidity, freezing, dystonia, and bradykinesia; "On" medication-related dyskinesias and significantly disabling "On–Off" medication motor fluctuations. One of the most important predictors of neurosurgical treatment response is the patient's response to levodopa. Patients who demonstrate a significant improvement in motor symptoms during "Off" versus

"On" levodopa medication state are most likely to benefit from surgery.

Tremor

In general, patients with distal tremor, either postural, intention/action, or resting tremor can be controlled with surgery. In contrast, the more proximal tremors are the most difficult to treat surgically [1–3]. Head, neck, and lower extremity tremors are also more difficult to treat than upper extremity tremors. Tremors involving the head/neck and axial regions usually require bilateral surgery.

Dystonia

Patients who are refractory to all the conservative measures, including medication trials and botulinum toxin injections, are potential candidates. Primary generalized dystonia [4–6], as well as patients with idiopathic cervical dystonia, can obtain the best motor benefits with bilateral internal globus pallidus DBS. Juvenile-onset idiopathic dystonia with age of onset >5 years and without multiple orthopedic deformities also has a good response to surgery.

Neuropsychological evaluation

Neuropsychological assessment is recommended as part of the preoperative assessment to determine candidacy for DBS. The neuropsychological assessment should include assessment of cognition, neuropsychiatric symptoms, social support, and goals for surgery. Patients with severe cognitive dysfunction or dementia on neuropsychological examination should be excluded from surgical intervention. Patients with mild cognitive impairment or a frontal dysexecutive syndrome may still undergo surgery but should receive extra counseling along with their family regarding the potential for increased risk of cognitive impairment and confusion post-surgery. Psychiatric conditions such as anxiety, depression, and mania must be identified and medically optimized preoperatively and an intraoperative anxiety counselor can be arranged. Neurosurgical intervention in patients with a delusional psychosis or severe personality disorder, such as borderline personality disorder, is generally not recommended.

Evaluation of associated medical conditions

Patients should be in stable overall health with respect to cardiac, pulmonary, and systemic conditions such

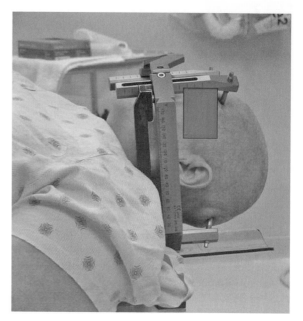

Figure 32.1. Patient in a Leksell frame on the operating table, illustrating the difficulty of accessing the airway with a frame in place.

as hypertension, diabetes, and cancer. Patients who require antiplatelet medications or coumadin must be able to tolerate complete withdrawal from these medications prior to surgery. Consultation with other medical specialists (e.g., cardiologists) may be required prior to proceeding with surgery in some patients.

Airway evaluation

Access to the airway is difficult once the frame is in place (Figure 32.1). A detailed evaluation of the airway is therefore essential. An awake intubation can be used in patients with cervical spine instability or severe cervical spine stenosis; intraoperative somatosensory evoked potential monitoring is useful for monitoring the integrity of the cervical spine cord during the procedure.

Conclusion

Deep brain stimulation surgery for Parkinson's disease requires a systematic approach to preoperative assessment. Understanding the medical and neuropsychological considerations of Parkinson's disease is essential for proper perioperative care.

References

1. **C. Berk, J. Carr, M. Sinden** *et al.* Thalamic deep brain stimulation for the treatment of tremor due to multiple sclerosis: a prospective study of tremor and quality of life. *J Neurosurg* 2002; **97**: 815–20.

2. **G. Deuschl, P. Bain**. Deep brain stimulation for tremor [correction of trauma]: patient selection and evaluation. *Mov Disord* 2002; **17**: S102–11.

3. **M. Kitagawa, J. Murata, S. Kikuchi** *et al.* Deep brain stimulation of subthalamic area for severe proximal tremor. *Neurology* 2000; **55**: 114–16.

4. **M. Krause, W. Fogel, M. Kloss** *et al.* Pallidal stimulation for dystonia. *Neurosurgery* 2004; **55**: 1361–8.

5. **A. Kupsch, S. Klaffke, A. A. Kühn** *et al.* The effects of frequency in pallidal deep brain stimulation for primary dystonia. *J Neurol* 2003; **250**: 1201–5.

6. **J. Y. Lee, M. Deogaonkar, A. Rezai**. Deep brain stimulation of globus pallidus internus for dystonia. *Parkinsonism Relat Disord* 2007; **13**: 261–5.

Functional neurosurgery

33 Airway crisis during deep brain stimulator placement

Ehab Farag

Deep brain stimulation (DBS) is the ultimate therapy for motor disease disorders like Parkinson's disease (PD) and dystonia. The anesthetic management of DBS is a challenging process. The patient needs to be sedated and comfortable but awake enough to conduct the proper neurologic examination and neurophysiologic recording for deep brain electrode insertion. Deep brain stimulation procedures are not without complications; here we describe one of the most common complications encountered during DBS.

Case description

The patient was a 70-year-old male with a past medical history of hypertension, hyperlipidemia, obstructive sleep apnea, and PD. The patient was scheduled for unilateral DBS electrode insertion in the subthalamic nucleus under sedation. After applying standard ASA monitors, sedation was started using propofol. Propofol was titrated between 50 and 100 mcg/kg/min to maintain required sedation. Systolic blood pressure was maintained ≤140 during the procedure with boluses of labetalol. Oxygen was administered via nasal canula at a rate of 3–4 L/min to maintain oxygen saturation ≥95%. The patient tolerated the insertion of the DBS electrode and identification of the subthalamic nucleus. During the closure phase of the procedure the sedation was restarted. The patient became agitated; boluses of propofol were given to deepen the level of sedation. The patient became apneic with a rapid decrease of oxygen saturation to 40% and a consequent decrease of the heart rate to 30 beats/min. Attempts to ventilate the patient using a face mask failed. The arrest code was called to the operating room due to the inability to intubate the patient. While his head was fixed in the DBS frame, a laryngeal mask airway (LMA) was inserted. Insertion of the LMA enabled successful ventilation and resuscitation. The closure of the procedure was accomplished under general anesthesia using sevoflurane via the LMA. At the

end of the procedure, the patient awoke neurologically intact. The patient was discharged the following day in a stable condition.

Discussion

Deep brain stimulation is considered the final therapy for medically refractory PD as well as other chronic neurologic disorders such as dystonia, depression, and chronic pain syndromes. The DBS procedure requires fixation of the patient's head to the stereotactic apparatus for accurate electrode placement. This can lead to substantial patient discomfort. Patient selection and preparation for the procedure are very important in order to minimize the perioperative complications. Aspirin and coumadin should be stopped. Blood pressure should be well controlled during the procedure to avoid the development of hematomas (subdural, subarachnoid, intraventricular, and intracrebral). Overall, the rate of hemorrhage has been estimated at 3–5% per patient [1]. The cessation of anti-Parkinsonian medications before the surgery (called "Off" period) can be very unpleasant, particularly for those patients with severe pain, dystonia, or depression. Benzodiazepines and long-acting narcotics should be avoided during the procedure to facilitate the proper electrode placement. The use of propofol for sedation during the procedure is not without complications. Propofol can induce respiratory depression and airway obstruction, as was seen in our case. Head fixation during the procedure usually renders endotracheal intubation very difficult. Placement of an LMA is the ideal method for managing the upper airway in emergency situations during DBS procedures.

We have noted that some patients receiving propofol experienced sneezing [1], which has already been documented by its manufacturer. Sneezing can be very troublesome to the patient and interferes with physiologic mapping during the DBS. In addition, sneezing may cause a sudden increase in intracranial pressure that may lead to intracranial hemorrhage. We have noted that age ≥64 is the single most important independent factor for complications during DBS [1]. Properties of dexmedetomidine make it well suited for sedation during DBS procedures. It has little effect on the patient's motor symptoms, respiratory functions, and upper airway. Dexmedetomidine creates an environment in which the patient feels comfortable and relaxed during the procedure [2–4].

Conclusion

Deep brain stimulation represents a significant anesthetic challenge for the anesthesiologist. Vigilance and awareness of the procedure's complications are the key elements for successful anesthetic management.

References

1. **R. Khatib, Z. Ehrahim, A. Rezai** et al. Perioperative events during DBS : the experience at Cleveland Clinic. *J Neurosurg Anesthesiol* 2008; **20**: 36–40.

2. **I. Rozet, S. Muangman, M. S. Vavilala** et al. Clinical experience with dexmedetomidine for implantation of deep brain stimulators in Parkinson's disease. *Anesth Analg* 2006; **103**: 1224–8.

3. **E. Farag**. Dexmedetomidine in the neurointensive care. *Discovery Medicine* 2010; **9**: 42–45.

4. **C. Trombetta, A. Deogaonkar, M. Deogaonkar** et al. Delayed awakening in dystonia patients undergoing deep brain stimulation. *J Clin Neurosci* 2010; **17**: 865–8.

34

Postoperative management of Parkinson's medications

Milind Deogaonkar

Deep brain stimulation (DBS) for Parkinson's disease (PD) has now become a routine therapeutic option. The success of surgery depends on proper patient selection, proper placement of electrodes, and postoperative programming. The management of anti-Parkinsonian medication in the postoperative period is affected by interaction of other perioperative medications with PD and the effects of DBS surgery.

Case description

A 62-year-old female with a 15-year history of PD was scheduled to have bilateral subthalamic nucleus (STN) DBS implantation. Her main symptoms were bilateral resting tremors, bradykinesia, rigidity, motor fluctuations, and dyskinesias. She had a unified Parkinson's disease rating scale motor score of 52, which improved to 26 after levodopa. She was on 1200 mg levodopa a day in divided doses and 4 mg ropinorole every day. Of note, she had a history of gastroesophageal reflux disease. Her anti-Parkinsonian medications were stopped as per the protocol the previous night. She underwent bilateral stereotactic STN DBS implants without any problems (Figure 34.1). Following the surgery she was observed to be very rigid and confused and did not open her eyes but was following commands. Her brain computed tomography scan was normal with some residual pneumocephalus. After she was given her regular medications the rigidity improved but she developed severe dyskinesias. After reducing the dose of her levodopa by half, the dyskinesias improved. During the night she developed symptoms of reflux and nausea and was given metoclopromide and some haloperidol for her agitation. Following this, she went into acute Parkinsonian crisis with severe rigidity and dystonic spasm. Her symptoms gradually improved once these medications were stopped. She was discharged after a stay of 3 days in the hospital.

Discussion

This case highlights the following points:

1. Importance of restarting PD medications soon after surgery.
2. Interactions between the STN DBS and levodopa.
3. Effect of postoperative neurologic changes and medication.
4. Interactions of other medication and Parkinsonism.

Importance of restarting PD medications soon after surgery

Parkinson's disease patients are off their routine PD medications for at least 12 hours before surgery. The reason for this medication stoppage is to aid in microelectrode recording and macrostimulation during surgery to confirm the proper placement of the DBS lead [1]. After completion of DBS surgery, which usually lasts anywhere between 4 to 8 hours, the patients need to be given the medications as soon as possible. Delay in restarting the medication can result in worsening of PD symptoms and severe dyskinesias and dystonias.

Interactions between the STN DBS and levodopa

Placement of DBS in the STN itself exerts an anti-Parkinsonian effect immediately after surgery. This can act synergistically with the anti-PD medications and can produce severe peak-dose dyskinesias. It is important to watch the patient closely and titrate the preoperative anti-PD medications in patients who have a significant micro-subthalamotomy effect [2, 3].

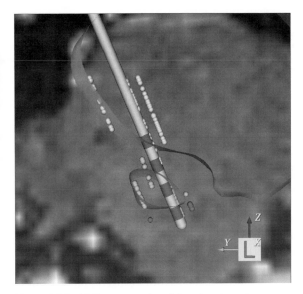

Figure 34.1. A 3-D representation of the microelectrode recording tracts and DBS lead implantation in STN.

Effect of postoperative neurologic changes and medication

The most common neuropsychiatric side effect in the immediate postoperative period following STN DBS is transient confusion with an incidence between 1% and 36% [4, 5]. Evidence of greater neuropsychological deficits prior to surgery is significantly associated with increased confusion following surgery [4]. Eyelid apraxia is also a commonly seen transient side effect of bilateral STN DBS [5]. This is transient and does not need any specific treatment but definitely affects the neurologic assessment in the postoperative period.

Interactions of other medication and Parkinsonism

Avoid any medications that have an antidopaminergic effect like haloperidol and metoclopramide and that can worsen the symptoms of PD patients or cause acute Parkinsonian crisis. The best antinausea medication for PD patients in the postoperative period is ondansetron; lorazepam in small doses works very well for confusion.

In summary, STN DBS has been demonstrated to be effective in alleviating the symptoms of medically refractory PD across multiple reports in the literature [5]. These results were confirmed by prospective series with double-blinded assessments and were largely sustained at 5-year follow-ups. Proper postoperative management can result in outstanding outcomes.

References

1. **A. R. Rezai, B. H. Kopell, R. E. Gross** et al. Deep brain stimulation for Parkinson's disease: surgical issues. *Mov Disord* 2006; **21**: S197–218.

2. **P. Krack, V. Fraix, A. Mendes** et al. Postoperative management of subthalamic nucleus stimulation for Parkinson's disease. *Mov Disord* 2002; **17**: S188–97.

3. **J. G. Nutt, S. L. Rufener, J. H. Carter** et al. Interactions between deep brain stimulation and levodopa in Parkinson's disease. *Neurology* 2001; **57**: 1835–42.

4. **J. G. Pilitsis, A. R. Rezai, N. M. Boulis** et al. A preliminary study of transient confusional states following bilateral subthalamic stimulation for Parkinson's disease. *Stereotact Funct Neurosurg* 2005; **83**: 67–70.

5. **A. R. Rezai, A. G. Machado, M. Deogaonkar** et al. Surgery for movement disorders. *Neurosurgery* 2008; **62**: 809–38.

35

Epilepsy surgery: intraoperative seizure

Oren Sagher and Shawn L. Hervey-Jumper

Epilepsy affects 5–10/1000 people in North America and is the second most common cause of mental health disability among young adults [1]. Despite advances in anti-epileptic drugs, 20–40% of all patients with epilepsy are refractory to medical management. For these patients, epilepsy surgery is an underutilized option.

Case description

The patient was a 20-year-old healthy male with a history of seizure disorder who was found to have a right frontal brain tumor. Although he had multiple events over a 6-month period characterized by brief loss of awareness, he now presented with a generalized seizure suffered while swimming. He was pulled out of the pool and after a brief post-ictal period, recovered to his neurologic baseline. He denied weakness, morning nausea or vomiting, speech changes, or headaches. Head computed tomography showed a posterior right frontal lesion, which on brain magnetic resonance imaging was non-enhancing and associated with minimal vasogenic edema. The lesion was located within the precentral gyrus and functional brain imaging confirmed its proximity to the primary motor cortex with the corticospinal tract fibers directly posterior to the mass lesion (Figure 35.1). The patient was admitted for a right frontal craniotomy with awake motor mapping and image-guided tumor resection.

The primary concerns of the anesthesiology team were: (1) management of intraoperative pain, particularly during Mayfield cranial pin placement, (2) management of the airway, (3) the potential for nausea and vomiting, and (4) intraoperative seizures during cortical stimulation. The patient was brought to the operating room and brief sedation was induced using a propofol and alfentanil infusion. He was placed in a Mayfield head-holder and his head coordinates were registered using the surgical navigational computer. A scalp block was performed using a combination of 1% lidocaine and 0.25% bupivacaine with 1:200 000 units epinephrine. A skin incision was made and craniotomy flap turned. Using image-guidance, the location of the tumor was identified. The propofol infusion was stopped for cortical mapping using electrocorticography and cortical stimulation. Polarity changes by somatosensory evoked potentials were found two gyri behind the tumor, suggesting that the tumor was anterior to the primary motor cortex. Electrical stimulation induced complex movements of the upper extremity at a low threshold, suggesting premotor cortex activation. Several small seizures were induced by stimulation, characterized by vocalization, facial twitching, and dystonic hand movements. These seizures were brief, and were controlled with cold saline irrigation of the brain surface. The patient's neurologic status was repeatedly assessed throughout the procedure and his pain was well controlled. The operation was completed uneventfully, and the patient retained normal speech and muscle strength at the end of the procedure.

Discussion

Epilepsy surgery is a well-established treatment option for patients with seizures originating from a single resectable focus. While temporal lobe resections are the most common surgical treatment for epilepsy worldwide, lesional resections have also shown favorable results, with 66% of patients seizure-free for at least 2 years [2]. Awake craniotomies are widely used in epilepsy surgery to facilitate intraoperative electrocorticography and cortical mapping, allowing precise identification of areas of the brain that control motor function and speech.

Prior planning and discussion are needed between surgeon and anesthesiologist for optimal patient positioning and room set-up. Communication is paramount, as the surgical team should be able to hear

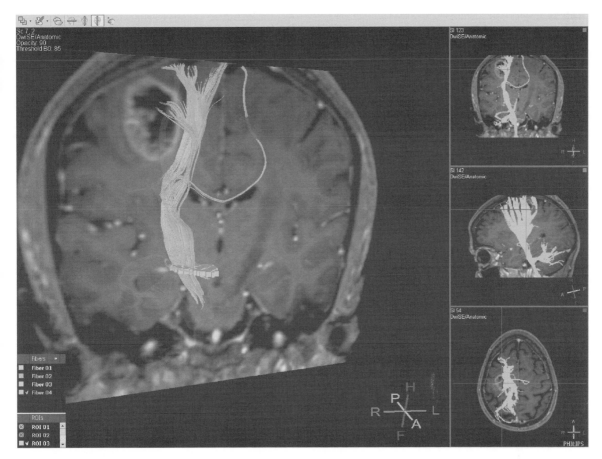

Figure 35.1. Functional magnetic resonance imaging with tractography shows corticospinal tract fibers running medially and posterior to the mass lesion.

both the patient and anesthesiologist clearly throughout the procedure. Lines and surgical drapes should be placed in such a way that allows for both access to and visibility of the patient. Furthermore, care should be taken early on in the procedure to ensure that the patient is comfortable, while allowing the patient's head to be positioned appropriately for surgical exposure.

Anesthetic complications and pitfalls associated with awake craniotomies for epilepsy surgery have been reviewed by Archer *et al.* and Skucas *et al.* [3, 4]. After reviewing 354 and 332 consecutive cases, respectively, they noted complications such as intraoperative seizures (3–16%), nausea and vomiting (0.9–8%), local anesthetic toxicity (0–2%), brain swelling (0.6–1%), and the need for conversion to general anesthesia due to airway and ventilation complications (1.8–2%) (Table 35.1).

The use of long-acting local anesthetic for nerve blocks helps avoid many problems associated with awake craniotomies. Nerve blocks should target the auriculotemporal, zygomaticotemporal, supraorbital, supratrochlear, lesser occipital, and greater occipital nerves on each side of the head, allowing for a complete ring of scalp analgesia. As the systemic absorption of long-acting local anesthetics, such as bupivacaine, affects the cardiovascular system and central nervous system, it is important to communicate to the surgeon at the beginning of the procedure the dosing limits of local anesthetics used. Toxic blood levels depress cardiac conduction resulting in arteriovenous blockage, ventricular dysrhythmias (often refractory to treatment), and arrest. Properly dosed and distributed, scalp blocks make intraoperative airway obstruction and nausea much less likely during the procedure, and are highly encouraged.

Table 35.1. Anesthetic considerations for awake craniotomies in epilepsy surgery.

Problems	Causes
Intraoperative pain	Inadequate analgesia causing pain may occur at time of rigid head-pin fixation, during temporalis muscle dissection, with traction on the dura close to the middle meningeal artery, and with traction of intracerebral blood vessels
Airway obstruction	May occur as the result of overzealous sedation to overcome pain when analgesia is suboptimal
Nausea and vomiting	Can be caused by surgical manipulation during dural opening, temporal lobe or amygdala manipulation, meningeal vessel handling, inadequate analgesia, or hypovolemia
Seizure	May occur as a result of decreased anticonvulsant levels, local anesthetic toxicity, or during cortical stimulation

Modified from Costello, Cormack, 2004 [7].

Direct cortical stimulation mapping has been shown to result in simple partial seizures in 5–20% of cases [5]. The propensity for intraoperative seizures is likely heightened in patients with a history of epilepsy. It is therefore of paramount importance for patients to be properly dosed with their anticonvulsants prior to surgery. It is advisable, for example, to allow patients access to their scheduled doses of anticonvulsants (with a sip of water) prior to surgery. In addition, it is useful for the anesthesiologist to know the patient's preoperative anticonvulsant blood levels (if the medications taken have an established efficacy range) as subtherapeutic drug levels greatly increase the probability of intraoperative seizures.

In the past, intraoperative seizures have been treated with intravenous benzodiazepines, barbiturates, and anticonvulsant boluses. The difficulty in relying on pharmacologic treatment of intraoperative seizures is that these medications may have unintended and often deleterious side effects. Benzodiazepines, for example, stop seizures effectively but often induce significant sedation that interferes with the mapping process. Phenytoin may also cause unintended problems, particularly when it is infused rapidly. Intravenous phenytoin is prepared with propylene glycol; therefore, its rapid intravenous administration can result in refractory hypotension, cardiac dysrhythmia, and even death [6]. Modern-day treatment of intraoperative seizures relies on the application of iced saline or Ringer's solution to the brain. This technique was initially described by Sartorius in 1998 [5] and has been quickly adopted by most centers, as it is able to rapidly and reliably terminate these seizures and eliminate the need for intravenously administered short-acting barbiturates or other anticonvulsant medications. The principal limitation of iced saline irrigation is related to occasional patient discomfort elicited by dural cooling.

Conclusion

In conclusion, epilepsy is a complex disease that imposes great disability on those affected. Epilepsy surgery is an underutilized treatment option and an awake craniotomy is sometimes warranted to allow precise cortical mapping. Although there are several pitfalls for which anesthesiologists should be aware, close monitoring, team communication, the safe and judicious use of long-acting local analgesia and prompt management of intraoperative seizures make for safe perioperative care.

References

1. S. Wiebe, W. T. Blume, J. P. Girvin *et al.* A randomized, controlled trial of surgery for temporal-lobe epilepsy. *N Engl J Med* 2001; **345**: 311–18.

2. J. Engel Jr. Surgery for seizures. *N Engl J Med* 1996; **334**: 647–52.

3. D. P. Archer, J. M. McKenna, L. Morin *et al.* Conscious-sedation analgesia during craniotomy for intractable epilepsy: a review of 354 consecutive cases. *Can J Anaesth* 1988; **35**: 338–44.

4. A. P. Skucas, A. A. Artru. Anesthetic complications of awake craniotomies for epilepsy surgery. *Anesth Analg* 2006; **102**: 882–7.

5. C. J. Sartorius, M. S. Berger. Rapid termination of intraoperative stimulation-evoked seizures with application of cold Ringer's lactate to the cortex. Technical note. *J Neurosurg* 1998; **88**: 349–51.

6. B. A. Boucher, C. A. Feler, J. C. Dean *et al.* The safety, tolerability, and pharmacokinetics of fosphenytoin after intramuscular and intravenous administration in neurosurgery patients. *Pharmacotherapy* 1996; **16**: 638–45.

7. T. G. Costello, J. R. Cormack. Anaesthesia for awake craniotomy: a modern approach. *J Clin Neurosci* 2004; **11**: 16–19.

Functional neurosurgery

Awake craniotomy and intraoperative neurologic decline

Oren Sagher and Shawn L. Hervey-Jumper

Awake craniotomy is routinely used in patients undergoing epilepsy surgery or surgery on eloquent areas of brain. The term "awake" may be considered a misnomer, as it includes a combination of local anesthesia, moderate sedation and analgesia, and the asleep–awake–asleep technique. This approach allows for intraoperative electrocorticography and cortical mapping, enabling identification of areas of the brain controlling motor function and speech. Awake craniotomy allows for optimal lesion resection with minimal postoperative neurologic dysfunction. However, there are associated complications that can contribute to both intraoperative and postoperative neurologic decline.

Case description

The patient was an otherwise healthy 27-year-old right-handed male with a history of psychotic depression who worked as a baggage handler at a local airline. He presented with a 6-month history of daily morning headaches after suffering a complex partial seizure. On brain magnetic resonance imaging, he was found to have a right frontal enhancing lesion. Given his normal motor examination, the patient initially elected to postpone surgical treatment. He was started on antiepileptic medications with close neuroimaging surveillance. After 6 months of follow-up, the lesion had increased in size. Because of his young age, normal preoperative motor examination, and tumor location within the posterior frontal lobe adjacent to the primary motor cortex, an awake craniotomy with image-guided resection and motor mapping was deemed to be the safest approach.

The primary concerns of the anesthesiology team were (1) preoperative airway assessment and management in the event of intraoperative airway obstruction, (2) intraoperative pain management, (3) management of intraoperative nausea and vomiting, and (4) close monitoring for signs of seizure or neurologic decline.

The patient was brought to the operating room and brief sedation was induced using a propofol and alfentanil infusion. His head was fixed in a Mayfield headholder and he was placed in the lateral position with the left side up. Head coordinates were then registered using the surgical navigational computer. Incisional and scalp blocks were performed using a combination of 1% lidocaine and 0.25% bupivacaine with 1:200 000 units epinephrine. Location of the tumor was mapped out on the scalp and the craniotomy flap was turned. Propofol infusion was stopped to accomplish cortical mapping by electrocorticography and cortical stimulation. A combination of direct visual inspection and image-guidance was used to localize the gyrus in which the tumor was located. The underlying brain was hyperemic, as well as swollen due to the underlying tumor. The motor region was then mapped with corticospinal fibers localized directly behind the region of the tumor. Resection of the tumor was planned using a subpial approach at medial and posterior margins. The patient's speech and motor status were repeatedly assessed. While removing tumor-infiltrated white matter posteriorly, the patient was noted to have significantly slowed responses of his left arm and leg, with an approximate 25% reduction in his preoperative strength. Resection was halted and the degree of resection assessed by stereotactic navigation. There was a small amount of residual tumor, but the decision was made to halt any further resection in order to avoid harm to nearby fibers passing from the primary motor cortex.

Discussion

Modern use of awake craniotomies began with the introduction of propofol and subsequently dexmedetomidine. These anesthetic agents facilitate intraoperative functional cortical mapping for indications that include surgery for intractable epilepsy, resection of lesions involving eloquent areas of cortex, as well as avoidance of general anesthesia for patients unable to tolerate it. Awake craniotomies allow surgical resection of tumors previously considered inoperable and allow for maximum resection while monitoring for neurologic damage. While the only absolute contraindication to the performance of awake craniotomy is patient refusal, relative contraindications include patient psychiatric illness, prone positioning, limited patient cooperation (due to cognitive deficits, emotional lability, diminished level of consciousness, or inability to overcome language barriers), significant preexisting neurologic damage that would preclude the ability to map or monitor neurologic function, or medical comorbidities that prevent the patient from lying still for long periods of time.

The decision to offer an awake craniotomy is made jointly by both the anesthesiologist and neurosurgeon. A preoperative anesthesia clearance appointment is recommended, during which potential contraindications should be considered. Careful airway assessment for predictors of difficult intubation is important in the event that there becomes a need for emergent general anesthesia. Preoperatively, anesthesiologists should also consider the degree of intracranial pressure, inquire regarding the type, frequency, and previous therapy for seizures, and assess the patient's overall degree of anxiety.

Most centers advise against the preoperative use of sedative medications on the day of surgery. Benzodiazepines have unpredictable effects on patient behavior and impair cortical mapping. Clonidine has been used in the past; however, the more highly selective alpha-2-adrenoreceptor agonist, dexmedetomidine, is now widely used to provide sedation, analgesia, and hemodynamic stability with minimal effect on cortical mapping and respiratory drive [1].

Optimal patient positioning in awake craniotomies ensures patient comfort, safety, and allows favorable conditions for functional mapping and lesion resection. The operating room should be set up to allow clear communication between members of the patient care team, visualization of the operative field and patient, and access to the patient for incident management [2].

There are three basic categories of anesthetic technique used in awake craniotomies: (1) local anesthesia used in isolation or in combination with sedation or periods of general anesthesia, (2) deep sedation, and (3) asleep–awake–asleep anesthesia, where gen-

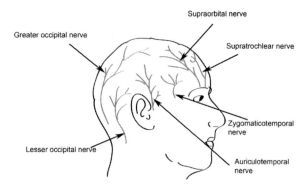

Figure 36.1. Diagram showing six sites for administering local anesthesia via bilateral block in awake craniotomy. Adapted from Piccioni, 2008 [8].

eral anesthesia is given followed by intraoperative awakening for cortical mapping and possibly lesion resection. Local anesthesia is best applied by bilateral block of the six scalp nerves: auriculotemporal, zygomaticotemporal, supraorbital, supratrochlear, lesser occipital, and greater occipital (Figure 36.1). The most commonly used local anesthetic includes a combination of bupivacaine and lidocaine (often with 1:200 000 units epinephrine, and occasionally sodium bicarbonate). Some studies suggest the use of levobupivacaine rather than bupivacaine because of its reduced peak plasma concentrations and a lower toxicity profile [2]. Ropivacaine is also an option.

Both sedation and asleep–awake–asleep techniques require that the anesthesiologist provide adequate sedation, hemodynamic control, and anesthesia while ensuring patient cooperation and alertness for intraoperative speech and motor testing. There are three anesthetic techniques that have been used to offer sedation: (1) neurolept anesthesia, (2) propofol-based anesthesia, and (3) dexmedetomidine-based anesthesia. Neurolept anesthesia involves the use of droperidol combined with a lipid soluble opiate (fentanyl, sufentanil, or alfentanil) and was the anesthetic technique used for early awake craniotomies [3]. This technique has largely fallen out of favor due to poor drug titratability, long duration of action, and cardiac effects. Neurolept anesthesia has been largely replaced by propofol-based techniques. Propofol is the most commonly used agent for awake craniotomies due to its easy titration, short duration of action, amnesic properties, and anti-emetic effects. Termination of propofol infusion 15 minutes before cortical mapping is typically sufficient. Herrick *et al.* compared neurolept and propofol-based anesthesia and noted

Table 36.1. Comparison of complications in awake craniotomy studies.

	Skucas[a]	Archer[b]	Gignac[c]	Herrick[d]	Danks[e]	Huncke[f]	Berkenstad[g]	Blanshard[h]	Sarang[i]
Airway problems	2	–	–	5/0	0/0	0	4	0.4	7/0/0
Hypoxemia	2	–	0/20/10	–	–	–	–	–	–
Hypertension	11	–	–	–	0/0	–	4	–	0/11/0
Hypotension	56	–	–	–	–	–	0	0.8	0/6/21
Tachycardia	14	–	–	10/35	–	–	0	–	–
Bradycardia	0.3	–	–	–	–	–	0	–	–
Seizures	3	16	10/30/10	0/41	0/20	0	8	8	0/6/0
Nausea/vomiting	0.9	8	50/30/70	10/18	–	0	0	0.8	–
Poor cooperation	2	2	20/0/10	–	–	0	4	–	0/3/5
Brain swelling	0.6	1	–	–	0/0	0	0	0	–
Local anesthetic toxicity	0	2	–	–	–	–	–	–	0/0/0

Adapted from Skucas, 2006 [5].
Values expressed as percentages.
(–), not reported.
[a] Retrospective review of 332 cases using unsecured airway and propofol infusion.
[b] Retrospective review of 354 cases using unsecured airways and fentanyl with droperidol.
[c] Prospective series of 30 cases, 3 groups with unsecured airways; fentanyl vs sufentanil vs alfentanil.
[d] Prospective series of 37 cases, 2 groups with unsecured airways; propofol vs fentanyl + droperidol.
[e] Prospective series of 21 cases, 2 groups with unsecured airways; midazolam + sufentanil + fentanyl vs propofol + midazolam + sufentanil + fentanyl.
[f] Prospective series of 10 cases, 1 group with airways secured by endotracheal intubation; volatile anesthetic + nitrous oxide +/− propofol +/− alfentanil.
[g] Prospective series of 25 cases, 1 group with unsecured airways; propofol+ remifentanil + clonidine.
[h] Retrospective review of 241 cases, unsecured airways.
[i] Retrospective review of 99 cases, 3 groups; unsecured airways propofol + fentanyl +/− midazolam +/− droperidol vs airways secured with LMA, propofol + fentanyl vs airways secured with LMA propofol + remifentanil.

increased intraoperative seizures and pain with neurolept anesthesia but higher incidence of transient respiratory depression in patients receiving propofol [4]. Propofol is generally used in combination with the opiates fentanyl or remifentanil. Recently, the highly selective alpha-2-adrenoreceptor agonist dexmedetomidine has gained popularity in awake craniotomies due to its ability to offer analgesia with easy arousal while causing minimal respiratory effects [1].

Despite improved anesthetic and operative techniques, neurologic changes can occur intraoperatively due to any number of known complications associated with awake craniotomies (Table 36.1). Repeated neurologic examinations during the resection allow for early detection of deficit caused by surgical trauma to the region of function or to fibers emanating from it. The surgical team can then make a determination about whether to halt resection or to proceed despite the deficit. A minor deficit is often tolerated, given its propensity to improve postoperatively. At that stage, it is of vital importance for the anesthesiologist to remain cognizant of the sedative properties of the anesthetic technique used, as sedation can often exacerbate the apparent focal neurologic deficit. During resection, some surgeons prefer to supplement monitoring with mapping of the white matter fibers. This stimulation mapping technique is similar to cortical mapping, and allows the surgeon to gain a better understanding of the proximity of important white matter tracts. Patients with preexisting motor deficits can be challenging to map and monitor, since it is more difficult to detect a change in the degree of deficit than it is to detect the presence of a new deficit. In general, the greater the presurgical deficit, the more difficult the monitoring is likely to be.

Other systemic complications of awake craniotomy may interfere with both mapping and monitoring. For example, respiratory complications resulting from airway obstructions can cause intraoperative hypoxemia and hypercapnia. Hypercapnia can result in brain swelling (0–1% of cases), thereby making surgical conditions difficult [5]. Respiratory complications occur in 0–7% of cases and are highest in obese patients and those receiving propofol-based techniques. Intraoperative seizures occur most commonly during cortical stimulation and can be controlled with cold Ringer's lactate irrigation [6]. The incidence is higher in patients receiving neurolept techniques (up to 41%) compared with propofol-based techniques (0–8%) [5]. Severe intraoperative pain makes for a very unpleasant patient experience and can limit neurologic assessment. Some institutions have adopted the use of remifentanil as the opiate of choice because it can be rapidly titrated. Local anesthetics at supratherapeutic doses or delivered directly intravenous can cause both cardiotoxicity and neurotoxicity. Although systemic toxicity is rare (<2%), one should recognize the early signs of this complication and take efforts to limit its occurrence [5]. Poor patient cooperation is seen in 0–20% of cases and is often associated with inadequate anesthetic [5]; this can often be managed after addressing the underlying cause. Finally, the need to convert to a general anesthetic does happen and has been reported in several large series to occur in 0.4–2% of cases [3, 7].

Conclusion

In conclusion, all patients who might benefit from awake neurologic testing during surgery should be considered for an awake craniotomy. Careful patient selection and preoperative consideration of potential contraindications, the use of scalp blocks, improved anesthetic agents, and clear communication among members of the patient's care team will minimize many potential complications and improve patient outcome and satisfaction.

References

1. **A. Y. Bekker, B. Kaufman, H. Samir** et al. The use of dexmedetomidine infusion for awake craniotomy. *Anesth Analg* 2001; **92**: 1251–3.

2. **T. G. Costello, J. R. Cormack**. Anaesthesia for awake craniotomy: a modern approach. *J Clin Neurosci* 2004; **11**: 16–19.

3. **D. P. Archer, J. M. McKenna, L. Morin** et al. Conscious-sedation analgesia during craniotomy for intractable epilepsy: a review of 354 consecutive cases. *Can J Anaesth* 1988; **35**: 338–44.

4. **I. A. Herrick, R. A. Craen, A. W. Gelb** et al. Propofol sedation during awake craniotomy for seizures: patient-controlled administration versus neurolept analgesia. *Anesth Analg* 1997; **84**: 1285–91.

5. **A. P. Skucas, A. A. Artru**. Anesthetic complications of awake craniotomies for epilepsy surgery. *Anesth Analg* 2006; **102**: 882–7.

6. **C. J. Sartorius, M. S. Berger**. Rapid termination of intraoperative stimulation-evoked seizures with application of cold Ringer's lactate to the cortex. Technical note. *J Neurosurg* 1998; **88**: 349–51.

7. **H. J. Blanshard, F. Chung, P. H. Manninen** et al. Awake craniotomy for removal of intracranial tumor: considerations for early discharge. *Anesth Analg* 2001; **92**: 89–94.

8. **F. Piccioni, M. Fanzio**. Management of anesthesia in awake craniotomy. *Minerva Anestesiol* 2008; **74**: 393–408.

Epilepsy surgery and awake craniotomy

Sumeet Vadera and William Bingaman

Awake craniotomies require a great deal of cooperation among all members of the surgical team, especially the surgeon and the anesthesiologist. It is important to be aware of the many obstacles that can be encountered during these procedures and how to successfully avoid complications. Here we describe a standard awake craniotomy case, the pitfalls that were encountered, and their effective management.

Case description

The patient was a 60-year-old right-handed male with a WHO Grade II astrocytoma diagnosed in 1991 and treated with gross total resection at that time. The patient presented with simple partial seizures of the right upper extremity and was noted to have persistent seizures despite an adequate trial of anticonvulsant therapy. Preoperative evaluation included magnetic resonance imaging (MRI) of the brain and video electroencephalography (vEEG). The MRI demonstrated an enhancing lesion in the left posterior frontal lobe suspicious for recurrent tumor (Figure 37.1a) and vEEG was concordant with seizure activity arising from this region. Surgical decision making involved plans to resect the lesion and area of cortex responsible for the seizures. As this involved functional sensorimotor cortex, the plan was for "awake" craniotomy with local anesthetic and intravenous sedation.

After the patient was transferred to the operating room table, he was turned to the lateral decubitus position with the left side positioned up. The patient's head was turned gently and placed on a foam donut (90 degrees perpendicular to the floor). The patient was allowed to become comfortable on the table and then sedated for application of a Mayfield head holder (Codman Inc) and insertion of an arterial line and bladder catheter. The head fixator was applied during intravenous sedation using a mixture of dexmedetomidine and propofol, and only after adequate local anesthesia at the pin sites was achieved. The head holder

was utilized to provide a reference for the stereotactic navigation system and was not fixed to the operating table during the procedure in order to prevent injury to the patient as he awakened. All pressure points were padded and double checked by all members of the operating room team.

The lesion was localized using the frameless stereotactic navigation system and a circumferential field block was performed using local anesthesia injection. Once an adequate level of sedation was achieved, the previous incision was opened by sharp dissection and the bone flap elevated using a high-speed air cranitome. The dura was opened after injecting local anesthetic along the middle meningeal vessels using a 25-gauge tuberculin syringe. The lesion was again localized with the frameless stereotactic system and visual inspection. At this point, intravenous sedation was discontinued, and the patient was awakened for serial neurologic exams and cortical mapping. During this 10–20 minute window, electrocorticography (ECoG) and somatosensory evoked potential identification of the rolandic fissure can be accomplished. As the patient awakens, the surgical team must be careful to anticipate and prevent patient head movement to avoid potential brain injury.

Somatosensory evoked potentials (SSEPs) were initially done using stimulation of the median nerve for central sulcus mapping. This mapping procedure was correlated with the expected position based on patient anatomy and stereotactic navigation. Intraoperative bipolar electrical stimulating electrodes were also used to define functional tissue including the peri-rolandic region and motor speech areas. During stimulation, current is gradually increased at the site tested until a positive motor or language response is seen or a maximum current of 15 milliamperes is reached. If no response is seen, the next site to be stimulated is chosen and the protocol repeated. Monitoring of the electroencephalogram using cortical subdural electrodes is performed during stimulation to detect

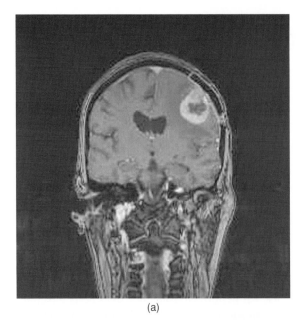

(a)

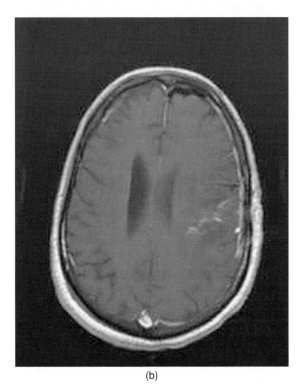

(b)

Figures 37.1a and 37.1b. Pre- and postoperative gadolinium-enhanced magnetic resonance imaging (MRI) of the brain in a patient with left frontal astrocytoma. (a) Preoperative coronal MRI with contrast demonstrating enhancing lesion in left frontal lobe just anterior to motor strip. (b) Postoperative contrast enhanced axial MRI demonstrating resection of lesion.

cortical afterdischarge potentials and seizures. If these occur, stimulation is stopped and ice cold saline irrigation is placed on the brain. Additionally, intravenous antiepileptic medications can be administered.

Finally, ECoG was performed to define the interictal irritative zone (that region of brain irritated by the lesion). In this case, an area just anterior to the precentral gyrus and adjacent to the lesion was noted on ECoG to demonstrate continuous spiking. At this point resection of the lesion and adjacent irritated cortex was begun with real time serial neurologic examination of the patient. This is the real advantage of "awake" craniotomy and maximizes the chances of resecting the entire lesion while avoiding neurologic deficit. Resection of the lesion proceeded with bipolar coagulation, subpial aspiration, and micro instruments. All pial vascular structures were preserved in order to avoid ischemic injury to adjacent functional cortex. During the resection, serial neurologic exams were conducted by a neurologist to ensure that functional cortex was not being injured. Gross total resection of the tumor was adequately achieved (Figure 37.1b) and the lesion was sent for frozen and permanent pathology. At this point, the patient was sedated and the wound was closed in the normal anatomic layers.

Upon awakening, the patient was noted to be at his neurologic baseline with no new deficits noted on exam.

Discussion

This case demonstrates some common adversities faced in epilepsy surgery during "awake" craniotomy. The first obstacle encountered during the procedure was the onset of simple partial seizures during awake cortical stimulation. Studies have shown that administration of ice-cold Ringer's lactate solution directly to the cortical surface is a rapid method to terminate cortical irritation and seizure onset [1]. Barbiturates and antiepileptic medications can also be used in these cases to assist with seizure cessation.

Electrocorticography was important in this case to localize the interictal irritative zone and delineate this region from areas of functional cortex. When continuous repetitive interictal spiking is measured, it is important to remove it to achieve an acceptable seizure-free outcome [2].

Functional mapping of motor cortex is widely considered the "gold-standard" technique to identify eloquent cortical areas. When combined with "awake" craniotomy and frequent neurologic examinations, the risks of new postoperative neurologic deficits are greatly decreased [3]. Even when these safety measures are employed, there is still the risk of temporary or permanent neurologic deficits arising postoperatively. These risks increase as the proximity of the "lesion" to eloquent cortex increases [4]. Although gross total resection was achieved in this case, some tumors that are located within eloquent cortex may be unresectable and a more limited debulking of tumor for tissue diagnosis and reduction of mass effect is performed [5]. Sedation in awake craniotomy usually is best performed using a mixture of dexmedetomidine and propofol. In order to allow the patient to be awake enough for neurologic testing, we usually give the patient minimal narcotics and benzodiazepines. The other benefit of giving minimal amounts of narcotics during the procedure is to avoid the depressant effect on the respiratory system with resultant hypercarbia and dangerous increase of intracranial pressure. The addition of dexmedetomidine to propofol decreases the amount of propofol needed for sedation and allows the maintenance of spontaneous respiration. The other benefit of dexmedetomidine is its inhibitory effect on hypercarbia-induced cerebral vasodilation and consequently intracranial hypertension. Patient education and a thorough discussion of the risks and benefits of such a procedure are important prior to surgical intervention being offered because of the potential complications that can be encountered during this procedure.

References

1. **C. J. Sartorius, M. S. Berger**. Rapid termination of intraoperative stimulation-evoked seizures with application of cold Ringer's lactate to the cortex. Technical note. *J Neurosurg* 1998; **88**: 349–51.

2. **A. Palmini, A. Gambardella, F. Andermann** *et al.* Intrinsic epileptogenicity of human dysplastic cortex as suggested by corticography and surgical results. *Ann Neurol* 1995; **37**: 476–87.

3. **A. R. Walsh, R. H. Schmidt, H. T. Marsh**. Cortical mapping and resection under local anaesthetic as an aid to surgery of low and intermediate grade gliomas. *Br J Neurosurg* 1990; **4**: 485–91.

4. **F. B. Meyer, L. M. Bates, S. J. Goerss** *et al.* Awake craniotomy for aggressive resection of primary gliomas located in eloquent brain. *Mayo Clin Proc* 2001; **76**: 677–87.

5. **R. C. Rostomily, M. S. Berger, G. A. Ojemann** *et al.* Postoperative deficits and functional recovery following removal of tumors involving the dominant hemisphere supplementary motor area. *J Neurosurg* 1991; **75**: 62–8.

38

Acute surgery: spinal and neurogenic shock

Ruairi Moulding and Scott T. McCardle

Spinal cord injury (SCI) is a devastating and life-threatening condition with an incidence of 27–81 cases/million/year in the USA, which equates to 10 000 new patients per year [1, 2]. There are two stages to the development of SCI. The primary injury leads to disruption of the neuronal tissue of the spinal cord via a variety of mechanisms including direct trauma, bony impingement or compression, mechanical stretching or interruption of the blood supply. These initial insults to the integrity of the spinal cord are compounded by the secondary injury. This secondary injury is a culmination of an intense inflammatory response leading to edema, cell death and may result in further nonreversible damage to the spinal cord.

Both spinal shock and neurogenic shock can result from a SCI. They are distinct entities. Spinal shock occurs with the loss of autonomic and reflex activity of the spinal cord caudal to the injury, resulting in the characteristic flaccid paralysis. This flaccidity, lasting up to 4 weeks, may lead eventually to spasticity with the loss of the descending inhibitory controls. Neurogenic shock is the phenomenon whereby patients with SCIs lose the sympathetic control of cardiovascular functions with only unopposed parasympathetic cardiac responses remaining.

Case description

The patient was a 26-year-old male with no significant medical history who presented to the emergency department by ambulance approximately 2 hours after diving 12 feet into a shallow pond in a rock quarry. The patient presented with a loss of sensation and motor control from the neck down. On examination he was in a cervical collar with sand bags for immobilization. He was in severe respiratory distress with a respiratory rate of 36 and his blood oxygen saturation (SaO_2) was 90% while breathing high-flow oxygen via a non-rebreathing mask. He had thready distal pulses with

poor capillary refill, cold peripheries and a central temperature of 36.5 °C. His noninvasive blood pressure on admission was 74/51 with a heart rate of 52 beats per minute. Computed tomography and magnetic resonance imaging showed complete cord transection at the C5–C6 level.

The patient was scheduled for an immediate posterior cervical decompression and stabilization by the neurosurgical service. The principal anesthetic concerns were (1) need for immediate tracheal intubation for respiratory insufficiency, (2) management of the airway in a patient with an unstable cervical injury with a full stomach, (3) prevention of secondary SCI, (4) the potential for labile hemodynamics secondary to the sympathectomy and lack of vasomotor tone below the level of the injury, (5) treatment of any concomitant injuries, and (6) prone positioning with an unstable cervical spine injury.

The patient was evaluated in the emergency room for other associated injuries and high-dose methylprednisolone was started. Prior to induction, atropine was given for vagolysis in preparation for the response to succinylcholine and concern for extreme bradycardia or asystole due to impairment of sympathetic cardioaccelerators. The potential for a difficult intubation was anticipated and a rapid sequence induction was performed using succinylcholine, inline stabilization, and cricoid pressure with video-assisted laryngoscopy. A grade I view was seen at laryngoscopy, an endotracheal tube was inserted, and the position checked.

Arterial and central venous catheters were inserted as well as a urinary catheter with monitoring of bladder and nasal temperatures. Large-bore intravenous (IV) access was obtained and fluid resuscitation instituted. The hemodynamic goal during the anesthetic was to prevent secondary SCI. First-line treatment of hypotension was with IV fluid, both crystalloid and colloid. Norepinephrine was administered to obtain a targeted mean arterial pressure of 85 mmHg.

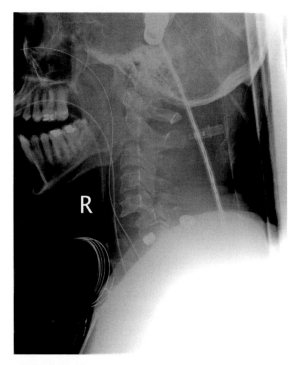

Figure 38.1. Cervical spine X-ray showing a fracture-dislocation of C5–C6 with risk of severe spinal cord compromise.

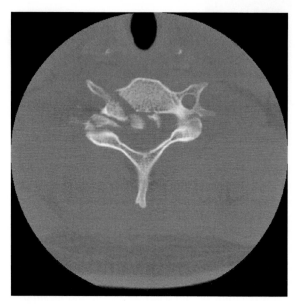

Figure 38.2. Computed tomography scan of C6 vertebral body compression fracture with fragments extending into the canal.

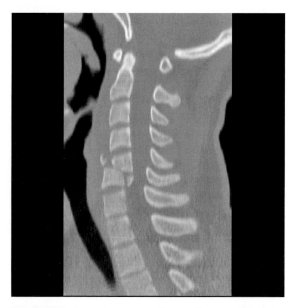

Figure 38.3. Computed tomography scan of compression fractures of C5 and C6 with severe canal stenosis. These findings are consistent with a hyperflexion type injury with retropulsed fracture fragments.

Positioning the patient prone required "log-rolling" in order to maintain spinal integrity and reduce further neurologic damage.

Maintenance of anesthesia included propofol and remifentanil infusions, in order to facilitate spinal cord monitoring with somatosensory and motor evoked potentials. Nitrous oxide was avoided due to the possibility of occult intracranial or thoracic injuries, where expansion of entrapped air could lead to devastating hemodynamic and neurologic complications. The case was completed with minimal blood loss and the patient was taken to the intensive care unit sedated, ventilated, and with a norepinephrine infusion for blood pressure control. Emergence and neurologic examination were not attempted due to hemodynamic instability.

Discussion

Spinal cord injuries occur most often in young adults with a 4:1 male to female preponderance. Nearly 80% of these injuries are related to either motor vehicle accidents or traumatic falls. The cervical spine is the most common level of injury and levels C1–2 and C5–7 are the most vulnerable (Figures 38.1–38.3) [3]. Traditionally, the leading cause of mortality in both the acute and chronic SCI patient has been due to respiratory and renal complications [4]. However, there is growing recognition that cardiovascular complicates may contribute significantly to early and late mortality [1].

Complete SCIs above the T6 level result in neurogenic shock related to sympathectomy and unopposed vagal tone below the level of the injury [4]. There is a direct link between severity of SCI at the cervical or high-thoracic level and severity of cardiovascular symptoms. Neurogenic shock can last for up to 5 weeks post-injury [1]. Incomplete SCIs and those below T6 may or may not develop cardiovascular compromise.

The characteristic components of neurogenic shock are hypotension (systolic blood pressure below 90 mmHg) and bradycardia. Although bradycardia is most common, other rhythm abnormalities may occur due to autonomic instability. Atrioventricular blocks, supraventricular tachycardias, ventricular tachycardias, and even cardiac arrest may all occur in the context of a severe SCI [1]. The bradycardia seen with SCI is due to the unopposed vagal tone and is amenable to treatment with vagolytics such as atropine, or transcutaneous pacing.

Sympathetic tone is an important factor in cardiovascular homeostasis and SCI patients may have reduced or absent control of coronary blood flow, cardiac contractility, and heart rate. Furlan and Fehlings [1] identified five elements of the autonomic circuits as potentially contributing factors: (1) disruption of the descending cardiovascular (or vasomotor) pathways; (2) morphological changes in the cardiac and vasomotor sympathetic preganglionic neurons; (3) sprouting and the potential formation of inappropriate synapses with spinal interneurons; (4) abnormal spinal afferents, and (5) development of altered sympathetic neurovascular transmission and smooth muscle responsiveness. As only the first element (disrupted descending pathways) may be present in the acute setting, this is the most likely contributing factor in the development of neurogenic shock.

A patient with neurogenic shock presents multiple clinical dilemmas for the anesthetic team. The care of patients with such devastating neurologic injuries is most appropriately handled at a Level I Trauma Center [2, 5]. However, the initial treatment and resuscitation is often started at a remote location. In all instances it is recommended to adhere to Advanced Trauma Life Support (ATLS®) guidelines [2]. Spinal cord injuries must be evaluated like all traumas that present to the emergency room, with stabilization of the patient and examination for any accompanying injuries. Patients with cervical spine injuries may have other spinal injuries remote from the primary site.

The timing of decompression and stabilization of spinal cord injuries may vary but surgery within 24 hours can improve neurologic outcomes [1, 5]. Surgery for spinal cord injury patients is not limited to alleviating cord compression or cervical instability but may be for other non-spinal injuries such as fracture repair or tracheotomy. The presence of hypotension in the context of a SCI should not preclude the physician from looking for alternative causes of the hypotension. Associated injuries such as pelvic, long bone, head, and visceral injuries are all potential causes of hypotension in the trauma patient.

High-dose methylprednisolone (30 mg/kg started within 8 hours of injury, and given over a 45-minute period, followed by 5.4 mg/kg/hour over subsequent 23 hours) has been shown in some spinal cord injuries to improve neurologic outcomes (but not necessarily mortality or quality of life) by the National Acute Spinal Cord Injury Study (NASCIS I, II, and III) [3]. However, these studies remain controversial, with higher rates of infection and gastrointestinal bleeding in the steroid treatment group.

Difficult intubation must be anticipated secondary to the need for cervical immobilization, the need for rapid sequence induction, use of cricoid pressure, prevertebral swelling secondary to hematoma, blood or debris in the airway, and distortion of the airway from maxillofacial trauma [3]. Alternative intubating devices including intubating laryngeal mask airways, video-assisted laryngoscopy, fiberoptic scope, and cricothyroidotomy equipment should be immediately available in the event that direct laryngoscopy proves unsuccessful.

It is important to maintain thermal homeostasis because hypothermia may worsen secondary injury. Care should be taken with warming SCI patients. Sympathectomy-induced vasodilatation may lead to hypothermia, however, lack of sweating below the level of injury may lead to iatrogenic hyperthermia from warming devices.

Intra-arterial blood pressure management is highly recommended to ensure adequate perfusion pressure for the spinal cord with a recommended mean arterial pressure of 85 mmHg [4]. It is important to note that secondary injury from hypoperfusion and hypoxia may extend the spinal cord damage cranially. Therefore, early recognition and aggressive treatment of neurogenic shock is recommended. Although intravenous fluids should be used initially, vasopressors may be needed to maintain adequate spinal cord perfusion pressure. Indeed SCI patients may be at greater risk of pulmonary edema through over-resuscitation and care should always be taken to use appropriate volumes of intravenous fluid. Central venous access may be required for resuscitation, evaluation of filling status and for infusions of vasopressors.

Conclusion

In conclusion, spinal cord injury is a devastating, life-threatening condition that produces a number of physiologic and anatomical derangements that must be acutely managed by the anesthetic team. The anesthetic goals should focus on establishing an airway (surgical, if necessary), and close hemodynamic and respiratory monitoring to maximize spinal cord perfusion to prevent secondary SCI. Furthermore, maintenance of an anesthetic that is amenable to a balance of appropriate surgical, neurophysiologic monitoring, and anesthetic considerations is paramount. The postoperative care of these patients might be extensive requiring multiple further anesthetics. Anesthesiologists must be familiar with the unique long-term complications of SCI such as spasticity, autonomic hyperreflexia, and chronic ventilator support that may alter anesthetic management.

References

1. **J. C. Furlan, M. G. Fehlings**. Cardiovascular complications after acute spinal cord injury: pathophysiology, diagnosis, and management. *Neurosurg Focus* 2008; **25**: E13.

2. **I. Miko, R. Gould, S. Wolf** *et al.* Acute spinal cord injury. *Int Anesthesiol Clin* 2009; **47**: 37–54.

3. **P. Veale, J. Lamb**. Anaesthesia and acute spinal cord injury. *CEACCP* 2002; **2**: 139–43.

4. **M. Denton, J. McKinlay**. Cervical cord injury and critical care. *CEACCP* 2009; **9**: 82–6.

5. **L. A. Wuermser, C. H. Ho, A. E. Chiodo** *et al.* Spinal cord injury medicine. 2. Acute care management of traumatic and nontraumatic injury. *Arch Phys Med Rehabil* 2007; **88**: S55–61.

Returning patient with autonomic hyperreflexia

Sherif S. Zaky

Patients with spinal cord injuries often return for subsequent surgeries. Loss of descending spinal cord inhibition and neuronal alterations of the cord itself may be associated with exaggerated sympathetic responses to what normally would be innocuous stimuli.

Case description

This patient was a 44-year-old male who sustained a motor vehicle accident 6 years previously that resulted in paraplegia secondary to T6 spinal cord injury. The patient also had a history of hepatitis C virus, thrombocytopenia, vascular insufficiency, and asthma. The patient developed gangrene of his left big toe extending to the medial side of his foot.

The patient presented to the operating room for debridement of his left foot with possible mid-tarsal amputation. He did not have sensation below T6, but he responded to painful stimulation below that level with jerky movements that would prevent proceeding with the surgery. The surgeon was concerned about the jerky movements and the possibility of autonomic hyperreflexia if the procedure was done under conscious sedation or local anesthesia, as was initially planned.

Although this could have been done under general anesthesia, the patient and anesthesia team preferred to do it under regional given the patient comorbidities such as reactive airway disease. However, neuraxial blockade was avoided in this patient due to the thrombocytopenia. Regional peripheral nerve block was therefore deemed more appropriate, so the sciatic nerve was blocked under ultrasound guidance in the popliteal fossa. Next, the saphenous nerve was blocked in the Sartorius canal, also with ultrasound guidance. The surgery was performed under the block and light sedation using midazolam without any complications or significant hemodynamic perturbations. The patient was discharged home the same day.

Discussion

Spinal cord injuries can be caused by either traumatic (e.g., motor vehicle accident, falls, water or skiing accidents) or nontraumatic causes (e.g., vascular events or neoplasms). Most of these patients survive to return for elective surgeries, most commonly urological and orthopedic procedures. After the initial injury, these patients go through different phases [1].

Initial consequences

The first response to spinal cord injury can be a brief but severe increase in sympathetic discharge leading to transient increase in afterload (on the order of minutes) that sometimes causes left ventricular failure, subendocardial infarction, and/or pulmonary edema. Following the acute response, neurogenic shock can occur in several days to 6–8 weeks after the initial injury and is characterized by hypotension, bradycardia, and unopposed vagal reflexes. The predominant parasympathetic tone can lead to severe bradycardia – even asystole – especially with tracheal intubation and suctioning [2].

The loss of sympathetic discharge leads to decreased preload and hypotension. Myocardial dysfunction may also play a role in the hypotension.

Delayed consequences

After the initial phase of spinal shock, changes in the neuronal connections occur in the spinal cord below the level of injury. Presynaptic boutons multiply and form chaotic, inappropriate reflexes. Interneurons excited by the afferent inputs synapse with preganglionic sympathetic neurons in the intermediolateral gray column. This will result in a widespread inappropriate sympathetic response, which lacks the usual descending inhibition from higher centers, leading to profound vasoconstriction [3–6]. Autonomic hyperreflexia is characterized by hypertension, headaches, pallor, or flushing above the level of injury and profuse sweating with sensory stimulation to areas below the level of the injury. Other symptoms include nausea, penile erection, pupillary changes, and Horner's syndrome. The reported incidence is variable due to lack of consensus on the definition of autonomic hyperreflexia, but it is thought to occur about 60–85% of the time after spinal cord injury at or above the T6 level [3, 7].

Anesthetic goals for patients with autonomic hyperreflexia

The main goal of anesthesia is to blunt or prevent this reflex. This can be achieved with either general or regional anesthesia. General anesthesia can be employed while maintaining adequate depth using potent volatile anesthetic, narcotics, and systemic sympatholytics to decrease the afferent sensory discharge. This usually requires a deeper level of anesthesia and frequently this can cause further hypotension and hemodynamic instability. The exact level or endpoint for anesthetic titration is not clear. Succinylcholine should be avoided from 2 days up to 1 year after the original injury due to increased risk of hyperkalemia secondary to denervation hypersensitivity.

Regional anesthesia, on the other hand, is preferred by many anesthesiologists as it more reliably blocks the afferent sensory signal before it reaches higher centers. This can be achieved with neuraxial (spinal or epidural anesthesia) or peripheral nerve blocks. In general, spinal anesthesia is more reliable than epidural anesthesia in preventing autonomic hyperreflexia. However, it might be impossible to determine the level of the block and the dose–response characteristics might not be the same in spinal cord injury patients [8, 9]. Peripheral nerve blocks using nerve stimulation might not give the sensory or the motor response that would be expected in normal patients, which can make it technically difficult. Epinephrine containing local anesthetic solutions should be avoided due to higher sensitivity of spinal cord injury patients to catecholamines.

Anesthetic management of the patient with a history of spinal cord injury

Before induction of anesthesia, obtaining large-bore intravenous access is recommended, followed by fluid preloading as these patients have reduced blood volume. Typically, 500–1000 mL of crystalloid is given to reduce the risk of hypotension associated with induction of general or neuraxial anesthesia [10]. Extra caution should be taken during positioning as pressure sores are more likely due to poor positioning. Anticholinergic drugs are commonly used, especially during the phase of neurogenic shock to avoid the risk of asystole due to unopposed parasympathetic tone. It is important to note that the risk of hypothermia is significantly higher due to impaired thermoregulation below the level of injury. The use of warming devices, especially surface warming, is essential.

Although gastric emptying is delayed in spinal cord injury patients, no significant increased risk of aspiration has been established; routine rapid sequence induction for the spinal cord injury patient is controversial.

If autonomic hyperreflexia occurs, it is typically brief and self-limiting. Initial management includes cessation of the stimulus and an increase in anesthetic depth. Labetalol, nifedipine, and nitroglycerin are the most commonly used drugs when pharmacologic management is required. Other medications that can be used include propranolol, esmolol, and midazolam [10]. Magnesium sulfate has also been successfully used for management of autonomic hyperreflexia in the chronic spinal cord injury patient [11].

Conclusion

The number of patients with autonomic hyperreflexia returning for various surgeries is increasing due to improved medical management of urinary tract and respiratory tract complications in patients with spinal cord injury [1]. Perioperative management of these patients requires knowledge of the risks associated with this phenomenon as well as the pathophysiology. Whether general or regional anesthesia is used, there will be specific challenges facing the anesthesiologist. Adequate preparation is usually the key for successful management.

References

1. **P. R. Hambly, B. Martin**. Anesthesia for chronic spinal cord lesions. *Anesthesia* 1998; **53**: 273–89.
2. **H. L. Frankel, C. J. Mathias, J. M. L. Spalding**. Mechanisms of reflex cardiac arrest in quadriplegic patients. *Lancet* 1975; **2**: 1183–5.

3. **N. B. Kurnick**. Autonomic hyperreflexia and its control in patients with spinal cord lesions. *Ann Internal Med* 1956; **44**: 678–86.

4. **A. Fraser, J. Edmonds-Seal**. Spinal cord injuries: a review of problems facing the anesthetist. *Anesthesia* 1982; **37**: 1084–98.

5. **A. V. Krassioukov, L. C. Weaver**. Reflex and morphological changes in spinal preganglionic neurons after cord injury in rats. *Clin Exp Hypertens* 1995; **17**: 361–73.

6. **A. V. Krassioukov, L. C. Weaver**. Episodic hypertension due to autonomic dysreflexia in acute and chronic spinal cord injured rats. *Am J Physiol* 1995; **268**: 2077–83.

7. **R. Lindan, E. Joiner, A. A. Freehafer** *et al*. Incidence and clinical features of autonomic dysreflexia in patients with spinal cord injury. *Paraplegia* 1980; **18**: 285–92.

8. **J. A. Stirt, A. Marco, K. A. Conklin**. Obstetric anesthesia for a quadriplegic patient with autonomic hyperreflexia. *Anesthesiology* 1979; **51**: 560–2.

9. **P. G. Loubser, W. H. Donovan**. Diagnostic spinal anesthesia in chronic spinal cord injury pain. *Paraplegia* 1991; **29**: 25–36.

10. **J. Goy**. Spinal injuries. In **Loach A**, ed. *Orthopaedic Anaesthesia*. London: Edward Arnold, 1994; 145–57.

11. **N. A. Jones, S. D. Jones**. Management of life threatening autonomic hyperreflexia using magnesium sulfate in a patient with a high spinal cord injury in the intensive care unit. *Br J Anesthesia* 2002; **88**: 434–8.

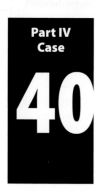

Spine surgery. Complex spine surgery

Preoperative evaluation

Julie McClelland and Ellen Janke

Indications for spinal surgery include congenital defects, tumors, infection, hematomas, trauma, arteriovenous malformations, herniated discs, and degenerative disease [1]. Operative treatment ranges from minimally invasive microsurgery to open procedures involving the entire spine. The preoperative evaluation provides the opportunity for assessment of patient, surgical, and anesthetic risks in order to formulate an appropriate anesthetic plan.

Case description

The patient was an otherwise healthy 27-year-old female, who presented with new onset of bilateral upper extremity weakness and sensory changes in the setting of 6 months of neck and upper back pain. Magnetic resonance imaging demonstrated a destructive paraspinal lesion involving the posterior elements of C7, T1, and T2 with pathologic fractures involving the right C7 lamina and T1–T2 spinous processes. Pathology from computed tomography-guided biopsy revealed hemangioma. The patient was admitted for C6–T2 laminectomy and C5–T4 posterior spinal fusion with endovascular embolization of the lesion preceding the case. Electrophysiologic monitoring with somatosensory (SSEP) and motor evoked potentials (MEP) was planned.

Review of the patient's drug history revealed chronic use of combined acetaminophen 500 mg and hydrocodone 5 mg, 6–8 tablets per day for pain control. Physical examination was notable for bilateral 4/5 strength of wrist flexion, extension and grip, with decreased sensation of both arms in the ulnar and radial nerve distributions. Cervical spine range of motion was limited due to pain; airway examination was otherwise normal. Laboratory tests included complete blood count, prothrombin and partial thromboplastin time, and type and crossmatch for four units of packed red blood cells. Two large-bore peripheral intravenous cannulae were inserted. A radial arterial line was established for continuous blood pressure monitoring and blood sampling.

Important anesthetic considerations in this case included (1) the airway (possible difficult intubation), (2) a prolonged procedure in the prone position, (3) an anesthetic technique allowing for optimal electrophysiologic monitoring and prompt emergence, (4) fluid management with regards to potential for large blood loss (despite embolization of mass), (5) adequate postoperative pain control, and (6) the potential for postoperative visual loss.

Anesthetic induction with fentanyl and propofol was followed by neuromuscular blockade with succinylcholine. The trachea was intubated with a 7.0 mm LITA (Laryngotracheal Instillation of Topical Anesthesia) endotracheal tube, using the Bullard laryngoscope. Anesthesia was maintained with isoflurane <0.5 minimal alveolar concentration (MAC), as well as propofol and sufentanil infusions. After turning the patient prone, SSEPs and MEPs were unchanged from baseline. Operative time was 9.5 hours with 2 liters of blood loss. Fluid replacement consisted of 3 liters of lactated Ringer's and 2 liters of albumin 5%. The patient's blood pressure was maintained within 30% of her baseline values, using volume resuscitation and vasopressor support. The case was completed uneventfully. Emergence was prompt and smooth; neurologic examination demonstrated a small but clear improvement of bilateral grip strength, exam was otherwise unchanged from that preoperatively.

Discussion

Co-morbidities associated with spinal disease range from acute traumatic spinal column instability or spinal shock to decreased cardiopulmonary function from chronic thoracic cage deformity [2]. Disease states and their anesthetic implications for spine surgery are summarized in Table 40.1.

Table 40.1. Anesthetic considerations for common diseases related to the spine.

Disease	Anesthetic consideration
Anklyosing spondylitis	Restricted movement of the sacroiliac joints and spine Vascular inflammation that may lead to aortitis and aortic insufficiency Pulmonary fibrosis Poor chest wall compliance
Carotid or vertebrobasilar insufficiency	Avoid extremes of cervical spine ROM when positioning Maintain SBP within 20% of baseline Maintain MAPs within patient-specific norms of autoregulation
Cervical spine ROM restriction (including instability)	Fiberoptic intubation, awake or asleep Other intubation adjuncts: Bullard larygoscope, intubating LMA, lightwand, Glidescope, C-MAC, etc.
Muscle weakness (including dystrophies, bedridden or wheelchair-bound)	Exaggerated hyperkalemic response to succinlycholine May be resistant to nondepolarizing NMBD May have compromised respiratory function; medical treatment should be optimized
Oncologic disease	Often not isolated to spine, may affect bone marrow, brain, heart, kidney, liver, or lungs Chemotherapeutic and radiation changes to organ systems
Rheumatoid arthritis	Increased difficulty for intubation (including cervical ROM, mouth opening and jaw protrusion) Atlantoaxial instability Chronic steroid use, may need stress dose Polypharmacy with rare drugs
Scoliosis	Restrictive lung disease → pulmonary HTN → RHF → cor pulmonale 10–25% patients have associated neuromuscular diseases and congenital anomalies including congenital heart disease Vital capacity reliable prognostic indicator of perioperative reserve Vital capacity <40% of predicted, patient likely to need prolonged ventilator support

Trauma	Acute phase:
	    sequelae of other injuries
	    spinal or neurogenic shock
	    assume cervical spine instability
	Post-acute phase T6 injuries and above:
	    autonomic hyperreflexia
	    poikilothermia (inability to regulate temperature)

HTN, hypertension; NMBD, neuromuscular blocker drug; LMA, laryngeal mask airway; MAP, mean arterial pressure; RHF, right heart failure; ROM, range of motion; SBP, systolic blood pressure.

General principles – preoperative history and physical examination

A comprehensive history and physical examination is a crucial component of preparation for complex spine surgery. Particular attention should be paid to the patient's baseline neurologic status and airway examination as well as to the disease process leading to the need for operative intervention. An accurate drug history is essential.

Cardiopulmonary function may be compromised in patients due to a primary disease process; secondary to restrictive chest wall disease from scoliosis, ankylosing spondylitis, or rheumatoid arthritis; or from conditions resulting in muscle weakness. Complex spine surgery may be considered intermediate risk

for cardiac events. Preoperative electrocardiogram and chest radiograph should be obtained if indicated by the patient's age and co-morbidities; however, if normal they do not exclude significant cardiopulmonary pathology. If cardiovascular disease is suspected or is otherwise difficult to evaluate due to exercise limitations, a chemically induced stress test may be considered. Pulmonary function testing may be useful to distinguish cardiac from pulmonary disease in the presence of symptoms such as dyspnea, especially if a thoracotomy is required (see below). An arterial blood gas obtained prior to anesthesia may be helpful. Prolonged ventilation postoperatively can be anticipated in some cases and should be discussed preoperatively with the patient.

The presence of renal and hepatic disease may influence drug dosing and other aspects of anesthetic management; if indicated by history and physical examination, evaluation of serum electrolytes, renal function, and hepatic function may help establish severity. The presence of diabetes has implications for multiple organ systems and the need for invasive monitoring.

In cases where considerable blood loss is possible, a hematocrit, platelet count, coagulation studies and type and screen are reasonable. Type and screen or type and cross may be indicated (see below, section on blood loss).

In all cases, medical treatment should be optimized preoperatively.

Airway/cervical spine instability

The airway examination may be notable for limited cervical spine range of motion as well as instability increasing the risk of spinal cord injury. In the case described above, neurosurgical evaluation deemed the cervical spine to be stable. However, the Bullard laryngoscope was used for intubation because it facilitates visualization without the need for excessive motion of an unstable spine. Other adjuncts for intubation in patients with a difficult airway from spine disease are listed in Table 40.1.

Positioning

The operative approach for complex spine surgery may be anterior, posterior, or lateral, alone or in combination. The anterior approach may be through the neck or the abdomen. For the latter, a general surgeon may be involved and a bowel prep required.

The prone position is associated with numerous complications, including decreased venous return, cervical spine injury, endotracheal tube malposition or obstruction, direct pressure injuries, visceral ischemia, macroglossia and oropharyngeal swelling, peripheral nerve injury, postoperative visual loss, and ischemic injury from arterial occlusion [3]. Use of the Mayfield head frame allows free access to the head and face; its application is highly stimulating and needs to be anticipated. Skeletal deformity may lead to difficulties in achieving optimal prone positioning. Postoperative visual loss is a rare complication and is discussed elsewhere in this volume. Strategies for avoiding complications as a result of prone positioning can be found in Table 40.2.

Table 40.2. Strategies for avoiding complications in the prone position.

Complication	Strategy
ETT obstruction/malposition	Reinforced tube
Direct pressure injury	Mayfield head frame Ensure eyes, chin, and nose are free from contact with any surface; check vigilantly Pad all pressure points Place breasts neutrally or medially Keep male genitalia free of compression from bolsters or thighs
Increased thoracic/abdominal pressure	Allow for chest excursion and free abdominal movement by using chest and thigh rolls and/or special mattress for OR table
Peripheral nerve injury	Avoid positions known to cause pain or paresthesias when patient is awake Pad axillary and ulnar neurovascular bundles Arms at sides when turning supine to prone Consider use of SSEP and MEP to monitor for brachial plexus ischemia Shoulder abduction <90 degrees and elbows placed in flexion
Swelling/dependent edema of the tongue and oropharynx	Judicious use of crystalloids for fluid replacement Check for ETT cuff leak prior to extubation
Vascular occlusion	Avoid extremes of cervical range of motion Watch for signs of jugular venous outflow obstruction

ETT, endotracheal tube; LITA tube, laryngotracheal instillation of topical anesthesia; MEP, motor evoked potential; OR, operating room; SSEP, somatosensory evoked potential.

The lateral position may be used for resection of tumors located anterior to the spinal cord. A thoracotomy may be required, with use of a double-lumen endotracheal tube to facilitate surgical exposure. The ability of the patient to tolerate one-lung ventilation should be ascertained preoperatively. Skeletal deformities may be important factors in positioning when the lateral approach is used.

Anesthetic technique

Anesthetic agents used for complex spine surgery must be compatible with neurophysiologic monitoring of central nervous system function (SSEP, MEP, electromyography) and permit rapid emergence for timely postoperative neurologic assessment. Motor evoked potential monitoring may preclude neuromuscular blockade; the presence of an endotracheal tube in unparalyzed patients can be hazardous. Blunting airway reflexes with local anesthetics topically or with appropriate nerve blocks, careful titration of opiates, and ensuring an adequate depth of anesthesia are essential.

In addition to standard monitors, spine surgeries often warrant continuous direct blood pressure monitoring with an arterial catheter. Maintenance of mean arterial pressures within the patient's presumed autoregulatory range potentially helps avoid spinal cord ischemia from hypotension and optimizes hemodynamic conditions for electrophysiologic monitoring. Direct arterial monitoring also allows for assessment of systolic pressure variation to help guide resuscitation efforts, and permits serial blood sampling for determination of hematocrit, plasma glucose, and arterial blood gas analysis. Preoperatively, parameters for intraoperative hemodynamic variables should be established and a blood transfusion trigger determined.

Fluid management/blood loss

The potential for blood loss during major spine surgery is significant, especially for multi-level and/or repeat procedures. In these cases, red blood cells should be cross-matched and made available for use in the operating room. Central venous catheterization may be indicated if massive transfusion is anticipated or if adequate peripheral access cannot be obtained. In cases not involving malignancy or infection a "cell saver" device may be used to scavenge and reinfuse the patient's blood intraoperatively, in an effort to reduce the volume of banked blood transfused. Induced hypotension and hemodilution are strategies that may be incorporated into the anesthetic technique to minimize blood loss, but the patients must be appropriately selected. For example, an elderly patient with degenerative disease and chronic hypertension may require higher systemic arterial pressures to ensure adequate spinal cord perfusion and thus is not likely to be a good candidate for deliberate hypotension. Other conditions precluding induced hypotension include myelopathy (in which spinal cord ischemia is ongoing) major cardiovascular disease and renal insufficiency (when hypoperfusion may worsen function). Antifib-

rinolytic agents such as tranexemic acid and alpha-aminocaproic acid may also be used to reduce blood loss intraoperatively. Finally, as in this case, preoperative embolization of a tumor or other vascular lesion may be used to minimize the likelihood of excessive surgical blood loss.

Prone positioning can result in edema of the airway and other dependent tissues. Minimizing intravenous infusion of crystalloid solution and use of colloid and blood may offset this problem because of the latter's relatively longer intravascular lifespan. Concerns about adverse effects on coagulation of hydroxyethyl starch solution (Hetastarch) limit its utility as a volume expander in the setting of complex spine surgery.

Perioperative pain control

Many patients with spine disease experience associated chronic pain. Polypharmacy and complex regimens are common, emphasizing the importance of a thorough drug history during preoperative evaluation. Nonsteroidal anti-inflammatory drugs may have been discontinued preoperatively for surgical reasons, contributing to acutely increased analgesic requirements. A good understanding of multimodal analgesia along with an appreciation for opiate tolerance helps to ensure appropriate perioperative pain management. Alpha-2-adrenergic receptor agonists (clonidine, dexmedetomidine) may be helpful intraoperatively and postoperatively. Consultation of a pain specialist can be invaluable in complex patients. It is imperative to discuss with patients reasonable expectations of pain control after surgery and to explore options such as epidural catheters placed under direct visualization by the surgeon for postoperative patient analgesia, and patient-controlled analgesic pumps [4].

Conclusion

Complex spine surgery presents unique challenges for the anesthesiologist with regard to airway management, positioning, monitoring, fluid management, and pain control. In an effort to achieve a successful outcome, preoperative evaluation should be thorough and consists of careful assessment of the risks associated with patient pathophysiology, anesthetic requirements, and the surgery itself.

References

1. **E. Ornstein, R. Berko**. Anesthesia techniques in complex spine surgery. *Neurosurg Clin N Am* 2006; **17**: 191–203.

2. **D. A. Raw, J. K. Beattie, J. M. Hunter**. Anaesthesia for spinal surgery in adults. *Br J Anaesth* 2003; **91**: 886–904.

3. **P. H. Petrozza**. Major spine surgery. *Anesthesiol Clin North America* 2002; **20**: 405–15, vii.

4. **J. P. Cata, E. M. Noguera, E. Parke** *et al.* Patient-controlled epidural analgesia (PCEA) for postoperative pain control after lumbar spine surgery. *J Neurosurg Anesthesiol* 2008; **20**: 256–60.

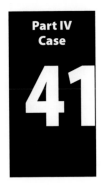
Spine surgery. Complex spine surgery

Loss of evoked potentials

Thomas Didier and Ellen Janke

Perioperative neurophysiologic monitoring is a useful tool for measuring the functional integrity of the central nervous system (CNS) during procedures that put this system at risk. Understanding the types of monitoring that are used – and how to address perioperative changes – is essential for delivering an effective and safe anesthetic that allows diagnosis of ischemia/hypoxia before irreversible damage occurs such that surgical and anesthetic management can be optimized.

Case description

The patient was a 56-year-old male, American Society of Anesthesiologists Class III, scheduled to undergo T9–T12 laminectomy and microsurgical correction of a T10–T12 dural ateriovenous fistula. He presented with 6 months of progressively decreased strength and sensation of his lower extremities. He underwent spinal angiography during which a complex multilevel arteriovenous fistula was visualized that was not amenable to embolization. The patient was therefore scheduled for operative repair. His past medical history was significant for chronic poorly controlled hypertension and traumatic brain injury with resultant expressive and receptive aphasia. Due to the risk of ischemic damage to the spinal cord and nerve roots, neurophysiologic monitoring with a general anesthetic was planned. Central nervous system function was monitored using somatosensory evoked potentials (SSEP), electromyography (EMG) and transcranial motor evoked potentials (MEP). Following uneventful induction, anesthesia was maintained with <0.5 minimum alveolar concentration of sevoflurane, a propofol infusion (70 mcg/kg/min) and a remifentanil infusion (0.2 mcg/kg/min). An hour and a half after surgical incision but before dural opening there were bilateral decreases in SSEPs of the lower extremities. This was followed by decreased MEP signals from the left foot 15 minutes later. Shortly after the opening of the dura, MEP signals were also lost at the right foot. Vasopressors were administered and the volatile anesthetic was discontinued, with compensatory increases in the propofol infusion rate. The temperature was confirmed as within normal limits. There was no appreciated surgical cause for the loss of signals. The signals did not return to baseline amplitude for the remainder of the operation. The patient's postoperative course was significant for profound weakness in the lower extremities on postoperative day 1. On postoperative day 2 magnetic resonance imaging showed abnormal cord signal from T6–T10. The patient's physical exam improved from postoperative days 3–6 and he was discharged with an examination unchanged from admission.

Discussion

The neurophysiologic monitors used in this case were monitors of CNS function, and can be described as follows:

Sensory evoked potentials

Sensory evoked potentials (SEPs) are measured electrophysiologic responses to somatosensory, visual, or auditory stimulation. They are obtained by stimulating a sensory system and recording the resulting response along a neural pathway. In this way the perioperative team can monitor the integrity of the sensory pathway continuously throughout operations that place the pathway at risk. The most commonly utilized SEP is somatosensory. Somatosensory evoked potentials (SSEPs) represent reproducible electrical activity of cortical and subcortical structures in response to a peripheral nerve stimulus. This provides monitoring along the dorsal column–medial lemniscus pathway, which transmits vibration, proprioception, and light touch. Stimulation is initiated at a peripheral nerve site, commonly the median, ulnar, posterior

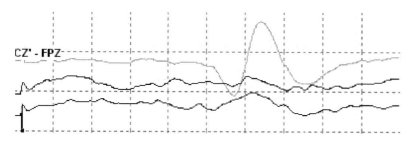

CZ' - FPZ

Figure 41.1. Somatosensory evoked potential (SSEP) signals. Example of the loss of SSEP signals of a posterior tibial nerve signal. The gray tracing is the initial signal and the black lines represent the signals with decreased amplitude and prolonged latency.

tibial, or peroneal nerve. Nerve impulses from these sites transmit signal to the dorsal horn ganglia at their respective root levels. The signal then propagates along the dorsal column to the medulla, where fibers synapse and decussate. The signal ascends along the medial lemniscus to the thalamus, the primary somatosensory cortex, and finally association cortices. The integrity of the signal can be monitored anywhere along the transmitted pathway. Signals monitored subcortically are more resistant to anesthetic influence [1]. Somatosensory evoked potentials are most commonly utilized for surgery involving the spinal cord and spinal column, especially in decompressive laminectomies and scoliosis repair. Somatosensory evoked potentials have also been utilized in carotid vascular surgery, aortic aneurysm repair, intracranial aneurysm repair, and intracranial mass lesion removal. The waveform of SEPs is described by latency, or time from stimulation to onset of peak of a response, and amplitude, the voltage of the response. A clinically significant change in SEPs is considered a 50% decrease in amplitude or a 10% increase in latency (Figure 41.1) [2].

There are a few important anesthetic considerations to understand in order to provide an adequate anesthetic that optimizes SSEP signals. Optimized baseline signals should be obtained under anesthesia but before surgical intervention occurs in order to best monitor for nerve damage during surgery. If signals are inadequate the anesthetic plan should be tailored to improve them before structures are vulnerable to surgical injury. Notably, if the patient has existing impaired spinal cord function, the baseline signals may be suboptimal. Both inhaled and intravenous anesthetics can impact the quality of SSEP signals obtained but intravenous agents have less effect than equipotent doses of inhaled agents. All inhaled agents increase latency and decrease amplitude of the signal with the exception of nitrous oxide, the effect of which is variable depending on the other anes-

thetics used. Somatosensory evoked potential signals are strongest when the total minimum alveolar concentration of the inhaled anesthetic is <1. Thiopental and propofol cause dose-dependent increases in latency and decreased amplitude that do not preclude intraoperative monitoring. In contrast, etomidate and ketamine both increase amplitude. Opioids cause an increase in latency and decrease in amplitude but these effects are not clinically significant. Alpha-2-adrenoreceptor agonists like dexmedetomidine have minimal effects on SSEPs. When using a balanced anesthetic technique the effects of multiple drugs are usually additive. Paralysis may be helpful in minimizing artifact and should be instituted if consistent with the other monitoring and surgical goals. In addition to the anesthetics utilized, hypothermia increases latency and has unpredictable effects on amplitude that do not preclude monitoring. Hypotension that extends below the autoregulatory threshold decreases amplitude but has little effect on latency [1].

Motor evoked potentials

Despite the usefulness of SSEPs, one of the shortfalls of this monitoring modality is the inability to monitor the tracts of the anterior spinal circulation. Motor evoked potentials allow surveillance of the corticospinal tract and therefore motor function. The primary motor cortex is stimulated either magnetically or electrically. The signal is then conducted to the brainstem where it decussates at the level of the pyramids in the medulla. The signal then travels down the corticospinal tract and exits the spinal cord through the ventral nerve root. After traveling through the peripheral nerves the signal is transmitted to the muscles causing contraction. There are various ways to measure responses to motor stimulation but the most common is the "all-or-none" criterion (Figure 41.2). In this method a clinically significant event is described as total loss of the

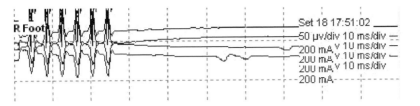

Figure 41.2. Motor evoked potential (MEP) signals. Example of decreased MEP signals. These were stimulated transcranially and monitored at the foot. The top tracings are the initial MEPs. The bottom portion is the MEP signal after an acute change. Note the loss of the inflection/deflection points in the middle of the tracing.

MEP signal. Since this method may not detect subtle deficits, other methods are being developed, though none has become standardized.

Prior to the use of MEPs, the only way to check motor function during surgery was to wake up the patient and ask him or her to move extremities. This is known as the "wake up test" and is still the gold standard for checking intraoperative motor function. Motor evoked potentials are usually induced transcranially in the intraoperative setting. Electrodes are placed on the scalp, directly over the motor cortex or directly on the spinal cord and then stimulated, inducing muscular contraction that corresponds to the area stimulated. Corresponding waveforms are then observed in the spinal cord, nerves, or muscles stimulated. Motor evoked potentials can also be stimulated magnetically, though this is impractical for intraoperative use. Motor stimulation requires much higher levels of stimulation than SSEPs and is monitored intermittently, unlike SSEPs, which can be monitored continuously. Additionally, MEPs are more technically challenging to obtain compared with SSEPs. Motor evoked potentials are commonly used in spinal cord/column surgery [2].

Motor evoked potentials are extremely sensitive to inhaled anesthetics. All inhaled agents induce dramatic decreases in MEP signal. Total intravenous anesthesia provides conditions that optimize MEP signals. Ketamine, opiates, propofol, and etomidate seem to have the least effect on MEPs. Dexmedetomidine, an alpha-2-adrenoreceptor agonist, causes no significant signal change in clinically used doses. Paralytic agents may be used but a twitch height of T1 in a train-of-four should be maintained at 30% of the control height [3]. Since this is clinically difficult if muscles are being monitored, paralytics are often avoided. As with SSEPs, it is vitally important to maintain a steady anesthetic level during the course of the operation. Contraindications to using MEPs include patients with deep brain stimulators and cochlear implants. Also, it is important that bilateral molar

bite blocks be placed to avoid tongue lacerations or hematomas.

Electromyography

Electromyography consists of monitoring muscle activity in response to either spontaneous or active nerve stimulation. Electrodes are placed either on the skin or directly in the muscle. Nerve propagation and therefore muscle activity is compromised with nerve stretching, compression, or pulling. This is manifested by continuous, repetitive EMG firing, called trains. Additionally, irregularity in the EMG can correlate with surgical proximity to the nerve and may manifest as spikes or bursts. With active nerve stimulation a peripheral nerve is stimulated and the muscular response is monitored. This is especially useful for surgical dissection to distinguish nerves from surrounding tissue. Surgeries in which EMG is commonly employed include posterior fossa craniotomies, spinal cord/column surgery and peripheral nerve surgery. Anesthetic considerations during EMG are primarily related to paralysis. Optimal conditions for EMG are created when no paralytics are used. If paralytics must be administered, three or four twitches should be present at all times. Additionally, conditions that affect the neuromuscular junction may limit the usefulness of EMG. These disorders include myasthenia gravis, botulinum toxin effects and muscular dystrophy.

Intraoperative changes

Careful monitoring and quick response to changes in neurophysiologic signals during spine surgery can prevent long-term morbidity. Loss of signals for even short periods represents an increased risk of postoperative deficits. Therefore, prompt attention should be given to any change detected. Thorough communication among the anesthesiologist, surgeon, and neurophysiologist is essential throughout the operation. Intraoperative changes that can cause a change in neuromonitoring signals include a change in the

Table 41.1. Response to the loss of evoked potentials.

Prompt communication with surgeon and neurophysiologist
Confirm that anesthetic is not a factor 　Decrease depth of anesthesia if necessary
Optimize oxygen delivery 　Increase mean arterial pressure 　Confirm adequate hemoglobin 　Administer 100% FiO$_2$
Rule out hypothermia
Consider small bolus of ketamine or etomidate to increase signal amplitude
Gold standard – wake up test

anesthetic level, temperature change (hypothermia), decreased oxygen delivery from systemic hypotension or regional hypoperfusion, electrical noise in the operating room, surgical ligation or ischemia. When there is an acute change in neuromonitoring signals the anesthesiologist should ensure that anesthetic factors are not the inciting cause (Table 41.1). First, ensure that the anesthetic level has been consistent. Then optimize oxygen delivery by increasing mean arterial pressure, confirm an adequate hemoglobin level, and increase inspired O$_2$ to 100%. Next, rule out hypothermia. Finally, consider a small bolus of etomidate or ketamine to increase signal amplitude. Throughout this procedure continuing communication with the surgeon is of the utmost importance. In the immediate postoperative period a brief neurologic exam completed by the anesthetic team should be documented in the anesthetic record. In these ways morbidity and mortality in complex spine surgery using neurophysiologic monitoring can be reduced.

References

1. M. Banoub, J. E. Tetzlaff, A. Schubert. Pharmacologic and physiologic influences affecting sensory evoked potentials: implications for perioperative monitoring. *Anesthesiology* 2003; **99**: 716–37.

2. A. A. Gonzalez, D. Jeyanandarajan, C. Hansen *et al.* Intraoperative neurophysiological monitoring during spine surgery: a review. *Neurosurg Focus* 2009; **27**: E6.

3. A. C. Wang, K. D. Than, A. B. Etarne *et al.* Impact of anesthesia on transcranial motor evoked potential monitoring during spine surgery: a review of the literature. *Neurosurg Focus* 2009; **27**: E7.

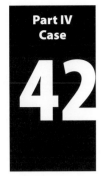
Spine surgery. Complex spine surgery

Effects of anesthesia on intraoperative neurophysiologic monitoring

Uma Menon and Dileep R. Nair

The primary objective in intraoperative neurophysiologic monitoring is to identify and prevent the development of new neurologic deficits or worsening of a preexisting neurologic injury to a patient who is undergoing surgery. Careful use of anesthetic regimens and knowledge of the effects of anesthesia on neurophysiologic modalities are critical for successful use of monitoring.

Case description

A 24-year-old right-handed female diagnosed with neurofibromatosis type I at age 3 years, presented with progressive right upper extremity weakness, new onset left upper extremity weakness and difficulty walking. She also complained of bilateral upper extremity numbness and perineal numbness. She was known to have scoliosis and multiple neurofibromas in the lumbar spine as well as cervical spine with previous surgical removal and gamma knife treatments. Prior magnetic resonance imaging of the cervical spine demonstrated bilateral neurofibromas at the level of C2 with no encroachment of the spinal canal. Also noted was a large (>3 cm) dumbbell neurofibroma with no cord compression. A repeat magnetic resonance imaging of the cervical spine at the time of current evaluation showed a large extramedullary mass centered within the right C2–3 and C3–4 neural foramina with extension into the central canal and moderate to severe mass effect on the cervical cord (Figure 42.1). She was scheduled for laminectomy at C2–3, C3–4 levels and removal of the right-sided extradural neurofibroma. The agents used for anesthesia were fentanyl, sevoflurane, nitrous oxide, and remifentanil. Somatosensory evoked potentials (SSEPs) and transcranial motor evoked potentials (MEPs) were recorded intraoperatively.

At baseline the right-sided SSEPs and MEPs were decreased in comparison to the left. Following the administration of a fentanyl bolus there was bilateral decrease in amplitude of all responses. However, due

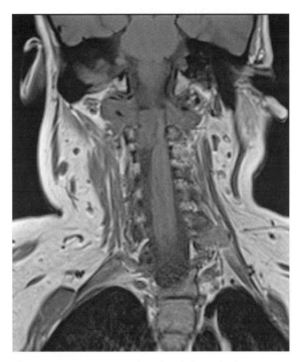

Figure 42.1. Demonstrates the right-sided extradural neurofibroma.

to the asymmetry present at baseline, it appeared that the anesthetic effect was unilateral. There was no surgical explanation for the change noted. Lowering of the sevoflurane levels and addition of nitrous oxide and remifentanil infusion resulted in return of the responses (Figure 42.2).

Discussion

Intraoperative neurophysiologic monitoring is an effective way of preventing injuries during neurosurgical procedures. However, the result of the monitoring depends on various factors, including temperature, blood flow, intracranial pressure, and especially the anesthetic agents that are used. Typically the effects of anesthesia and changes in other body parameters

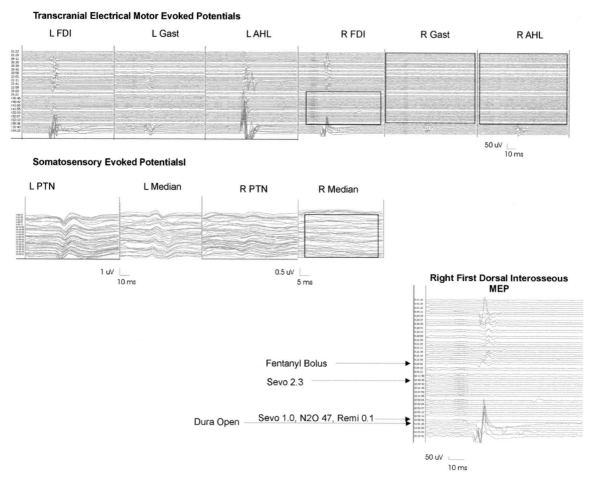

Figure 42.2. Shows an apparent asymmetric change in both right-sided motor evoked potentials (first dorsal interosseous muscle, gastrocnemius, and adductor hallucis longus) as well as posterior tibial and median nerve sensory evoked potentials. These findings are explained by the presence of a baseline decreased amplitude on right-sided responses from the extradural neurofibroma. The apparent loss of responses on the right was associated with the administration of fentanyl bolus producing a bilateral decrease in amplitudes but in the face of the preexisting asymmetry the change appears as a unilateral loss of responses. No clear intraoperative surgical manipulation could explain these findings.

on neurophysiologic tests are bilateral unlike the findings of this case. The changes produced appeared unilateral only because of a preexisting lesion. Bilateral changes especially in tests used as a control for the monitoring (such as median nerve SEPs in thoracolumbar level surgery) should suggest the possibility of effects of anesthetics or other body parameters. However, bilateral changes do not exclude the possibility of a significant change from surgery, but unilateral changes typically suggest that the effect is not anesthetic (with the exception highlighted in this case). Different evoked potentials have different sensitivities to anesthesia (visual evoked potentials > SSEPs > brainstem auditory evoked potentials (BAEPs)). The

effect of anesthetic agents on the recordings increases with the number of synapses in the pathway being monitored. This is related to the effect of anesthetic agents on synaptic transmission and axonal conduction. This is why cortical SSEPs are more affected by anesthesia than are the subcortical responses.

The following is a brief overview of the various anesthetic agents and their effects on neurophysiologic monitoring [1].

Inhalational agents

Use of halogenated agents causes a dose-related reduction of amplitude and prolonged latency of SEPs whereas BAEPs are minimally changed, except at high doses when they are lost. Transcranial electrical MEPs (particularly single pulse) on the other hand can be completely abolished with doses of 0.5 minimum alveolar concentration (MAC). Nitrous oxide at equipotent doses to the halogenated agents can also cause a dose-related reduction in amplitude and prolongation of latency of cortical SEPs. Additionally, the effects of nitrous oxide are also dependent on the other agents used concurrently.

Intravenous anesthetic agents

Intravenous anesthetic agents include barbiturates, benzodiazepines, etomidate, propofol, and ketamine. In general barbiturates do not produce much change of SEPs. Thiopental, which is commonly used for induction, can produce transient reduction in amplitude and prolonged latency of cortical SEPs. However, MEPs can be completely abolished with barbiturates and are to be avoided if such monitoring is required. With single doses of midazolam, a commonly used benzodiazepine, there is minimal effect on evoked potentials, but with continuous infusions it can reduce the latency and amplitude of SEPs. The MEP responses, however, are significantly reduced with the use of midazolam. Etomidate is a unique anesthetic agent in that it causes enhancement of SEP and MEP responses. It may be an agent to consider in a difficult setting, but with awareness of the idiosyncratic reaction of adrenal suppression and increased mortality with prolonged infusion. Opioids used for total intravenous anesthesia include fentanyl, remifentanil, sufentanil, and alfentanil. These intravenous opioid agents typically have little effect on evoked potentials even at very high doses making them quite useful during intraoperative monitoring. The current case represents an exception. Ketamine is another agent with some unique properties in that it can enhance the cortical evoked potential responses. Dexmedetomidine is a selective alpha-2-adrenoreceptor agonist, which is used as an intravenous adjunct to any of the general anesthetics and which does not cause a significant change in SEP or MEP recordings up to doses of 0.6 ng/mL [2].

Neuromuscular blocking agents

Use of neuromuscular blocking agents can affect the ability to record myogenic responses from a variety of monitoring modalities such as transcranial MEPs, free-running electromyography, direct nerve stimulation evoked motor responses, pedicle screw stimulation, and cortical stimulation motor mapping. On the other hand these agents can improve the recordings of SEPs and MEPs by reducing noise produced by muscle activity.

Conclusion

Almost all of the anesthetic agents can cause depression of the evoked potentials if given at sufficiently high doses and therefore a suitable combination of anesthetic agents should be chosen in discussion with the surgeon, anesthetist, and the monitoring team. Consideration should be given that the agent(s) chosen have the least effect on the evoked potentials with the least possible stable dose without causing any patient discomfort. A team approach with good communication between the neurophysiologist, anesthesiologist, and surgeon is very important to the success of neurophysiologic monitoring and its clinical utility [3, 4].

References

1. A. C. Wang, K. D. Than, A. B. Etame *et al.* Impact of anesthesia on transcranial electric motor evoked potential monitoring during spine surgery: a review of the literature. *Neurosurg Focus* 2009; 27: E7.

2. E. Bala, D. I. Sessler, D. R. Nair *et al.* Motor and somatosensory evoked potentials are well maintained in patients given dexmedetomidine during spine surgery. *Anesthesiology* 2008; 109: 417–25.

3. M. L. James. Anesthetic considerations. In Husain A. M., ed. *A Practical Approach to Neurophysiologic Monitoring.* 1st edn. New York: Demos Medical Publishing, 2008.

4. T. B. Sloan, E. J. Heyer. Anesthesia for intraoperative monitoring of the spinal cord. *J Clin Neurophys* 2002; 19: 430–43.

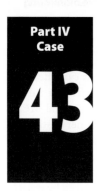

Neurofibromatosis type 1 and spinal deformity

George A. Mashour

Neurofibromatosis type 1 (NF1) is one of the most common genetic disorders of the nervous system, affecting approximately 1 in 3000 individuals. The most typical manifestations are multiple neurofibromas and melanogenic abnormalities (both of neural crest origin), but the phenotype may also include skeletal abnormalities.

Case description

The patient was a 39-year-old female with a history of NF1 and four previous spine surgeries, the last of which occurred at the age of 16. She presented with a history of progressive difficulty walking, as well as numbness, tingling, burning, and spasm in her lower extremities. Imaging revealed a kyphotic deformity and severe angulation at the junction of the cervical and thoracic spine (Figure 43.1); she was also diagnosed with a pseudomeningocele. The patient was admitted for correction of the deformity and her cervical spine was stabilized with a halo device. Electrophysiologic monitoring with somatosensory and motor evoked potentials was planned.

The primary concerns of the anesthesiology team were (1) management of the airway in the halo, (2) the potential for significant blood loss given the history of multiple spine surgeries, and (3) anesthetic maintenance consistent with effective neurophysiologic monitoring. In preparation for an awake fiberoptic intubation, glycopyrrolate was administered as an antisialogogue; subsequently, the patient's heart rate increased to the 160s. Tachycardia was treated with esmolol and a dexmedetomidine infusion was started for both sedation and sympatholysis. Nebulized and atomized lidocaine was administered for airway topicalization, with additional boluses of fentanyl for sedation. During the awake fiberoptic intubation, systolic blood pressures rose to >200 mmHg. After confirming endotracheal intubation, a central venous catheter was placed in the femoral vein and balanced anesthe-

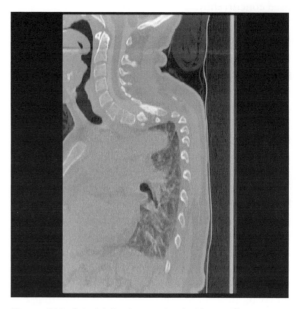

Figure 43.1. Spinal deformity associated with neurofibromatosis type 1 (NF1). Note the marked angulation of the spine at the cervicothoracic junction.

sia was maintained with dexmedetomidine, sufentanil infusion, and isoflurane at 0.5 minimum alveolar concentration. The case was completed uneventfully with approximately 1 liter estimated blood loss; emergence was smooth and the patient was neurologically intact.

Discussion

Neurofibromatosis type 1 (also known as von Recklinghausen's disease) is an autosomal dominant disorder with nearly complete penetrance and highly variable expressivity. It results from a mutation of the *NF1* gene on chromosome 17, which encodes the tumor suppressor neurofibromin. Although in this case the patient's mother had a diagnosis of NF1, spontaneous mutation of the gene without family history occurs in approximately 50% of patients. Melanogenic abnormalities such as café-au-lait macules, freckling, and hyperpigmentation occur earlier in life, while tumor formation usually manifests in puberty. Neurofibromatosis type 2 is a clinically and genetically distinct entity. Neurofibromatosis type 2 is more rare than NF1, with an incidence of approximately 1 in 40 000. Neurofibromatosis type 2 also has an autosomal dominant mode of transmission and is characterized by vestibular schwannomas (often referred to as acoustic neuromas), as well as meningiomas.

Patients with NF1 may present for surgical procedures involving peripheral nervous system tumors (neurofibromas, malignant peripheral nerve sheath tumors), central nervous system tumors (benign optic gliomas, astrocytomas), scoliosis or other skeletal abnormalities, and a host of other disorders. Because the phenotype is so highly variable, a thorough and systematic approach to the patient with NF1 is essential (Table 43.1) [1].

The airway was of particular concern in this patient. In addition to the obvious difficulties presented by cervical spine immobilization, neurofibromas may also develop in the trachea and respiratory tree [2, 3]. Patients with tracheobronchial tumors may be asymptomatic for many years and may present with normal chest radiographs. Recent history of dyspnea, cough, dysphagia, dysarthria, stridor, or change of voice should be especially concerning in a patient with NF1. The need for an awake fiberoptic endotracheal intubation because of the halo, in conjunction with the rare but real possibility of airway tumors, led us to choose dexmedetomidine as a mode of sedation that would help preserve respiratory drive. Furthermore, dexmedetomidine has also been demonstrated to be a useful adjunct for spine surgery that does not significantly interfere with neurophysiologic recording [4].

The marked increases in heart rate and blood pressure during the preparation and performance of fiberoptic intubation were initially concerning. The vagotonic effects of fentanyl, alpha-2 agonist sympatholytic properties of dexmedetomidine, and what appeared to be adequate airway topicalization with lidocaine did not attenuate the hemodynamic response. Approximately 6% of patients with NF1 have hypertension, but there is also a well-known association with pheochromocytomas (another neural crest derivative). Refractory hypertension in a patient with NF1 should therefore prompt consideration and diagnostic evaluation of pheochromocytoma. In the current patient, the blood pressure stabilized after the airway was secured.

Table 43.1. Anesthetic considerations of neurofibromatosis type 1 (NF1).

System	Comments
Airway	Neurofibromas of the tongue, pharynx, or larynx may interfere with tracheal intubation Suspicion is raised by history of dysphagia, dysarthria, stridor, or change of voice
Respiratory system	Intrapulmonary neurofibroma, pulmonary fibrosis may produce cough and dyspnea Right ventricular failure may be present Scoliosis or kyphosis may compromise lung function
Cardiovascular system	Raised arterial pressure usually essential hypertension but consider pheochromocytoma or renal artery stenosis Hypertrophic cardiomyopathy may occur Mediastinal tumors may result in superior vena caval obstruction
Nervous system	A variety of peripheral nerve tumors and intracranial tumors are common Increased incidence of epilepsy and learning disorders Cerebrovascular disease may co-exist Hydrocephalus Cognitive impairment
Gastrointestinal tract	Intestinal tumors may present with pain, gastrointestinal hemorrhage or perforation Carcinoid tumors occur in duodenum and may result in jaundice and carcinoid syndrome
Genitourinary system	Neurofibromas may cause ureteric/urethral obstruction
Musculoskeletal system	Vertebral deformities or spinal cord tumors may make spinal/extradural techniques difficult Pseudoarthroses

Modified with permission from Hirsch *et al.*, 2001 [1].

Conclusion

In conclusion, NF1 patients are complex and present for a variety of neurosurgical interventions. Given the multisystem involvement and variable phenotype, a systematic approach to the NF1 patient is necessary for safe perioperative care.

References

1. **N. P. Hirsch, A. Murphy, J. J. Radcliffe.**
Neurofibromatosis: clinical presentations and

anaesthetic implications. *Br J Anaesth* 2001; **86**: 555–64.

2. **K. L. Irion, T. D. Gasparetto, E. Marchiori** *et al.* Neurofibromatosis type 1 with tracheobronchial neurofibromas: case report with emphasis on tomographic findings. *J Thorac Imaging* 2008; **23**: 194–6.

3. **S. S. Moorthy, S. Radpour, E. C. Weisberger**. Anesthetic management of a patient with tracheal neurofibroma. *J Clin Anesth* 2005; **17**: 290–2.

4. **E. Bala, D. I. Sessler, D. R. Nair** *et al.* Motor and somatosensory evoked potentials are well maintained in patients given dexmedetomidine during spine surgery. *Anesthesiology* 2008; **109**: 417–25.

44

Major vascular complication during spine surgery

Zeyd Ebrahim and Jia Lin

The incidence of vascular injury during major spine surgery is low. However, when this catastrophe occurs, as outlined in this case, it presents a major challenge to the anesthesia team. Anesthesiologists involved in the care of patients undergoing complicated spine surgery should be cognitive of this infrequent but serious complication [1, 2].

Case description

A 75-year-old female was scheduled for removal of instrumentation at L4–S1 and re-exploration of a previous posterior lumbar inter-body fusion. Her current symptoms included lower extremity weakness and pain. She had a history of well-controlled hypertension, hyperlipidemia, anxiety, depression, tobacco use (quit 25 years prior), morbid obesity (body mass index 36.1), lumbar stenosis and spondylolisthesis, and was status post arthrodesis and segmental instrumentation (about 6 months prior). Her functional class was at the level of FC III.

There was no significant abnormality seen on physical examination. The laboratory values revealed normal basic metabolic panel, complete blood count, and coagulation tests; her electrocardiogram and chest X-ray were unremarkable. Magnetic resonance imaging showed lumbar stenosis and spondylolisthesis. Stress echocardiogram was negative for myocardial ischemia, revealed normal left and right heart function and normal valve structures.

The patient was taken to the operating room with a peripheral intravenous catheter *in situ*. Standard ASA monitors were applied. Anesthesia was induced with fentanyl, propofol, and rocuronium. After induction, an arterial line and an additional 16G peripheral catheter were placed. The patient was positioned prone on the Jackson table with all pressure points padded and the abdomen hanging unimpeded. Maintenance of anesthesia was achieved with 1.0 minimum alveolar concentration (MAC) of isoflurane, and 40% oxy-

gen air mixture and IV continuous infusion of sufentanil. Rocuronium was administered as needed following neuromuscular blockade monitoring.

The first arterial blood gas after the start of the procedure revealed a pH of 7.44; $PaCO_2$: 30 (end-tidal CO_2 ($ETCO_2$) between 26 and 30); PaO_2: 210 (FiO_2: 0. 43); HCO_3: 20; Base excess: −3 and Hct: 34. The first 5 hours of the procedure were uneventful and the patient was stable. The surgeon confirmed for the anesthesia team that the old hardware had been removed and that he was performing an extended dissection and evacuating the disk space.

A sudden drop in blood pressure, oxygen saturation, bispectral index and $ETCO_2$ were noticed. The arterial line wave form was almost flat. It was noted that the blood pressure dropped from 100s/60s mmHg to systolic pressure of 30s; $ETCO_2$ dropped to <10 mmHg.

The breath sounds were clear, bilateral, and equal. The ventilator did not show any change in the peak airway pressure of 27 cmH_2O and the arterial line was flushed and aspirated to ensure patency. However, upon inquiry the surgeon confirmed excessive blood loss.

After the initial evaluation and examination, the inspiratory FiO_2 was changed to 1.0; phenylephrine 1000 mcg in divided doses was given. Fluid blouses and blood were transfused but with little effect on the low blood pressure. Help was called to the operating room and epinephrine 1 mg was given which increased the blood pressure to 100s/60s and heart rate increased to 120s. However, the effect was temporary.

While the patient was being resuscitated, the surgeon quickly closed the incision and the patient was turned to the supine position. A left subclavian central access was quickly established and a vascular surgeon was called for an evaluation of an intra-abdominal vascular injury. A large amount of bright red blood in the abdomen was noted. The aorta was then cross clamped at the supraceliac level. Further exploration

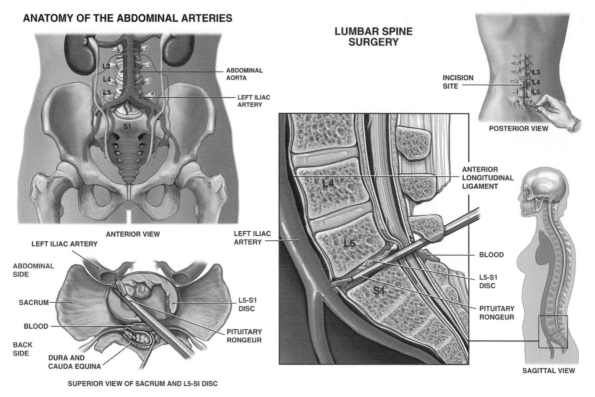

Figure 44.1. Iatrogenic injury to iliac artery during L5–S1 lumbar spine surgery. Reprinted with permission. Illustration Copyright © 2010 Nucleus Medical Art, All rights reserved. www.nucleusinc.com.

of the abdomen revealed a severely calcified aorta and a posterior wall injury at the very proximal left common iliac artery just at the level of aortic bifurcation. The aorta was reconstructed with a bifurcated graft.

The intraoperative course was also complicated by significant coagulopathy from massive blood loss and transfusion. Total estimated blood loss was approximately 10 liters. Intraoperative partial thromboplastin time (PTT) was 150.8 and the platelet count was 29K.

The patient was transferred to the intensive care unit (ICU) with stable vital signs, reasonable urine output, and improving coagulopathy. The initial laboratory values in the ICU were: PTT: 39.4, International Normalized ratio (INR): 1.4, fibrinogen 104, and a platelet count of 194. Coagulopathy was further corrected overnight.

The postoperative course was complicated by nonoliguric renal failure, pneumonia, and urinary tract infection. Following an ICU stay and prolonged hospital course, the patient was discharged to a rehabilitation facility on postoperative day 29.

Discussion

Iatrogenic major vascular injury during lumbar spine operations is a rare and potentially fatal complication. The incidence is about 1–5/10 000; mortality is about 38–65% in cases of arterial laceration. Risk of injury can be explained by the close anatomical relationship between the retroperitoneal vessels and the vertebral column (Figure 44.1). Vessels that can be injured include the left common iliac artery and vein, abdominal aorta and superior rectal artery.

Variable clinical manifestation is one of the main reasons for the apparent low incidence of vascular injury, which is thought to be underestimated. The diagnosis can be delayed or overlooked if the acute hemorrhage is retroperitoneal. With formation of a pseudoaneurysm or arteriovenous fistula, diagnosis can be delayed for weeks or even years.

Therefore, a high degree of suspicion of vascular injury should always be maintained with unexplained hypotension. In addition, in these cases there is no correlation between the real blood loss and that viewed in the surgical field. As always, communication between the anesthesia and surgical team is extremely important. Also, this case highlights the importance of having the blood products available before starting any complex spine surgery [3, 4, 5].

The role of central venous monitoring is always debated in the context of major spine surgery. However, central venous pressure readings in the prone position may not reflect accurate data and large bore intravascular access and invasive blood pressure monitoring are probably more important in the hemodynamic management of these cases.

Conclusion

In conclusion, anesthesia for complex spine surgery requires invasive monitoring, large-bore intravenous access, and awareness of the potential for disaster.

References

1. **E. F. Reilly, N. S. Weger, S. P. Stawicki**. Vascular injury during spinal surgery. *OPUS 12 Scientist* 2008; **2**: 7–10.

2. **B. Düz, M. Kaplan, C. Günay** *et al.* Iliocaval arteriovenous fistula following lumbar disc surgery: endovascular treatment with a stent-graft. *Turk Neurosurg* 2008; **18**: 245–8.

3. **U. Nilsonne, A. Hakelius**. On vascular injury in lumbar disc surgery. *Acta Orthop Scandinav* 1965; **35**: 329–37.

4. **W. R. Smythe, J. P. Carpenter**. Upper abdominal aortic injury during spinal surgery. *J Vasc Surg* 1997; **25**: 774–7.

5. **J. Inamasu, B. H. Guiot**. Vascular injury and complication in neurosurgical spine surgery. *Acta Neurochir* 2006; **148**: 375–87.

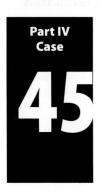
Spine surgery. Complex spine surgery

Complex spine surgery for a Jehovah's Witness

Matthew Martin and Vijay Tarnal

Jehovah's Witness (JW) is an evangelical Christian denomination best known to physicians for beliefs regarding the refusal of all blood product transfusions. Based on their interpretation of the bible, Jehovah's Witnesses believe that acceptance of any blood once it has left the body is "in violation of Gods Law" [1]. This is a challenge from both a clinical and ethical standpoint during complex spine surgeries.

Case description

The patient was a 54-year-old female with a history of obstructive sleep apnea, hyperlipidemia, and scoliosis who presented for T10–L5 posterior spinal fusion. She previously had undergone a posterior lumbar fusion, but recently experienced progressive back and hip pain as well as new-onset difficulty with walking. Imaging of the patient's thoracolumbar spine showed significant progression of her scoliosis, cephalad to her previous fusion (Figure 45.1). The procedure was scheduled for 7.5 hours with somatosensory and motor evoked potentials. A detailed preoperative discussion focused on the anesthetic management, the potential for significant blood loss, and the patient's wishes should profound anemia occur.

The primary concerns for the anesthesiologist were (1) the potential for significant intraoperative blood loss in a Jehovah's Witness, especially given the size and duration of the procedure, and (2) a balanced anesthetic technique in the setting of somatosensory and motor evoked potential monitoring. After uneventful induction and placement of an endotracheal tube, dexmedetomidine and sufentanil infusions were started. Using a SAFESET™ reservoir monitoring kit, a radial arterial catheter was placed for hemodynamic monitoring and arterial blood gas analysis. Since the patient had poor venous access, a right internal jugular central venous catheter was placed. The patient was placed in a Mayfield headrest and positioned prone, with appropriate precautions to prevent

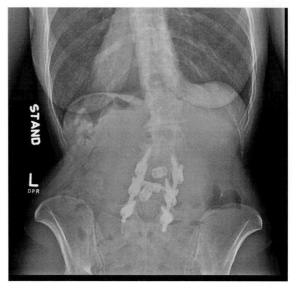

Figure 45.1. Scoliosis of thoracolumbar spine, cephalad to the patient's previous fusion.

pressure on the inferior vena cava. Balanced anesthesia was maintained using dexmedetomidine, sufentanil, and a propofol infusion; systolic blood pressure was maintained within 20% of the patient's baseline. The patient's preoperative hematocrit was 42%. Based on the clinical status and blood loss, arterial blood gas analyses were done using the SAFESET™ reservoir, which meant no additional blood loss due to frequent sampling. The arterial blood gas analysis was used not only to assess respiratory and metabolic state but also the hematocrit.

The antifibrinolytic drug aminocaproic acid was infused during the case to reduce blood loss. The case was completed without complications with an estimated blood loss of 2200 mL. At the completion of the case, the patient's final intraoperative hematocrit was 27%. After a smooth emergence and tracheal extubation, the patient was transferred to the recovery room hemodynamically stable and neurologically intact.

Discussion

The Jehovah's Witness faith was founded in the late nineteenth century out of the controversy stemming from the interpretation of the bible by Catholic and Protestant denominations. It was not until 1945 that it was determined that blood transfusion should be forbidden because it violated God's law. Complex spine procedures on the Jehovah's Witness patient pose a significant challenge for the anesthesiologist. Blood conservation must be planned for and discussed with the patient and surgical team preoperatively. Several strategies have been described in the literature in the last 50 years including: proper patient positioning, autologous blood donation and transfusion, normovolemic hemodilution, artificial blood products, and blood salvage [2]. Other options include pharmacologic therapies such as desmopressin, aminocaproic acid, and recombinant factor VII. It must be stressed that different Jehovah's Witnesses may follow different beliefs – it is therefore crucial to discuss and document the patient's wishes thoroughly prior to any procedure.

One mainstay of spine surgery is proper patient positioning. By leaving the abdomen free in the prone position, there is decreased inferior vena cava pressure and thus decreased venous plexus filling around the spinal cord. There is also a theoretical benefit of decreased vertebral venous pressure and reduced intraoperative blood loss from decreased bone bleeding [3].

Preoperative autologous donation utilizes the patient's own blood, which is usually harvested prior to the operation, allowing the patient to intrinsically replace the lost blood. This has been utilized for procedures with high potential for blood loss, but has shown only modest benefits. The technique is also associated with many of the same risks of allogenic blood transfusion, including infection. Some Jehovah's Witnesses will accept this technique, but most will not accept any blood (even their own) once it has left the body.

Acute normovolemic hemodilution utilizes the same principles as above, but only shows very modest (if any) benefit in blood conservation. This technique requires the anesthesiologist to remove the patient's blood and replace the volume with crystalloid or colloid. The concept is that the hemoglobin content of the "lost blood" would be less if the blood were dilute. The removed whole blood would then be re-infused at the completion of the case. Again, most Jehovah's Witnesses would oppose this treatment, as their blood would leave the body.

Perioperative blood salvage employs strategies of taking the patient's own blood and re-infusing it after washing and purifying. This "cell-saving" technique has been used in some Jehovah's Witnesses as the circuit can be maintained in-line with the patient's circulation. The cell-salvage technique is now widely used for procedures in which significant blood loss is anticipated. The risks, although low, include infection, coagulopathy, and air embolism. The benefits of cell salvage far outweigh the risks.

Another option is the use of pharmacologic therapy to reduce blood loss. Desmopressin can be used, which is thought to increase serum levels of von Willebrand factor, which forms a complex with Factor VIII and increases coagulation. While the potential for reduction in blood loss during spine surgery exists, there have been conflicting results throughout the literature. Aminocaproic acid is a lysine analog that works as an antifibrinolytic and has been shown to reduce blood loss during complex spine procedures. With the removal of Aprotinin from the market in 2007, aminocaproic acid has been widely used for many cardiac and complex spine procedures.

Erythropoietin is a blood-stimulating hormone normally synthesized in the kidney that stimulates red blood cell production in the bone marrow. It is usually accepted by Jehovah's Witness patients and has been shown useful in blood conservation [4]. This therapy is usually started weeks to months in anticipation of major surgery. Elevated hemoglobin levels can be advantageous preoperatively, but increased cardiovascular complications have been described in patients using erythropoietin with hemoglobin levels greater than 13 g/dL.

Finally, the use of "hypotensive anesthesia" to reduce blood loss can be an effective blood conservation strategy in the Jehovah's Witness population. This has been described for many years as a way to reduce blood loss by up to 40% during complex spine procedures [5]. Although this technique has been widely accepted as an effective technique for reduction in blood loss, there are potential risks associated with hypotension in the prone position. One potential complication, which has seen a recent surge of attention, is postoperative visual loss. The etiology can be the result of ischemic optic neuropathy, of which both anemia and hypotension may be contributing factors [6].

The risk is significant enough such that the American Society of Anesthesiologists recommend that any patient undergoing a "lengthy" spine surgery in the prone position should be warned about this complication. One guideline is to keep the systolic blood pressure maintained within 20% of the patient's baseline. It is prudent to exclude patients from induced hypotensive anesthesia if they have significant cardiovascular co-morbidities such as hypertension, cerebrovascular disease, and coronary artery disease.

Conclusion

In conclusion, while complex spine procedures in the Jehovah's Witness patient may be challenging, successful outcomes can be achieved. With active preoperative assessment, communication, blood conservation strategies, proper positioning and meticulous surgical and anesthetic technique, complex spine surgeries are possible in the Jehovah's Witness population.

References

1. *The Watchtower*, September 15, 1961, p. 558.

2. **T. R. Kuklo, B. D. Owens, D. W. Polly Jr.** Perioperative blood and blood product management for spinal deformity surgery. *Spine J* 2003; **3**: 388–93.

3. **T. C. Lee, L. C. Yang, H. J. Chen**. Effect of patient position and hypotensive anesthesia on inferior vena caval pressure. *Spine* 1998; **23**: 941–7.

4. **T. K. Rosengart, R. E. Helm, J. Klemperer** *et al.* Combined aprotinin and erythropoietin use for blood conservation: results with Jehovah's Witnesses. *Ann Thorac Surg* 1994; **58**: 1397–403.

5. **J. W. Brodsky, J. H. Dickson, W. D. Erwin** *et al.* Hypotensive anesthesia for scoliosis surgery in Jehovah's Witnesses. *Spine* 1991; **16**: 304–6.

6. **L. A. Lee, S. Roth, K. L. Posner** *et al.* The American Society of Anesthesiologists Postoperative Visual Loss Registry: analysis of 93 spine surgery cases with postoperative visual loss. *Anesthesiology* 2006; **105**: 652–9.

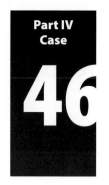

Diplopia following spine surgery

Alaa A. Abd-Elsayed and Ehab Farag

Visual disturbances are known to occur after spine surgery. Although postoperative visual loss will be discussed in the next case, here we describe a case of postoperative diplopia.

Case description

A 34-year-old woman presented to the clinic with post-laminectomy kyphosis and subsequently underwent posterior fusion and fixation in the prone position. The patient received 7000 mL of crystalloids and 1465 mL of colloids during surgery. The patient developed facial edema and reported diplopia on the first postoperative day. Examination and history revealed no obvious cause for the developed diplopia, which resolved completely after 2 days without treatment.

Discussion

Abducens nerve palsy, which causes diplopia without any other neurologic signs, is reported to be the most common cranial nerve palsy [1]. Abducens nerve palsy was reported to be a complication of different procedures such as lumbar puncture, shunt surgery, maxillary osteotomy, cranial trauma, and skull traction [2–6]. The sixth, ninth, tenth, and twelfth cranial nerves have a vertical or oblique course in the cranium making them the most vulnerable nerves to stretch injuries with the abducens nerve being the most at risk of injury [2]. Barsoum *et al.* reported a case of apparent abducens nerve palsy after only 5 lb of traction at lumbar spinal surgery [2]. The cause of the palsy was thought to be stretching of the cranial nerve by skull traction.

Abducens nerve palsy has also been recognized as a complication of lumbar puncture [7]; the reason for this was attributed to caudal displacement and neurotoxic spinal arachnoiditis. All the causes of diplopia that were reported in the literature were investigated in our case but none seemed to apply. We speculate that the diplopia in our patient was caused by fluid overload during surgery, as the patient received enough volume to cause facial edema and thus possibly abducens nerve stretch.

Conclusion

Prone spine cases are associated with postoperative visual disturbances. The present case suggests that diplopia in this context may be a self-limiting process due to sixth nerve stretch after fluid overload.

References

1. **C. Wilkins, G. D. MacEwen**. Cranial nerve injury from halo traction. *Clin Orthop Relat Res* 1977; **126**: 106–10.

2. **W. K. Barsoum, J. Mayerson, G. R. Bell**. Cranial nerve palsy as a complication of operative traction. *Spine* 1999; **24**: 585–6.

3. **M. J. Botte, T. P. Byrne, R. A. Abrams** *et al.* Halo skeletal fixation: techniques of application and prevention of complications. *J Am Acad Orthop Surg* 1996; **4**: 44–53.

4. **A. R. Hodgson**. Halo-pelvic traction in scoliosis. *Isr J Med Sci* 1973; **9**: 767–70.

5. **K. K. Jain**. Aberrant roots of the abducent nerve. *J Neurosurg* 1964; **21**: 349–51.

6. **E. A. Miller, P. J. Savino, N. J. Schatz**. Bilateral sixth-nerve palsy. A rare complication of water-soluble contrast myelography. *Arch Ophthal* 1982; **100**: 603–4.

7. **G. L. Clifton, E. R. Miller, S. C. Choi** *et al.* Lack of effect of induction of hypothermia after acute brain injury. *N Engl J Med* 2001; **344**: 556–63.

Postoperative visual loss in spine patients

Goodarz Golmirzaie and Laurel E. Moore

Postoperative visual loss (POVL) is a rare but catastrophic complication of spine surgery. The extremely low incidence has made its study and prevention a challenge for neuroanesthesiologists.

Case description

The patient was a 62-year-old female who presented for a revision L4–5 foraminotomy and L4–S1 transverse lumbar interbody fusion. Her past medical history was significant for obesity (body mass index = 39), longstanding hypertension, depression, and systemic lupus erythematosus. The patient had a history of recurrent deep vein thrombosis and pulmonary embolus, thought to be secondary to a hypercoagulable state related to lupus. The patient's activity was limited secondary to chronic low back pain. Her preoperative laboratory values were normal with a hematocrit of 40%; vital signs included a baseline blood pressure of 140/85.

The 6-hour surgery was uneventful. Systolic blood pressure was kept in the range of 90–95 mmHg for >75% of the procedure. The lowest systolic blood pressure recorded was 65. The estimated blood loss was 1500 mL and the hematocrit nadir was 25%. Fluids included 1000 mL of 5% albumin and 3000 mL of lactated Ringer's solution. Urine output for the case was 450 mL. She was recovered in the postanesthesia care unit and subsequently transferred to the neurosurgical intensive care unit for routine observation. That evening she reported that she could not see out of her left eye.

Discussion

To understand POVL it is necessary to understand the anatomy of the optic nerve and its vascular supply (Figure 47.1). The optic nerve can be divided into four portions, including the intracranial (optic chiasm to the optic canal within the lesser sphenoid wing), the intracanalicular (within the optic canal), the posterior or intraorbital (optic foramen to the lamina cribrosa) and the anterior or intraocular (from the lamina cribrosa to the optic disk). The lamina cribrosa is a perforated membrane overlying the posterior scleral foramen through which the optic nerve, as well as central retinal artery and vein, enter the eye.

The retina and optic nerve are supplied by branches of the ophthalmic artery [1]. Once the ophthalmic artery passes through the optic foramen it branches into several vessels including the central retinal artery and a series of posterior ciliary arteries. The intraorbital optic nerve is supplied by a pial plexus which in turn is supplied by branches of the central retinal artery. The most anterior portion of the optic nerve is supplied primarily by short posterior ciliary arteries. The posterior aspect of the optic nerve is supplied by end-vessels that are comprised of easily compressed centripetal pial vessels, thus placing this region of the optic nerve at particular risk for ischemia.

Mechanism of injury

There are multiple causes of POVL, including cortical infarction, direct injuries to the eye and ischemic injuries to the retina and optic nerve. The most common permanent injuries are ischemic in nature including central retinal artery occlusion (CRAO) and ischemic optic neuropathy (ION). Ischemic optic neuropathy can be further subdivided into posterior ischemic optic neuropathy (PION) and anterior ischemic optic neuropathy (AION). While CRAO and AION have been historically associated with cardiac surgery, PION has more recently attracted attention in the medical literature and lay press because of its perceived increase in frequency following complex spine surgery [2]. However, the current literature suggests that the incidence for spine cases is dropping. According to Shen *et al.* the incidence of POVL after spine cases is approximately 3/10 000, which is lower

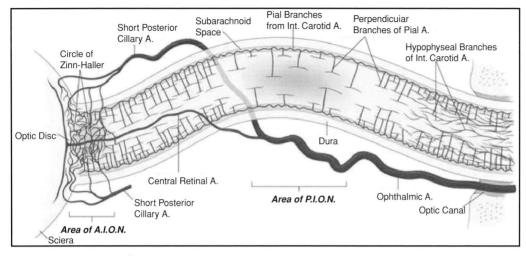

Figure 47.1. Anatomy and vascular supply of the optic nerve. Reproduced with permission from *Neurosurg Focus* 2007; 23 (5); E15.

than previously published incidences of approximately 2/1000 [3, 4].

Central retinal artery occlusion

Central retinal artery occlusion generally presents with painless monocular visual loss following emergence from anesthesia. In cardiac surgery, the cause of CRAO is generally thought to be embolic [1]. When it occurs during spine surgery, it is most commonly associated with direct compression of the globe, thus the term "headrest syndrome" [4]. Intraocular pressure has been demonstrated to increase in prone patients [4]. If this increase in pressure is further augmented by direct compression of the globe by improper head position, the intraocular pressure may exceed central retinal artery pressure and retinal ischemia may result. In the American Society of Anesthesiologists (ASA) visual loss registry, 10/93 cases of POVL following spine surgery were thought to be secondary to CRAO [4]. This subgroup of patients was less likely to have been positioned in a Mayfield head holder and 9/10 had signs of injury to structures around the eye [4]. Significant visual recovery is rare following CRAO [4].

Ischemic optic neuropathy (anterior and posterior)

Anterior ischemic optic neuropathy is generally associated with cardiac surgery [1]. In the last several years, PION has become increasingly recognized after com-

plex surgical spine procedures [3, 5]. Whether the optic nerve injury is anterior or posterior to the lamina cribrosa, patients present with painless binocular or (less commonly) monocular visual loss. The severity of the visual loss can range from visual field deficits to complete loss of light perception. Recognition of the problem postoperatively can be immediate or delayed by several days. Unlike CRAO there is no evidence of external eye injury. There is usually a reduced or absent pupillary light reflex [2]. Anterior ischemic optic neuropathy and PION can be differentiated based on fundoscopic examination. The initial fundoscopic examination in AION shows an edematous disc, whereas with PION the initial fundoscopic exam is generally normal and subsequently deteriorates [1].

Intuitively the etiology of ION would appear to be related to pre-existing vascular disease and reduced oxygen delivery to the optic nerve. However, the etiology is probably more complex than this. There are reports of ION occurring in patients with normal perfusion pressures and normal hematocrits [4]. There have also been reports of ION occurring in children [3, 4]. This would suggest that there is a certain population of patients that is at greater risk of developing ION, either based on the vascular supply, the anatomical structure of the eye, or deficiencies in autoregulation of blood flow to the optic nerve. Supporting this, patients with ION often have bilateral disease [4]. In the ASA registry, 66% of patients had bilateral visual loss [4]. In most patients with POVL secondary to ION, there was no evidence of injury to other vascular beds (heart, liver, etc.), suggesting that the intraorbital optic nerve may be particularly vulnerable to ischemic injury.

Anatomically there appear to be patients identified as having a "disc at risk" for AION. These patients have an unusually small disc and small opening in Bruch's membrane, resulting in crowding of the optic nerve fibers as they pass through this restricted space [6]. In the setting of ischemia this creates a vicious cycle in which early edema of the optic nerve produces greater compression of the nerve and its vascular supply, which in turn further reduces oxygen delivery [6].

Similarly, another possible mechanism for PION might be a form of orbital "compartment syndrome." The intraorbital optic nerve is enclosed by dura and thus has little room for expansion. Should there be swelling of the posterior optic nerve related to increasing venous pressure in the prone position or from large volumes of crystalloid, the edema could result in compression of sensitive vascular structures.

Finally, there are several case reports of sildenafil and AION in adult males with erectile dysfunction and in children treated for pulmonary hypertension [4].

Risk factors for postoperative visual loss

Because of the rare incidence of POVL, prospective studies evaluating risk factors are limited. There are many seemingly intuitive risk factors for POVL that are described in the literature including prone positioning, prolonged procedures, hypotension, anemia, and the need for blood transfusion [4]. Premorbid systemic diseases such as diabetes, hypertension, peripheral vascular occlusive disease, and hypercoagulable states have also been correlated with POVL [4, 5]. In a population-based study by Patil *et al.*, it was demonstrated that hypotension, anemia, and peripheral vascular disease were potential risk factors for POVL with odds ratios of 10, 4.3, and 6.4 respectively [5]. Of these many potential risk factors, however, two in particular are consistently supported: prolonged surgery (more than 6 hours) and large blood loss (more than 1 liter) [4]. In the ASA POVL registry, 94% of spine patients had surgeries that were longer than 6 hours and 82% had operations that had an estimated blood loss of one liter or more [4].

Prevention of postoperative visual loss

Since the etiology of POVL remains poorly understood, prevention remains difficult. However, there are some clinical precautions that may reduce the possibility of POVL based on current evidence. The first is ensuring that the eye is free of pressure while the patient is prone. Careful initial positioning with subsequent eye checks (and documentation) every 15 minutes should be routine for all prone cases. Furthermore, whenever possible the head (and thus orbit) should be positioned at or above the level of the heart to optimize venous drainage and improve perfusion pressure to the retina and optic nerve.

In addition to these precautions, the following are recommendations summarized in the ASA practice advisory [7] developed in 2005 by a task force comprised of anesthesiologists, spine surgeons, and neuro-opthalmologists. These do not constitute practice standards but are recommendations developed after an extensive literature review and survey of practicing physicians.

1. Anemia, atherosclerotic disease, and obesity may be associated with POVL, but at present they cannot be considered predisposing factors.
2. Factors that classify patients as "high risk" include procedures that are prolonged (greater than 6.5 hours), associated with large blood loss, and performed in the prone position.
3. The use of an arterial line is recommended for patients with chronic hypertension, but the task force could not make recommendations with regards to induced hypotension based on the evidence they had at the time.
4. There was no consensus on a "minimal acceptable hemoglobin."
5. A combination of crystalloid and colloid is recommended to replace significant blood loss.
6. While neuroanesthesiologists as a group felt that the extensive use of alpha-agonists decreased oxygen delivery to the optic nerve, no consensus was achieved on this point.
7. Staging long procedures was one strategy discussed.
8. No proven treatment exists for POVL but the panel agreed that anemia should be treated, hypotension corrected, and oxygen administered to patients with suspected POVL. All patients should have an ophthalmologic consultation.
9. Finally, practitioners should consider including discussion of POVL in the informed consent process.

Management of postoperative visual loss

Our patient with POVL had two major risk factors: she had an estimated blood loss of 1.5 liters and she had a prolonged surgery. Furthermore, she was relatively hypotensive for prolonged periods. In this particular case the patient recovered most of her vision prior to being discharged from the hospital. In general only 50% of patients with ION have significant visual recovery [4].

Unfortunately there is no proven treatment for POVL. In the setting of acute POVL the correction of anemia and hypotension should be considered. An ophthalmologic consultation may be helpful in determining the cause of POVL and a formal fundoscopic examination should be performed and documented. It is reasonable to obtain magnetic resonance imaging to rule out an unusual etiology for the blindness such as cortical infarction or pituitary apoplexy. Administration of acetazolamide (to reduce intraocular pressure) and CO_2 inhalation (to increased blood flow to the retina and optic nerve) have not been shown to change outcome in POVL.

Conclusion

In conclusion, POVL is a rare complication with an approximate incidence of 3/10 000 for spine procedures and 9/10 000 to 5/100 for cardiac surgeries [3, 4]. When it does occur it is a devastating event for the patient. While the incidence of CRAO may be decreased with careful attention to the orbit, ION is less clear in its etiology and thus more difficult to prevent. Many risk factors have been proposed yet our understanding of the etiology of ION remains inade-quate. Clearly there are both patient and perioperative factors involved. Until we have a better understanding of these risk factors, careful attention to the eyes, staged procedures, vigilance with regard to intraocular pressure (venous drainage) and the optimization of oxygen-carrying capacity are the best preventative measures available.

References

1. **E. L. Williams, W. M. Hart, R. Tempelhoff.** Postoperative ischemic optic neuropathy. *Anesth Analg* 1995; **80**: 1018–29.

2. **L. M. Buono, R. Foroozan.** Perioperative posterior ischemic optic neuropathy: review of the literature. *Surv Ophthalmol* 2005; **50**: 15–26.

3. **Y. Shen, M. Drum, S. Roth.** The prevalence of perioperative visual loss in the United States: a 10-year study from 1996 to 2005 of spinal, orthopedic, cardiac, and general surgery. *Anesth Analg* 2009; **109**: 1534–45.

4. **L. A. Lee, S. Roth, K. Posner** *et al.* The American Society of Anesthesiologists Postoperative Visual Loss Registry: analysis of 93 spine surgery cases with postoperative visual loss. *Anesthesiology* 2006; **105**: 652–9.

5. **C. G. Patil, E. M. Lad, S. P. Lad** *et al.* Visual loss after spine surgery: a population-based study. *Spine* 2008; **33**: 1491–6.

6. **S. S. Hayreh.** Ischemic optic neuropathy. *Prog Retin Eye Res* 2009; **28**: 34–62.

7. **American Society of Anesthesiologists Task Force on Perioperative Blindness.** Practice advisory for perioperative visual loss associated with spine surgery: a report by the American Society of Anesthesiologists Task Force on Perioperative Blindness. *Anesthesiology* 2006; **104**: 1319–28.

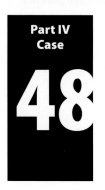

Spine surgery. Complex spine surgery

Prone cardiopulmonary resuscitation

Justin Upp and Sheron Beltran

Neurosurgical procedures are very rarely performed in a straightforward supine position. As such, there are significant challenges associated with the management of cardiopulmonary arrests that are not found in other surgeries.

Case description

A 69-year-old female with a history of renal cell carcinoma developed new back pain and radiculopathy. Magnetic resonance imaging of the lumbar spine revealed a pathologic lumbar compression fracture with tumor encroachment upon the neural foramen bilaterally. The patient presented to the operating room for a complex anteroposterior corpectomy 24 hours after embolization of the mass. Induction of general endotracheal anesthesia with thiopental and succinylcholine was uneventful. Maintenance anesthesia consisted of a low concentration of sevoflurane with remifentanil and propofol infusions to facilitate motor and somatosensory evoked potentials. Adequate intravenous access and an arterial line were obtained before the patient was positioned prone for the posterior portion of the case. This initial stage of the procedure was complicated by 1900 mL of blood loss for which the patient was appropriately resuscitated. After completion, the patient was placed in a modified lateral position for retroperitoneal exposure of the anterior lumbar spine. This portion of the case was complicated by aortic injury and brisk blood loss. A vascular surgical team was summoned to repair the aorta, but despite aggressive resuscitation with crystalloid, albumin, fresh frozen plasma, platelets, and 29 units of packed red blood cells, the patient developed pulseless electrical activity (PEA) arrest. Resuscitation efforts continued while the wound was packed and the patient was repositioned supine to facilitate external cardiac compressions. The wound continued to bleed during the unsuccessful resuscitation effort.

Discussion

This case was one of two at our institution in which exposure to the surgical site of bleeding was poorly accessible due to the need to perform cardiopulmonary resuscitation (CPR) in the supine position [1]. Although this case was performed in the lateral position, it sparked an ongoing dialog and exploration into the possibility of prone CPR during complex spine procedures.

In the operative setting, cardiac arrest necessitating CPR is an event that fortunately occurs infrequently. When it does occur, however, patients undergoing neurosurgery may be in a variety of surgical positions which are suboptimal for the performance of adequate chest compressions. Repositioning a prone patient to the supine position often requires additional personnel, equipment (bed or stretcher) and may make surgical exposure to a bleeding vessel inaccessible to repair. Additionally, it requires time to reposition, which is crucial during an arrest. Throughout the 1960s there was a significant amount of research into cardiopulmonary support and resuscitation eventually leading to the adoption of CPR by the American Heart Association (AHA), and culminating in Basic Life Support (BLS) and Advanced Cardiac Life Support (ACLS).

There has been strong evidence supporting the use of CPR in the supine position, however, a paucity of evidence exists regarding its application in other positions. Publications by McNeil in 1989 were the first descriptions that effective CPR could be conducted in the prone position [2]. His proposal of prone CPR was originally written to address commonly encountered issues with CPR outside the hospital, including a hesitancy of bystanders to administer mouth-to-mouth ventilation as well as aspiration risks. Although these risks may not be applicable in the operative theater during spine surgery with controlled ventilation and a secure airway, the concept of CPR in the prone position does offer an alternative to conventional CPR.

The obvious goal of closed chest compressions, whether supine or prone, is forward blood flow from the heart and thoracic cavity into the systemic circulation. However, the mechanism by which this successful blood flow occurs is less obvious. There are two proposed physiologic models of CPR: the cardiac pump mechanism and the thoracic pump mechanism [2].

The cardiac pump mechanism is the traditional model explaining blood flow during CPR. Direct external compression of the sternum causes direct mechanical compression of the heart. This increases intraventricular pressure and, when combined with atrioventricular valve closure, leads to an artificial cardiac output. These findings have recently been confirmed through transesophageal echocardiography by Higano [3]. During CPR there was echocardiographic evidence of ventricular compression, atrioventricular valve closure, and regurgitation through the mitral valve all indicating a greater increase in ventricular pressure over atrial pressure. After compression ceases, rebound of the thorax transmits negative pressure resulting in venous return, atrioventricular valve opening, and diastolic coronary filling.

The thoracic pump model differs from the cardiac pump mechanism in that direct compression of the cardiac chambers is not thought to be necessary to generate forward blood flow. The thorax as a whole acts as a pump when external compression increases intrathoracic pressure. The more rigid aorta and arterial structures resist collapse, but are compressed causing increased arterial pressure. Venous structures of the thorax collapse under thoracic pressure preventing retrograde blood flow. It is also believed that retrograde blood flow is prevented by valves in the subclavian and jugular veins. After compression of the thorax is released, negative intrathoracic pressure promotes venous return similar to that described in the cardiac pump model [4].

There is no consensus on the optimal way to perform prone CPR, as the AHA only recommends prone CPR when the supine position is inaccessible. Prone CPR is not currently taught in BLS or ACLS courses. Prone CPR has been described in multiple ways, but the evidence mostly consists of case reports and other small nonrandomized studies. The method of conducting compressions varies according to several factors including patient's age, number of rescuers performing CPR, presence and/or location of surgical

incision, the type of bed or operating table that the patient rests on, and the presence of a definitive airway.

In infants, prone CPR can be performed much the same way as supine CPR, with both hands wrapped around the thorax. Rather than bilateral thumbs compressing the sternum, the rescuer would compress the thoracic spine. Compressions can also be accomplished by compressing of the thoracic spine with the fingers of one hand while providing counter pressure with the other. For larger children and adults there are also multiple ways of performing compressions. Compressions have been performed with and without counter pressure. Counter pressure can be accomplished by using another rescuer to support the sternum, or a firm surface with either a saline or sandbag beneath the patient's sternum. Compressions have been described to be effective in the midline two-thirds up the patient's spine between the scapulae. Compressions can also be performed at the same level with both hands placed laterally if there is a mid-line incision.

Despite prone CPR first being described in the literature over 30 years ago, there still remains a paucity of evidence supporting its efficacy. There is no published trial to date addressing prone CPR outcomes, however, a few small trials exist supporting the physiologic feasibility of prone CPR. Mazer et al. conducted a study on six patients in the intensive care unit (ICU) after they suffered circulatory arrest and failed ACLS after 30 minutes. Patients underwent supine CPR for 15 minutes followed by 15 minutes of prone CPR. The means of the systolic, diastolic, and mean arterial pressures were recorded during the 30 minutes of supine and prone CPR. After the patients were enrolled in the trial no other ACLS drugs were given other than 1 mg of intravenous epinephrine every 3 minutes. To conduct prone CPR, patients in this trial were placed on a CPR board with counter pressure provided by a sandbag placed under the sternum. The rescuers performed compressions in the midline from T7–T10 vertebral bodies at a rate of 60–100 compressions/minute. During prone CPR they found a statistically significant increase in mean systolic blood pressure as well as calculated mean arterial pressure. Mean diastolic pressure was also increased, however, this finding was not statistically significant [5].

Wei et al. conducted a similar study on 11 ICU patients. After failing ACLS and expiring, both prone and supine CPR were performed for 1 minute each. Systolic and diastolic blood pressures were recorded by invasive measurement. Prone CPR was found to yield higher mean systolic and diastolic blood pressures than those obtained by standard supine CPR with results reaching statistical significance [6].

Conclusion

In conclusion, current BLS and ACLS guidelines make recommendations with the purpose of achieving effective resuscitation over a broad variety of locations and scenarios. These recommendations do not currently include prone CPR. The operating room differs from other resuscitative settings, as it is a more controlled environment. The patient will already have a definitive airway and intravenous access established, thereby eliminating potentially the largest drawbacks of prone CPR: the hindrance of airway and intravenous catheter acquisition.

During resuscitation it is well established that early defibrillation is associated with better outcomes, and effective and continuous CPR aids in successful defibrillation. In this respect prone CPR may have a theoretical advantage over supine CPR in prone surgeries, as the time from initiation of ACLS to external cardiac compression may be reduced. However, it must be mentioned that no data exist on prone defibrillation success rate or improved outcomes. Current data do support the hemodynamic effectiveness of prone

CPR and, possibly, a more significant finding was that none of the hemodynamic parameters were less than the averages during supine CPR [5, 6]. Intraoperative scenarios in which the patient is in the prone position, as in cases of spinal surgery, are unique settings for which prone CPR may be well-suited as a resuscitation technique.

References

1. **S. L. Beltran, G. A. Mashour**. Unsuccessful cardiopulmonary resuscitation during neurosurgical procedures: is the supine position always optimal? *Anesthesiology* 2008; **108**: 163–4.

2. **E. L. McNeil**. Re-evaluation of cardiopulmonary resuscitation. *Resuscitation* 1989; **18**: 1–5.

3. **S. T. Higano, J. K. Oh, G. A. Ewy** *et al.* The mechanism of blood flow during closed chest cardiac massage in humans: transesophageal echocardiographic observations. *Mayo Clin Proc* 1990; **65**: 1432–40.

4. **C. F. Babbs**. New versus old theories of blood flow during CPR. *Crit Care Med* 1980; **8**: 191–5.

5. **S. P. Mazer, M. Weisfeldt, D** *et al.* Reverse CPR: A pilot study of CPR in the prone position. *Resuscitation* 2003; **57**: 279–85.

6. **J. Wei, D. Tung, S. H. Sue** *et al.* Cardiopulmonary resuscitation in prone position: a simplified method for outpatients. *J Chin Med Assoc* 2006; **69**: 202–6.

49 Open spine stabilization with polymethylmethacrylate augmentation

Mariel Manlapaz and Greta Jo

Open spine stabilization with polymethylmethacrylate (PMMA) augmentation procedures requires significant attention during anesthetic management due to the complication of PMMA embolization. We present a case of hemodynamic instability due to embolization during surgery as well as its management.

Case description

A 54-year-old male with a T12 burst fracture presented for a second stage posterior instrumentation of T9–L4. His past medical history included a T12 corpectomy and T11–L1 instrumentation by a transthoracic approach, osteoporosis, deep vein thrombosis, and mild left ventricular dysfunction.

After induction, the trachea was intubated with a 7.5 mm endotracheal tube and maintained on isoflurane and sufentanil infusion. An arterial line, central line and 14-gauge intravenous catheter were placed. Two hours after incision, the patient was found to have frequent premature ventricular contractions associated with a drop in blood pressure. At that time, the surgeons were augmenting T9, L3, and L4 with PMMA. The premature ventricular contractions were not sustained and the blood pressure responded to 100 mcg boluses of phenylephrine. Meanwhile, several blood samples were sent and the fluids were opened. Differential diagnoses considered included transient effects of PMMA, bone/marrow embolism, cement monomer toxicity, and anaphylactoid reaction.

Fifteen minutes later, the patient developed sustained ventricular tachycardia. The blood pressure dropped along with his oxygen saturation and end-tidal CO_2. The patient was moved from the prone to the supine position and given epinephrine, amiodarone, and vasopressin. He was then maintained on norepinephrine, epinephrine, and amiodarone infusions. Myocardial ischemia, pulmonary embolism (PE) from deep venous thrombosis or PMMA, and anaphylactoid/anaphylaxis reaction were considered.

An intraoperative transesophageal echocardiogram was performed, showing global hypokinesis of the right and left ventricle, patent foramen ovale, and thrombus in the pulmonary artery.

Vascular medicine recommended a heparin bolus and infusion, cardiology agreed with the diagnosis of PE, and cardiothoracic surgery recommended that the patient proceed with an embolectomy. Repeat TEE in the cardiothoracic operating room did not show a PE and the plans for embolectomy were aborted. Further work-up included a cardiac catheterization showing non-stenotic coronary vessels, moderate right and left ventricular dysfunction, no PE in the main pulmonary artery or first and second branches. An inferior vena cava filter was then placed. A computed tomography scan of the chest showed high attenuation embolized material, presumably PMMA in the superior and inferior vena cavae, right cardiac chambers, and the right pulmonary artery. A repeat transthoracic echocardiogram showed a 2 cm right ventricular mass above the tricuspid valve and 3+ tricuspid regurgitation. Because the patient had persistent respiratory problems, the decision was made for surgical intervention: pulmonary embolectomy, closure of the patent foramen ovale, and tricuspid valve repair. Upon opening the cardiac chambers, PMMA was found traversing the right ventricle, right atrium and pulmonary artery (Figures 49.1–49.3). At a follow-up visit, the patient was back to his baseline cardiac and mental status.

Discussion

This patient had osteoporosis, a systemic skeletal disease characterized by low bone mass and microarchitectural deterioration of bone tissue, with a consequent increase in bone fragility and susceptibility to fractures. Such people are susceptible to painful vertebral body compression fractures. Treatment options include medical management, open surgical

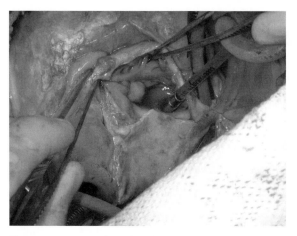

Figure 49.1. Intracardiac polymethylmethacrylate in the right atrium, right ventricle, and pulmonary artery.

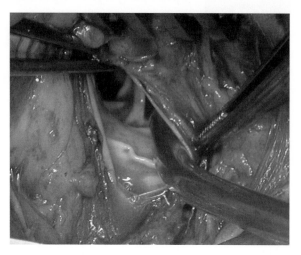

Figure 49.2. Intracardiac polymethylmethacrylate in the right atrium, right ventricle, and pulmonary artery.

stabilization, and percutaneous vertebral augmentation using vertebroplasty or kyphoplasty.

Polymethylmethacrylate is used in vertebroplasty and kyphoplasty and can be used in open surgical stabilization. Vertebroplasty restores stability through a percutaneous bone cement injection via high-pressure filling. Kyphoplasty is another percutaneous procedure, restoring vertebral body height. Kyphoplasty involves low-pressure filling by first producing a void with a balloon and then creating an internal cast. A fundamental difference between the two is that in vertebroplasty, filling is done until the cement leaks, making the volume and pattern unpredictable. For kyphoplasty, filling is done until the cavity is full, making the volume and pattern more predictable [1, 2].

While there are multiple reports in the literature regarding cement leaks with vertebroplasty and kyphoplasty, reported cases of cement leakage during open surgical stabilization are rare. The rate of cement leaks during percutaneous intervention is high

and is seen in up to 73% of vertebral bodies treated, with venous leaks reported in up to 24% of vertebral bodies treated. With leaking comes the risk of cement embolism. In a study by Choe *et al.* [1], cement PE was seen in 4.6% of 65 patients who had percutaneous vertebroplasty or kyphoplasty [1]. Causes of cement embolism include insufficient polymerization of PMMA at the time of injection, poor needle position with respect to the basivertebral vein, or overfilling of the vertebral body. This allows migration of the embolus into the inferior vena cava and the venous system. Anticoagulation prevents thrombus formation on the emboli, but it does not reduce right ventricular afterload nor improve the resulting ventilation/perfusion defect. Generally, 4–11 mL of cement per level is recommended. Less volume should be given for multiple levels. For this patient, 15 mL of PMMA was used [3, 4].

An option to avoid such complications is to concurrently use a venogram to visualize venous outflow

Figure 49.3. Length of polymethylmethacrylate embolus.

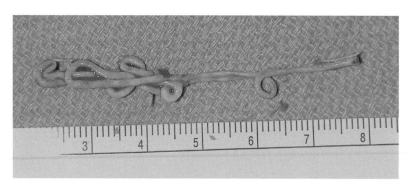

from the vertebra at the time of injection. A venogram can be performed through a bone needle and requires injection of a small volume of dilute, low osmolar nonionic contrast agent. Furthermore, biplane fluoroscopy during PMMA application can improve visualization and the surgeon can stop injection if cement exudes [5].

Conclusion

The incidence of cement leakage is high with percutaneous vertebral augmentation. The case presented here is PMMA venous leakage and PE during open surgical stabilization. Cardiopulmonary presentation is either immediate or delayed and can be catastrophic. Consider a chest X-ray, echocardiogram (transthoracic or transesophageal), and computed tomography scan as diagnostic tools. If strongly symptomatic, consult cardiothoracic surgery for possible embolectomy.

References

1. **D. H. Choe, E. M. Marom, K. Ahrar** et al. Pulmonary embolism of polymethyl methacrylate during percutaneous vertebroplasty and kyphoplasty. *Am J Roentgenol* 2004; **183**: 1097–102.

2. **D. R. Fourney, D. F. Schomer, R. Nader** et al. Percutaneous vertebroplasty and kyphoplasty for painful vertebral body fractures in cancer patients. *J Neurosurgery* 2003; **98**: 21–30.

3. **J. Hodler, D. Peck, L. A. Gilula** et al. Midterm outcome after vertebroplasty: predictive value of technical and patient-related factors. *Radiology* 2003; **227**: 662–8.

4. **C. Vasconcelos, P. Gailloud, N. J. Beauchamp** et al. Is percutaneous vertebroplasty without pretreatment venography safe? Evaluation of 205 consecutives procedures. *AJNR* 2002; **23**: 913–17.

5. **F. M. Phillips, F. Todd Wetzel, I. Lieberman** et al. An in vivo comparison of the potential for extravertebral cement leak after vertebroplasty and kyphoplasty. *Spine* 2002; **27**: 2173–8.

50 Extubating the trachea after prolonged prone surgery

Vijay Tarnal and Robert Scott Kriss

Respiratory complications *after* tracheal extubation are three times more common than complications occurring *during* tracheal intubation [1]. Airway difficulties after complex spine surgeries in prolonged prone position can cause catastrophic complications including severe hypoxia and death. This case will discuss the importance of an appropriate extubation strategy in light of the known postoperative complications of prolonged prone positioning.

Case description

The patient was a 22-year-old male with severe scoliosis scheduled for a T3–ilium fusion with vertebral column resections. The case was scheduled for 9 hours. He presented with a history of cerebral palsy complicated by significant cognitive deficits, seizures, and diffuse spasticity. His spinal curvature was so severe and painful that he was unable to sit in his wheelchair and was required to lie flat at all times. Imaging revealed a severe levoconvex rotary scoliosis of the thoracolumbar spine, approximately 103 degrees from T3–L4, and associated rib cage deformity. The patient had an uncomplicated left hip surgery 5 years previously. Electrophysiologic monitoring with somatosensory and motor evoked potentials was planned.

Given the severity of the scoliosis, the primary concerns of the anesthesiology team were (1) difficulty in positioning supine for laryngoscopy and intubation, (2) respiratory difficulties, (3) difficult prone positioning, (4) the potential for significant blood loss given the complexity of the planned procedure, (5) a balanced anesthetic technique consistent with effective neurophysiologic monitoring, and (6) difficulty with extubation following the prolonged prone surgery. For preoxygenation and induction of anesthesia, the patient was positioned on the operating table in a semi-upright position and pressure areas protected with foam pads. With loss of consciousness, the patient was mask ventilated while the operating table was repositioned for laryngoscopy and intubation. Following an uncomplicated tracheal intubation, balanced anesthetic technique using dexmedetomidine, sufentanil, and desflurane at 0.4 minimum alveolar concentration (MAC) was maintained. The case was completed in 11 hours without significant surgical intraoperative complications. The estimated blood loss was approximately 28% of the patient's total blood volume and he required four units of packed red blood cells in order to achieve a target hematocrit between 24 and 27%. The sufentanil infusion was stopped 90 minutes before the case was completed. The patient was positioned supine and a "cuff-leak test" was done, which was positive for leak around the endotracheal tube. Because of the long duration of the procedure in prone position involving significant blood loss, as well as preoperative mental status, a delayed extubation was planned. The patient was transported to the recovery room and started on pressure support ventilation. The trachea was subsequently extubated over a Cook Airway Exchange Catheter 2 hours after arrival in the postanesthesia care unit. The patient tolerated the airway exchange catheter, and maintained his own airway, with a SaO_2 >94% on 8 L/min of humidified oxygen. The repeat arterial blood gas analysis following extubation was within normal limits. Analgesia was administered using intravenous morphine, titrated to effect.

Discussion

Prone positioning during anesthesia is required to provide operative access for a wide variety of surgical procedures. This position is not only associated with predictable changes in physiology but also a number of complications [2]. The airway complications and management strategies are discussed in this chapter. For a patient to be positioned prone there is a potential risk of airway loss and for this reason, a definitive airway is established using an endotracheal tube. The complications that result from this position are typically due to application of either direct or indirect pressure to dependent parts of the body resulting in significant injuries to the upper airway.

Problems with extubation

1. Prone position can result in extensive facial edema, macroglossia, including the swelling of soft palate, pharynx, and arytenoids. Excessive flexion of the head and endotracheal tube obstructs the lingual and pharyngeal venous drainage. This can result in postoperative upper airway edema. Long operative time, blood loss, and administration of large volumes of crystalloid can make the facial and upper airway edema progressively worse [2, 3].
2. Although rare, the prone position can result in stretching and compression of the salivary ducts leading to painful swelling of the submandibular glands especially if the head is rotated [4]. This distorts the anatomy and the swelling of the soft tissue of the floor including the tongue can lead to partial or complete obstruction of the pharynx.
3. Tracheal extubation can also lead to an increase in systemic and intracranial pressures. Coughing, laryngospasm, and upper airway obstruction can occur after extubation.

Tracheal re-intubation poses significant challenges compared with the initial, elective intubations. The patients are more likely to be hypoxic, hypercapnic, and combative. Furthermore, oral secretions and vomit can make the glottic view more difficult. To manage such difficult airway scenarios, the anesthesiologist should have strategies for alternative airway techniques. The American Society of Anesthesiologists Task Force on Management of the Difficult Airway recommends that the anesthesiologist should have a preformulated strategy for extubation of a difficult airway [5]. The preformulated extubation strategy will depend, in part, on the surgery, the condition of the patient, and the skills and preferences of the anesthesiologist. A safe extubation strategy should aim to minimize risks and discomfort, maintain adequate oxygenation, ventilation and if the need arises, re-intubate without any complications. In complex spine surgeries, the main advantage of immediate recovery and extu-

bation is to allow earlier neurologic examination and establishment of a baseline to guide further examination. This also comes with early extubation risks of hypoxemia, hypercarbia, and compromised respiratory and hemodynamic status.

Airway assessment prior to extubation

Numerous attempts have been made to recognize and assess tracheal and oropharyngeal edema prior to extubation. The leak test and visual inspection of airway swelling are the most common risk assessment tests for extubation.

1. The "cuff-leak test" is performed by deflating the tracheal tube balloon, occluding the tracheal tube and assessing the air movement around the endotracheal tube [6]. Although not specific for predicting stridor, it appears that no or low leak volumes of air are reliably associated with an increased risk of upper airway obstruction. In such situations a decision to delay the extubation is prudent.
2. Flexible fiberoptic endoscopic exam should be used to directly assess edema and other causes of upper airway obstruction if any uncertainty exists with a cuff-leak test.
3. The spirometer on modern anesthesia machines can also be used to quantify leakage. It is calculated by the difference in the inspired and expired volumes.

Strategies for difficult extubation

1. Tracheal tube exchange catheter. If there is any appreciable risk of post-extubation airway obstruction, a tracheal tube exchange catheter should be used. In the event of airway obstruction, re-intubation can be achieved by introducing an endotracheal tube over the exchange catheter.
2. Laryngeal mask airway, flexible fiberoptic bronchoscope and Aintree catheter. The laryngeal mask airway has also been used with limited success. A flexible bronchoscope using the laryngeal mask airway and Aintree intubation catheter can also be used. There is an increased risk of bleeding due to upper airway edema making the technique difficult and challenging.
3. Deferred extubation in the recovery room or intensive care unit should be planned in the event

Table 50.1. Criteria for extubation following complex spine surgery in prone position.

Defer extubation	Consider extubation
Inability to open eyes and not obeying commands	Awake and obeying commands
Agitated or combative	Regular spontaneous breathing
Poor respiratory efforts	
O_2 saturation <94% on high flow O_2	O_2 saturation >94% on high flow O_2
Hypercarbic (PaCO$_2$ > 50 mmHg)	Normocapnic (PaCO$_2$ > 30 mmHg <50 mmHg)
Hemodynamically unstable	Hemodynamically stable
Hypothermic (<36 °C)	Normothermic
	Neuromuscular blockade completely reversed (TOF > 90%, sustained head lift and strong hand grip)
Operating time >10 hours	Operating time <10 hours
Blood transfusion >4 units	Blood transfusion of <4 units
Evidence of facial edema and macroglossia	
Negative "cuff-leak test"	Positive "cuff-leak test"
Evidence of pharyngeal and laryngeal edema on flexible fiberoptic bronchoscopy	No evidence of pharyngeal and laryngeal edema on flexible fiberoptic bronchoscopy

that the patient does not meet extubation criteria listed in Table 50.1. Extubation should be performed in a location where a full range of equipment, appropriate personnel, and all preparations (including surgical airway equipment) are available.

Conclusion

In conclusion, given the numerous complications unique to patients undergoing complex spine surgeries in the prone position, a systematic approach to extubation should begin as early as possible to optimize safe perioperative care.

References

1. **T. Asai, K. Koga, R. S. Vaughan**. Respiratory complications associated with tracheal intubation and extubation. *Br J Anaesth* 1998; **80**: 767–75.

2. **H. Edgcombe, K. Carter, S. Yarrow**. Anaesthesia in the prone position. *Br J Anaesth* 2008; **100**: 165–83.

3. **B. Kwon, J. U. Yoo, C. G. Furey** *et al.* Risk factors for delayed extubation after single-stage, multi-level anterior cervical decompression and posterior fusion. *J Spinal Disord Tech* 2006; **19**: 389–93.

4. **P. Hans, J. Demoitie, L. Collignon** *et al.* Acute bilateral submandibular swelling following surgery in prone position. *Eur J Anaesthesiol* 2006; **23**: 83–4.

5. **American Society of Anesthesiologists Task Force on Management of the Difficult Airway**. Practice guidelines for management of the difficult airway: an updated report by the American Society of Anesthesiologists Task Force on Management of the Difficult Airway. *Anesthesiology* 2003; **98**: 1269–77.

6. **R. J. Adderley, G. C. Mullins**. When to extubate the croup patient: the "leak" test. *Can J Anaesth* 1987; **34**: 304–6.

51 Perioperative peripheral nerve injury

Lisa Grilly, George A. Mashour and Chad M. Brummett

Neurosurgical procedures are often performed with patients in the prone, lateral, and other non-supine positions. This creates the risk of perioperative neurologic deficit due to peripheral nerve injury (PNI).

Case description

A 55-year-old female presented for scoliosis correction with posterior instrumentation at T5–L5. The case was performed under general anesthesia with neurophysiologic monitoring of somatosensory evoked potentials, motor evoked potentials, and electromyography. After induction and endotracheal intubation, the patient was positioned prone on a Jackson frame with her head in a Mayfield holder. Bilateral upper extremities were padded and positioned above the head. Baseline monitoring was established and anesthetic maintenance consisted of 50% nitrous oxide and isoflurane (minimum alveolar concentration 0.3–0.4), as well as sufentanil and dexmedetomidine infusions. During the surgery, there were episodes of diminished motor evoked potentials of the right upper extremity, which reversed with repositioning and additional padding of the arm. During periods of acute blood loss there was also concern about hypotension affecting the monitoring, which was discussed among the surgery, anesthesia, and neurophysiology monitoring teams. The case lasted a total of 9 hours and estimated blood loss was 2 liters. The patient received one unit of packed red blood cells and one unit of fresh frozen plasma. At the end of the case the trachea was extubated without complication. Right upper extremity weakness was found immediately after emergence. The initial postoperative neurologic examination showed 2/5 right hand grip, 2/5 right wrist extension, 1/5 right biceps, 1/5 right triceps, and 3/5 right deltoid strength. The patient was presumed to have a right brachial plexus injury and was started on dexamethasone. Neurology and physical therapy were consulted after admission to the neurosurgical intensive care unit. The patient's right upper

extremity strength gradually improved to a maximum of 4/5 throughout by postoperative day 8, and she was discharged that day to an acute rehabilitation center.

Discussion

Perioperative peripheral nerve injury can be a devastating complication, resulting in motor dysfunction and the sequelae of lower motor neuron disease. Nerve injuries comprise approximately 15% of claims in the most recent American Society of Anesthesiologists closed claims analysis [1], a proportion unchanged from a prior study [2]. The lack of improvement over approximately a 10-year period indicates the need for a better understanding of both the etiology and prevention of PNI. Mechanisms for peripheral neuropathy include compression, stretch, ischemia, metabolic abnormalities, and direct trauma. The "double crush" hypothesis of Upton and McComas suggests that the nerve is subject to two insults that lead to neuropathy, the first insult rendering it less tolerant of the second [3]. In the surgical milieu, this would imply that preoperative co-morbidities might make peripheral nerves more vulnerable to perioperative adverse events that might otherwise be tolerated.

A recent study by Welch et al. demonstrated that diabetes mellitus, hypertension, and tobacco use were preexisting patient factors that were associated with PNI [4]. All three of these risk factors may compromise microvascular circulation, rendering peripheral nerves more susceptible to modes of perioperative injury associated with ischemia. General and epidural anesthesia were also found to be associated with PNI, in contrast to monitored anesthesia care, spinal anesthesia, and peripheral nerve block [4]. What may be most striking with respect to the present case is that, among approximately 20 surgical services, neurosurgery had one of the strongest associations with PNI. It is important to note that the nerve injuries reported in this investigation were *not* due to a surgical or preexisting neurologic etiology, but were likely related to positioning and patient co-morbidities. Neurosurgery was associated with a 2.7-fold risk of PNI (95% confidence interval 1.4–5.1); only cardiac surgery was comparable with a hazard ratio of 2.8 (95% confidence interval 1.3–5.7).

Conclusion

The present case and the recent study by Welch *et al.* [4] demonstrate that neurosurgical procedures are associated with significant risk for PNI. These injuries are distressing for patients and may mask or exacerbate underlying pathology related to the central nervous system. Vigilance with respect to positioning and appropriate padding of pressure points is critical, especially in patients with diabetes mellitus, hypertension, and a history of tobacco use. Neurophysiologic monitoring may aid in the intraoperative detection of injury and should be taken seriously. Evidence of PNI should prompt an evaluation by neurology, as well as the involvement of physical and occupational therapy.

References

1. **F. W. Cheney, K. B. Domino, R. A. Caplan, K. L. Posner**. Nerve injury associated with anesthesia: a closed claims analysis. *Anesthesiology* 1999; **90**: 1062–9.

2. **D. A. Kroll, R. A. Caplan, K. Posner, R. J. Ward, F. W. Cheney**. Nerve injury associated with anesthesia. *Anesthesiology* 1990; **73**: 202–7.

3. **A. R. Upton, A. J. McComas**. The double crush in nerve entrapment syndromes. *Lancet* 1973; **18**: 359–62.

4. **M. B. Welch, C. M. Brummett, T. D. Welch** *et al.* Perioperative peripheral nerve injuries: a retrospective study of 380,680 cases during a 10-year period at a single institution. *Anesthesiology* 2009; **111**: 490–7.

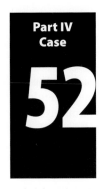
Unstable cervical spine

David L. Adams and David W. Healy

Each year in the USA there are approximately 10 000 new cases of spinal injury and the cervical spine is most commonly affected. Young adult males have the highest incidence of injury, with motor vehicle accidents accounting for 50% of cases; violent assault, falls, and sporting injuries account for the remainder.

The incidence of cervical spine injury in blunt trauma is approximately 2–4%. The incidence is increased if there is an associated head injury with a Glasgow Coma Scale (GCS) score of <8 or if there is a focal neurologic abnormality. Up to 10% of patients with a cervical spine injury will suffer a neurologic deterioration while in the hospital. The term *secondary injury* refers to a deterioration or new injury following the initial injury. The mechanism of injury responsible for the deterioration is often unclear. Secondary neurologic injuries occurring in the perioperative period are important as they are potentially avoidable.

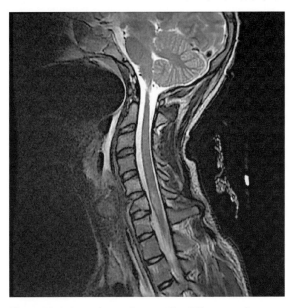

Figure 52.1. Injured cervical spine with a C6 fracture and spinal cord contusion revealed by magnetic resonance imaging (T2 weighted).

Case description

A 27-year-old male was an unrestrained front-seat passenger in a motor vehicle accident. He was extracted from the vehicle and immobilized on a spinal board, with rigid cervical collar, sandbags and tape. On evaluation in the emergency room he was found to have head and facial injuries with bleeding from the nose and mouth. His GCS score was 12 (M5, V4, E3). There was bruising to the anterior chest wall and abdominal distention with a heart rate of 125 beats per minute and a blood pressure of 90/55 mmHg. Due to hemodynamic instability and a deteriorating level of consciousness, urgent airway control was deemed necessary. The anterior portion of the cervical collar was removed, manual in-line stabilization (MILS) maintained and cricoid pressure was applied. The trachea was intubated following a rapid sequence induction with propofol and succinylcholine. In an attempt to maintain cardiovascular stability he received intra-

venous crystalloid and a bolus dose of phenylephrine around the time of anesthetic induction. Definitive imaging of the head and spine was deferred until after the patient had undergone urgent surgical management of his abdominal injuries. On the first postoperative day he was suitably stable to undergo imaging and was found to have a fracture at C6 with spinal cord contusion revealed by magnetic resonance imaging (Figure 52.1).

Discussion

The key aspects of anesthesia care for this patient were (1) rapid definitive airway control, (2) protection of neural structures from secondary injury, and (3) adequate intravenous access and fluid resuscitation. Endotracheal intubation with controlled ventilation is a common aspect of the initial care of patients with severe trauma. This may be essential for airway protection and ventilation following neurologic deficit, or be required for the operative management of other injuries. The anesthesia provider must maintain the mechanical integrity of the spinal cord by limiting neck movement, as well as ensure adequate spinal cord perfusion by avoiding hypotension and subsequent tissue hypoxia. The immobilization of the spine in trauma patients until injuries have either been excluded or definitively treated remains a cornerstone of modern trauma care. The introduction of spinal immobilization techniques in pre-hospital care has dramatically reduced the incidence of secondary spinal cord injury. The most effective technique is with a backboard, rigid collar, sandbags, and tape. These techniques reduce cervical spine motion to approximately 5% of the normal range.

It has been demonstrated that basic airway maneuvers such as chin lift, jaw thrust, and placement of both oral and nasal airways cause movement of cervical spine segments. This is seen in both the intact and injured cervical spine and is not completely prevented by the application of cervical collars. The use of immobilization techniques reduces but does not eliminate spinal movement associated with basic airway interventions. Even mask ventilation may lead to cervical spine displacement. The application of cricoid pressure has not been shown to cause significant movement of cervical spine segments in either stable or unstable models.

In injured, as well as uninjured patients, direct laryngoscopy causes significant motion of cervical spinal segments, particularly in the upper cervical spine. Manual in-line stabilization has been found to be the most effective method of limiting cervical spine distraction during direct laryngoscopy, though it does not eliminate movement altogether [1]. Historically, other methods have been attempted but result in increased movement at laryngoscopy.

While MILS limits the motion of injured spinal segments, it can worsen the view during direct laryngoscopy. However, this view is better than that obtained in those patients immobilized with collar, sandbag, and tape [2]. The use of a collar significantly limits neck extension and mouth opening, which are essential for optimizing the view obtained at laryngoscopy. During direct laryngoscopy one may remove the anterior part of the cervical collar while maintaining MILS. The consequences of failed airway control and resultant hypoxia can be devastating, and if an

adequate view of the glottis cannot be obtained, it is considered permissible to relax manual stabilization to the degree required to intubate the trachea. The use of adjuncts such as the gum elastic bougie should be encouraged in such circumstances to minimize neck movement. The use of both straight and curved laryngoscope blades causes a comparable amount of spine movement and there is no evidence to favor one blade over the other.

In an attempt to optimize the view at laryngoscopy while maintaining MILS, alternative airway instruments have been evaluated. The intubating stylets (e.g., Bonfils, Lightwand) and indirect video laryngoscopes (e.g., Bullard, Glidescope) have been studied in patients in spinal immobilization. These techniques allow a view of the glottis that does not rely upon neck extension and the alignment of the airway axes. Additionally, it has been suggested that less force may be required during the procedure. The use of the Bullard, in particular, has been shown to result in less cervical movement that direct laryngoscopy [3], but the other methods (notably the Glidescope) cause the same degree, or greater, of cervical distraction. In general, these techniques have been found to take longer than direct laryngoscopy even in practiced hands. The increased time to intubation can be attributed to the increased complexity of passing an endotracheal tube out of the line of sight. The use of extraglottic airway devices, such as the laryngeal mask airway cause less cervical spine movement than direct laryngoscopy. However, their placement may specifically displace a destabilized upper cervical segment. The clinical relevance of this remains uncertain.

Flexible fiberoptic laryngoscopy causes the least movement and angulation of the spine [4], and in the elective situation has become the method of choice. A higher degree of skill is required when compared with other techniques, and even in experienced hands the time taken for intubation is increased. In North America anesthesiologists have expressed a preference for this technique in patients with suspected spinal injuries, although some of the same practitioners question their own competence with the technique. Even in alert, cooperative patients, oxygen desaturation during attempts at awake fiberoptic intubation is well reported and is clearly an undesirable event in the setting of acute neurologic injury. Furthermore, blood or other debris in the airway can make the use of the fiberoptic laryngoscope extremely difficult. In this setting, the lightwand is beneficial and is associated with less

Table 52.1. Key management points in a patient with suspected cervical spine injury.

Cervical spine injury occurs in 2–4% of victims of blunt trauma, and is particularly associated with head injury. This incidence is increased if the Glasgow Coma Scale is <8 or there is a focal neurologic deficit
"Basic" airway techniques such as chin lift, jaw thrust and mask ventilation can also cause cervical displacement
The presence of a cervical collar limits mouth opening and consistently worsens the view obtained at laryngoscopy. The anterior part of the collar may be removed to facilitate direct laryngoscopy
The use of manual in-line stabilization limits, but does not completely prevent, the movement of injured spinal segments during airway interventions, but is still the technique of choice compared with the other methods
No single intubation technique has been shown to be superior to any others. The available evidence suggests a favorable safety profile with all techniques. Achieving rapid airway control while minimizing hypoxia and hypotension should be primary goals

cervical spine mobility than direct laryngoscopy or the Glidescope.

The degree of movement and angulation in spinal segments with any of these intubation techniques is of uncertain clinical significance. While flexible fiberoptic laryngoscopy causes the least amount of movement, it is not always the most appropriate technique. In the emergency room setting, timely placement of an endotracheal tube with prevention of hypoxia is vital and the technique should be chosen with consideration of the clinical state of the patient, as well as the skill and experience of the laryngoscopist.

The evidence does not support the use of any one technique over another [5]. All types of laryngoscopy have a favorable safety profile and the incidence of proven neurologic deterioration attributable to airway management is extremely low. Table 52.1 summarizes key points in the management of patients with cervical spine injury.

References

1. **M. C. Gerling, D. P. Davis, R. S. Hamilton** et al. Effects of cervical spine immobilization technique and laryngoscope blade selection on an unstable cervical spine in a cadaver model of intubation. *Ann Emerg Med* 2000; **36**: 293–300.

2. **K. J. Heath.** The effect on laryngoscopy of different cervical spine immobilization techniques. *Anaesthesia* 1994; **49**: 843–5.

3. **R. H. Hastings, A. C. Vigil, R. Hanna** et al. Cervical spine movement during laryngoscopy with the Bullard, Macintosh and Miller laryngoscopes. *Anesthesiology* 1995; **82**: 859–69.

4. **J. Brimacombe, C. Keller, K. H. Künzel** et al. Cervical spine motion during airway management; a cinefluoroscopic study of the posteriorly destabilized third cervical vertebrae in human cadavers. *Anesth Analg* 2000; **91**: 1274–8.

5. **E. T. Crosby.** Airway management in adults after cervical spine trauma. *Anesthesiology* 2006; **104**: 1293–318.

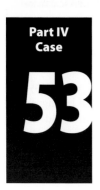

Part IV Case

Spine surgery. Cervical spine and airway issues

53 Cervical spine limitations

David L. Adams and David W. Healy

Cervical spine mobility is central to the conventional safe management of the airway. The term *cervical spine limitations* (CSL) refers to a range of limitations to neck mobility including limited extension, flexion or both, and known or suspected unstable cervical spine conditions requiring immobilization with a cervical collar or halo. Limitations of cervical spine mobility are common in patients presenting for neurosurgery, but are not confined to this group; the incidence across all adults at a tertiary care center in the USA has been estimated at approximately 8% [1]. Congenital causes include Klippel–Feil syndrome (characterized by fusion of two or more cervical vertebrae) and Goldenhar syndrome (a type of mandibular hypoplasia associated with underdeveloped vertebrae, often in the neck). Acquired causes are mainly degenerative diseases (osteoarthritis, degenerative disc disease), inflammatory processes (rheumatoid arthritis, ankylosing spondylitis), trauma, and prior surgical fusion (see Table 53.1).

Case description

A 68-year-old male with severe ankylosing spondylitis sustained a fracture through the C6 vertebral body following a fall. Despite an initial period of immobilization in a halo jacket, he experienced persistent pain and deformity, and was therefore scheduled for a C3–T4 posterior instrumentation and vertebral column resection. In addition to the ankylosing spondylitis, the patient's medical history was significant for hypertension, type 2 diabetes with peripheral sensory neuropathy, peripheral vascular disease, and symptomatic gastroesophageal reflux disease. Physical examination showed mild symmetrical sensory neuropathy in both feet, but no motor deficit. Airway examination demonstrated a marked cervical kyphosis ("chin-on-chest-deformity") with severe limitation of both flexion and extension. Although the patient was edentulous, mouth opening was limited, the Mallampati class was

Table 53.1. Causes of cervical spine limitations.

Congenital
Klippel–Feil syndrome
Goldenhar syndrome
Diffuse idiopathic hyperostosis (DISH)
Acquired
Osteoarthritis
Degenerative disc disease
Fracture/trauma
Surgical fusion
Scoliosis
Rheumatoid arthritis
Ankylosing spondylitis

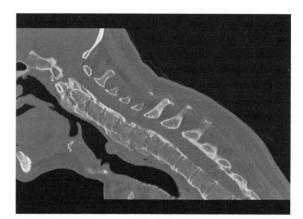

Figure 53.1. Sagittal plane computed tomography image of the cervical spine showing a transverse fracture through C6 and typical appearances of a "bamboo spine."

IV, and there was limited mandibular protrusion. The thyromental distance was 3 cm. A computed tomography (CT) image is shown in Figure 53.1.

In view of the potential difficulties with airway management and presence of symptomatic reflux disease, an awake fiberoptic intubation technique was chosen. A peripheral venous line and a radial arterial catheter were placed under local anesthesia and gly-copyrrolate 200 mcg was administered intravenously. Topicalization of the airway with 4% lidocaine was then started in preparation for awake fiberoptic intubation. The patient was connected to standard monitors, including invasive blood pressure, and oxygen was administered at 2 liters per minute through nasal canulae. Once adequate airway anesthesia had been achieved, a remifentanil infusion was started at 0.01 mcg/kg/minute, and oral fiberoptic intubation was commenced. The remifentanil infusion was adjusted to a maximum of 0.05 mcg/kg/minute, guided by the arterial blood pressure, respiratory rate, and the degree of sedation. Supplementary airway anesthesia was provided in a "spray-as-you-go" technique. Intubation of the trachea and placement of a size 7.0 cuffed tracheal tube were uneventful with no episodes of desaturation and no significant deviation in the blood pressure from baseline. The patient was awake and comfortable and a gross assessment of neurologic function was carried out before the induction of general anesthesia.

The patient was positioned in the prone position with care taken to avoid cervical spine extension and to preserve the alignment of the cervico-thoracic spine, to the extent that was possible given the underlying deformity. The blood pressure was maintained at pre-induction values at all times. At the end of surgery, the patient once again demonstrated neurologic integrity; however, extubation was deferred until the following morning, to allow for airway edema to resolve and a leak around the tube cuff to develop. There were no airway sequelae following extubation.

Discussion

Ankylosing spondylitis is a seronegative spondyloarthropathy strongly associated with the HLA-B27 genotype. Recurrent painful inflammatory flares involve the axial skeleton and sacroiliac joints, leading to progressive bony fusion of adjacent vertebral segments causing the characteristic fixed kyphotic "bamboo spine." Ankylosing spondylitis also affects other parts of the musculoskeletal system and has associations with diseases in many organ systems (see Table 53.2).

The rigidity of the fused spine makes it vulnerable to damage and fractures can occur following apparently minor injuries. Hyperextension of the cervical spine is commonly associated with fractures at the C5–

Table 53.2. Common clinical features and disease associations of ankylosing spondylitis.

Musculoskeletal system
Spinal fusion and rigidity ("bamboo spine")
Atlanto-axial instability
Sacroiliitis
Peripheral arthritis (hips, knees, temperomandibular, costovertebral, and costochondral joints)
Achilles tendonitis
Plantar fasciitis
Other systems
Neurologic – Spinal cord and nerve root compression, vertebrobasilar insufficiency
Cardiovascular – Aortic valve insufficiency and cardiac conduction defects
Pulmonary – Upper lobe fibrosis
Gastrointestinal – Inflammatory bowel disease
Occular – Anterior uveitis
Skin – Psoriasis
Genitourinary – Prostatitis

6 level. Common causes include falls and motor vehicle accidents. Iatrogenic causes also should be considered; poor patient positioning in the operating room can easily cause neurologic damage in these vulnerable patients.

The purpose of the preoperative airway assessment is to predict, as accurately as possible, the degree of difficulty that will be encountered during mask ventilation and tracheal intubation. The failure to intubate combined with failure to adequately ventilate is rightly feared by anesthesiologists. It should be remembered that prolonged or forceful attempts to perform direct laryngoscopy and intubation may cause trauma to either the airway or to the cervical spine and cord, particularly in a patient with preexisting cervical spine pathology.

The assessment of the range of cervical spine motion is a routine part of preoperative airway evaluation. Many patients with CSL will have a reduced range of extension at the occipito-atlanto-axial (OAA) complex, which is vital for maximal mouth opening. Therefore, these patients may demonstrate a reduced interincisor distance, an increased Mallampati score, and reduced mandibular protrusion. The Mallampati classification (with the head in the neutral position, and tongue maximally protruded) can be modified in normal patients to include an assessment of mouth opening and tongue protrusion at maximal cranio-cervical extension (Extended Mallampati Score) [2]. The Extended Mallampati Score increases the positive predictive value of the examination and reduces false positives. In normal patients the facilitation of mouth opening afforded by extension at the OAA complex can decrease the modified Mallampati score; this may not be seen in patients with CSL.

The incidence of difficult or impossible mask ventilation in patients with CSL when compared with normal controls is increased. A Mallampati classification of III or IV, limited jaw protrusion and a thyromental distance of less than 6 cm are features that can be found in association with CSL, and have been found to be predictive of difficult or impossible mask ventilation [3]. The incidences of difficult laryngoscopy [4] and difficult intubation [5] are more common in patients with CSL. It has also been demonstrated that significant increases in the incidences of *both* difficult laryngoscopy *and* intubation are found in CSL due in part to the difficulty in positioning the patient.

Patients with a known or potentially unstable cervical spine and those in cervical collars or halo traction will generally be immobilized in the neutral position. Intubation difficulties in these patients are principally related to the lack of extension at the OAA complex. In patients that do not require immobilization in the neutral position, the conventional positions for direct laryngoscopy are with the head extended at the OAA complex, or with the head extended at the OAA complex *and* the cervical spine flexed at the thoraco-cervical junction (the "sniffing position"). The sniffing position gives rise to a greater degree of extension at the OAA complex [6], and in patients with limited cervical spine extension (and in the obese), this has been shown to be particularly advantageous [7].

When difficulty with direct laryngoscopy is anticipated, a number of options are available to the anesthesiologist. There is an increasing role for novel direct and indirect video-assisted airway management devices in enabling the practitioner to "look around the corner" to facilitate tracheal tube placement. The common incidence of difficult mask ventilation in patients with CSL should lead to caution when considering these techniques, as their use usually requires induction of general anesthesia. There are some descriptions of their use in unanesthetized,

spontaneously breathing patients – but these are case reports and very small case series.

Awake fiberoptic intubation is the most popular technique for definitive airway control in patients with an unstable or limited cervical spine. This method was performed in this case as it involved an elective procedure, which gave adequate time for careful preparation. Even in an emergent situation the method of awake fiberoptic intubation should be considered on a risk–benefit basis. Awake fiberoptic intubation also allows the assessment of gross neurologic function after tracheal tube placement. It is therefore desirable to use a technique which allows adequate patient comfort and airway control, while avoiding over sedation during the intubation process. The technique requires patient cooperation and adequate airway topicalization. Our patient was pre-treated with glycopyrrolate, which reduces secretions and dries the mucosa of the upper airway. This enhances the speed and effectiveness of topical lidocaine, and has the added benefit of preventing a bradycardia which may occur with the subsequent use of remifentanil. There are numerous described techniques for the topicalization of the airway and the conduct of awake fiberoptic intubation. These are technical skills that are best learned at the bedside under the instruction of an experienced practitioner.

Remifentanil was used as an adjuvant during the awake fiberoptic intubation. It is rapidly titratable and suppresses the urge to cough and gag, while verbal contact with the patient can be maintained. Infusion should be started at very low rates and titrated gently to effect. A loading dose should be avoided as it can cause apnea, so infusions should start several minutes before airway instrumentation to allow the achievement of steady-state plasma drug levels. Rapidly increasing the rate of infusion can cause over-sedation and subsequent apnea and desaturation. It is therefore not recommended. Unanticipated hypotension, hypoxia and over-sedation are adverse events that are well reported, and the presence of two practitioners at the time of intubation should be encouraged. While one anesthesiologist conducts the fiberoptic intubation, the second can administer sedation while monitoring the patient's level of consciousness, blood pressure, and oxygenation.

The patient presented in this case demonstrated several of the features that predict difficulty in airway management. Furthermore, the "chin-on-chest-deformity" would have prevented the formation of a surgical airway. Awake flexible fiberoptic intubation is considered to be the gold standard in this challenging patient group.

References

1. **G. A. Mashour, M. L. Stallmer, S. Kheterpal** *et al.* Predictors of difficult intubation in patients with cervical spine limitations. *J Neurosurg Anesthesiol* 2008; **20**: 110–15.

2. **G. A. Mashour, W. S. Sandberg**. Craniocervical extension improves the specificity and predictive value of the Mallampati airway evaluation. *Anesth Analg* 2006; **103**: 1256–9.

3. **S. Kheterpal, R. Han, K. K. Tremper** *et al.* Incidence and predictors of difficult and impossible

4. **I. Calder, J. Calder, H. A. Crockard**. Difficult direct laryngoscopy in patients with cervical spine disease. *Anaesthesia* 1995; **50**: 756–63.

5. **K. Karkouti, D. K. Rose, D. Wigglesworth** *et al.* Predicting difficult intubation: a multivariable analysis. *Can J Anaesth* 2000; **47**: 730–9.

6. **I. Takenaka, K. Aoyama, T. Iwagaki** *et al.* The sniffing position provides greater occipito-atlanto-axial angulation than simple head extension: a radiological study. *Can J Anaesth* 2007; **54**: 129–33.

7. **F. Adnet, C. Baillard, S. W. Borron** *et al.* Randomized study comparing the "sniffing position" with simple head extension for laryngoscopic view in elective surgery patients. *Anesthesiology* 2001; **95**: 836–41.

mask ventilation. *Anesthesiology* 2006; **105**: 885–91.

Spine surgery. Cervical spine and airway issues

Rheumatoid disease

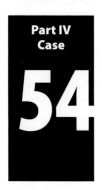

David L. Adams and David W. Healy

Rheumatoid arthritis (RA) is a progressive symmetrical, deforming inflammatory polyarthropathy with numerous extra-articular features. It is a common condition, with prevalence in the USA of approximately 1%, affecting females three times more commonly than males. The skeletal effects of RA are characterized by an inflammatory synovitis with progressive destruction of cartilage. Over time, ankylosis of joints occurs, causing stiffness and reduced range of motion. The small joints of the hands and feet are most commonly involved; however, any joint can be affected. The cervical spine complications of RA can lead to instability and limitation of motion, and surgery is commonly required for stabilization and correction of deformity. The cervical instability and limitation of movement (including prior surgical stabilization) must be carefully considered before anesthetizing this patient group.

Case description

A 62-year-old female with seropositive rheumatoid arthritis presented for anterior cervical discectomy and fusion for long-term progressive pain and upper extremity myelopathy. The patient described worsening intermittent tingling and increasing, symmetrical, arm weakness. Airway examination in the neutral position revealed reduced mouth opening (<3 cm), a Mallampati class III examination, and severely limited neck extension. Blood pressure was 140/90 mmHg and body weight was 60 kg.

Preoperative imaging consisted of plain radiographs and magnetic resonance imaging of the cervical spine. These demonstrated spinal stenosis at C5/6 due to a posterior disc bulge, and erosive changes at the occipito-atlanto-axial (OAA) complex, typical of severe rheumatoid disease.

In view of the degree of cervical spine pathology, an awake fiberoptic intubation was planned. This was performed uneventfully and a neurologic examination

after tracheal tube placement showed that no deterioration had occurred. General anesthesia was then induced.

The patient was positioned supine and the head was supported on a Mayfield ring. Great care was taken to ensure that the neck was in a neutral position. The intraoperative course was uneventful with maintenance of blood pressure at or around pre-induction values.

At the end of the case, the patient was awakened but remained intubated to allow neurologic status to be re-evaluated before extubation. This was satisfactory and the airway was then assessed for the presence of swelling and edema with the endotracheal tube cuff deflated. No significant leak was detected so the decision was made to leave the trachea intubated and sedated and transferred to the neurosurgical intensive care unit. Twelve hours later the trachea was uneventfully extubated after the airway swelling had improved.

Discussion

This case illustrates several important issues that must be considered when identifying the airway management options for patients with cervical spine pathology. A careful history and examination are vital to establish the range of symptom-free neck movement and elucidate symptoms and signs of possible nerve impingement or spinal cord compression. Closely allied to this is a formal examination of the airway.

The effect of RA on the cervical spine is typified by a combination of structural instability and stiffness [1]. The instability is due to progressive erosion of bone and ligaments, and the stiffness due to chronic inflammation, thickening, and calcification. This case exhibited both features. In addition to limiting neck extension and causing potential instability, RA may disrupt both the temporomandibular joints and

Normal

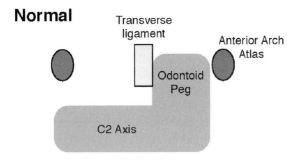

Subluxation

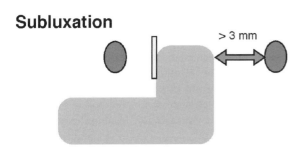

Figure 54.1. Diagram representing the radiological changes associated with degradation of the transverse ligament and resulting atlantoaxial subluxation.

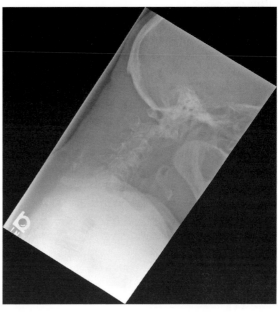

Figure 54.2. Lateral C spine X-ray demonstrating atlantoaxial subluxation.

laryngeal cartilage articulations. Pain on mastication or mouth opening may indicate temporomandibular joint disease. A history of increasingly hoarse voice may suggest disease affecting the arytenoid cartilages. Along with the cervical stiffening and bony degeneration associated with RA, atlantoaxial instability is of particular concern. Ligamentous degradation around the OAA complex, particularly of the transverse ligament, can lead to atlantoaxial subluxation. The transverse ligament of the axis links the lateral masses of the atlas and loops around the odontoid process holding it firmly in contact with the anterior arch of the atlas. With degradation of this ligament the odontoid process becomes free to move, bringing the axis with it resulting in atlantoaxial subluxation. The displaced odontoid process can compress the spinal cord or medulla and damage the vertebral arteries.

It is well known that atlantoaxial instability can be completely asymptomatic, but there is little consensus regarding mandatory cervical spine imaging for patients with RA undergoing surgery. A reasonable approach is to obtain flexion and extension views of the cervical spine preoperatively for all patients with neurologic symptoms and for those taking regu-

lar steroids or disease-modifying antirheumatic drugs (e.g., methotrexate). The normal distance between the anterior edge of the odontoid process and the posterior border of the anterior arch of the atlas should be less than 3 mm; any increase is pathological (Figure 54.1). Imaging was obtained preoperatively in this case. The best way to identify a widening of the atlanto-odontoid space is on a lateral cervical X-ray taken in flexion (Figure 54.2); alternatively it can be imaged by computed tomography scans (Figure 54.3) or magnetic resonance imaging.

When considering the airway options for a patient with disease at the OAA complex an appreciation of the importance of this area in overall airway management is essential. Extension at the OAA complex is important for both basic airway management such as "chin lift" and mask ventilation as well as to facilitate direct laryngoscopy. Neck extension may be limited by disease or iatrogenic externally applied stabilization (e.g., manual in-line stabilization). The efficacy of the sniffing position, to facilitate the view at direct laryngoscopy, is thought to be due to its ability to maximize the degree of extension at the OAA complex. Adequate mouth opening is important for successful airway management, for which neck extension is essential [2].

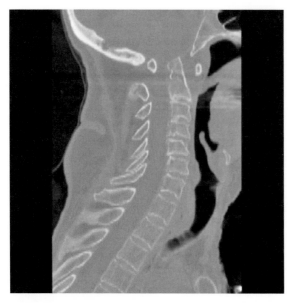

Figure 54.3. Computed tomography demonstrating atlantoaxial subluxation.

Rheumatoid arthritis can also cause pathological changes in the lower cervical spine. During cervical spine extension, there can be posterior disc protrusion and buckling of the ligamentum flavum. These changes may cause cord impingement in the neutral position. Therefore, any additional extension (and to a lesser extent, flexion) may increase spinal cord compression. Cord injury may be produced by mechanical deformation, ischemia or both.

To prevent damage to neurologic structures it is desirable to maintain the cervical spine in a neutral position. This may be different for each patient and care should be taken to enlist the patient's cooperation in finding the most comfortable neck position. Some practitioners advocate positioning the patient for surgery before the induction of general anesthesia, though this may present difficulties, particularly if the patient is to be in the prone position. The prone position often causes a degree of cervical spine extension, which should be minimized as much as possible.

Awake fiberoptic intubation is the most popular technique for definitive airway control in patients with an unstable or limited cervical spine [3]. This method is associated with the least amount of cervical spine movement, and in our patient, extension was completely avoided at the OAA complex. Preoperative assessment of this patient demonstrated limited mouth opening, and a Mallampati class III assessment,

strongly indicative of limited extension at the OAA complex. In very severe temporomandibular joint disease it may be impossible to pass an oral endotracheal tube and the nasal route should instead be used. Direct laryngoscopy in our patient could have either caused cord injury at the site of an unstable OAA complex, or failure to achieve an adequate view of the glottis due to a severe limitation of spinal extension. A role has been suggested for indirect video laryngoscopy in this clinical setting, but its efficacy is unproven beyond an improvement in glottic view [4].

This patient was awakened at the end of the procedure, and a further neurologic examination performed. The examination was comparable with that performed before induction of anesthesia, though it should be appreciated that this can only ever be a crude assessment of neurologic function. Most practitioners would wait until this gross assessment of neurologic function had been completed before extubating the trachea, as a worsening of function may precipitate the need for urgent imaging or re-operation. At the preoperative visit patients should be warned that they may awake with a "breathing tube" in place and asked to perform simple tasks on command (e.g., "Squeeze hands" etc.). They should be reassured that they will be comfortable and relaxed and the tube will soon be removed.

The trachea in this case, however, was not extubated at the end of the procedure. This was due to the absence of a leak around the deflated tracheal tube cuff, suggesting airway edema and soft tissue swelling. This should always be considered at the end of cervical spine surgery and cases in which the patient has been positioned in the prone or head-down position [5]. Such patients should remain intubated and re-sedated if necessary and periodically re-evaluated for evidence of resolution of the swelling. The head-up position and the use of corticosteroids may accelerate the resolution of edema.

Conclusion

This case typifies some of the challenges encountered by the anesthesiologist when managing the airway in a patient with rheumatoid arthritis and limited cervical spine motion. Careful preoperative evaluation and planning are essential; adequate time and personnel should be allocated to securing the airway in a controlled and safe manner. Finally, it should be noted that extubation is a high-risk time for these patients and that a plan should be made to ensure this is performed safely and at the appropriate time.

References

1. **A. MacArthur, S. Kleimann**. Rheumatoid cervical joint disease – a challenge to the anaesthetist. *Can J Anaesth* 1993; **40**: 154–9.

2. **I. Calder, J. Calder, H. A. Crockard**. Difficult direct laryngoscopy in patients with cervical spine disease. *Anaesthesia* 1995; **50**: 756–63.

3. **E. T. Crosby**. Considerations for airway management for cervical spine surgery in adults. *Anesthesiol Clin* 2007; **25**: 511–33.

4. **A. D. Watts, A. W. Gelb, D. B. Bach** et al. Comparison of Bullard and Macintosh laryngoscopes for endotracheal intubation of patients with a potential cervical spine injury. *Anesthesiology* 1997; **87**: 1335–42.

5. **H. C. Sagi, W. Beutler, E. Carroll** et al. Airway complications associated with surgery on the anterior cervical spine. *Spine* 2002; **27**: 949–53.

Preoperative evaluation

Nicholas F. Marko and Robert J. Weil

Preoperative evaluation of patients presenting for transphenoidal resection of pituitary tumors is a very complex process, requiring careful assessment of the patient's symptoms and the proper preoperative laboratory tests. The pituitary tumor can be a secretory tumor or a nonsecretory tumor. The following cases will highlight the proper preoperative evaluation for different types of pituitary tumors.

Case description 1

History: A 32-year-old male was referred for evaluation of a possible neuroendocrine disorder. The patient had a 7-year history of hyperlipidemia managed with a statin medication as well as hypertension that had been controlled with a diuretic and an ACE-inhibitor. He had required multiple increases in the dosages of these medications over the past several years. The patient reported no acute symptoms and had no new complaints. On careful questioning he reported that he had limited exercise tolerance (he could only walk 2–3 blocks without resting) and had daily "arthritis in my back, knees and shoulders." He felt that this was because he had always been "a big man," and he noted that he has had limited success with attempts at weight control with diet and exercise in the past. He knows he should exercise more because he has been told he is a "borderline diabetic." He denied headache, recent, unintentional weight changes, heat or cold intolerance, polyuria, polydypsia, or galactorrhea. His medical history was remarkable for hypertension and hyperlipidemia, as well as sleep apnea since age 25 for which he used nightly continuous positive airway pressure (CPAP) therapy. His only surgical history was bilateral carpal tunnel release 2 years ago, "because I type all day at work." His medications included hydrochlorothiazide 25 mg QD, lisinopril 20 mg QD, and atorvastatin 40 mg QD. He was a nonsmoker.

Examination: He was a 32-year-old man in no distress, although he appeared mildly diaphoretic. He was

178 cm tall and weighed 95.5 kg (BMI 30). He was neurologically intact, including no visual field deficits, no cranial neuropathies, and no other focal neurologic deficits. His skin appeared thickened and his facial features were coarse. Scars from his carpal tunnel surgery were noted bilaterally, and his radial pulses were difficult to palpate because his hands and wrists were large. The remainder of his physical exam was unremarkable and was notable for the absence of galactorrhea, buffalo hump, or abdominal striae.

Radiology: Gadolinium-enhanced magnetic resonance imaging (MRI) demonstrated a 7-mm, well-circumscribed area of diminished enhancement within an otherwise-normal anterior pituitary gland. There was no compression of the optic apparatus and no hydrocephalus. The remainder of the MRI was unremarkable.

Laboratory evaluation: Laboratory tests were obtained as shown in Table 55.1. Normal values are indicated in parentheses.

Diagnosis: Acromegaly – growth hormone secreting pituitary microadenoma.

Discussion: Acromegaly is the clinical syndrome associated with abnormally elevated growth hormone (GH) levels. It is a slowly progressive disease, so there is often a period of years between the onset of symptoms and the final diagnosis. Patients with acromegaly classically exhibit coarse facial features, acral enlargement, and thickened skin [1]. These changes give rise to several classic associated findings, including carpal tunnel syndrome (often bilateral) and obstructive sleep apnea. Joint arthropathies and calcific spinal disc disease are also common in patients with acromegaly. Cardiovascular manifestations include hypertension, cardiomyopathy, ventricular hypertrophy, arrhythmias, and cerebrovascular disease, while endocrinologic findings include diabetes and hyperparathyroidism. Patients are also prone to malignancy, particularly those of the colon and pancreas. Because of these effects of GH excess on

Table 55.1. Laboratory results for patient in case description 1.

CBC:	Normal	FSH:	2 mU/mL (0–10 mU/mL)
BMP:	Fasting glucose 112 mg/dL (<100 mg/dL)	LH:	1 mU/mL (<7 mU/mL)
Prolactin:	15 ng/μL (2–17 ng/μL)	GH:	2.8 ng/mL (0–3 ng/mL)
TSH:	0.750 μU/mL (0.500–5.500 μU/mL)	IGF-1:	937 ng/mL (117–329 ng/mL)
Free T4:	1.0 ng/dL (0.7–1.8 ng/dL)	Total cortisol, 07:00	17 mcg/dL (3.4–26.9 mcg/dL)

Low-dose (1 mcg) ACTH (cortrosyn) stimulation test: $t_0 = 17$ mcg/dL, $t_{30\,min} = 29$ mcg/dL, $t_{60\,min} = 29$ mcg/dL (>18 mcg/dL within 60 minutes after cortrosyn administration).

	Oral glucose tolerance test					
	Baseline (t_0)	30 min (t_{30})	60 min (t_{60})	90 min (t_{90})	120 min (t_{120})	150 min (t_{150})
GH (ng/mL)	2.8	3.2	3.6	3.1	2.8	2.6
Glucose (mg/dL)	112	198	186	172	161	152

(Normal: GH <1.0 by t_{150}; Glucose <100 by t_{150}.)

multiple organ systems, patients with acromegaly have significantly increased mortality versus the general population [1]. Acromegalics have a standardized mortality ratio of 1.72 (95% CI: 1.62–1.83), a 32% increased risk for all-cause mortality, and a death rate of 50% by the age of 60 in untreated patients. However, with successful treatment resulting in sustained GH levels <2.5 ng/mL and normalization of insulin-like growth factor 1 (IGF-1) levels, the standardized mortality ratio returns to 1.1 (95% CI: 0.9–1.4).

The classic clinical syndrome of acromegaly is GH hypersecretion, but GH levels alone are unreliable in diagnosing hypersecretory states because GH secretion is pulsatile and may vary throughout the day. The single, best screening test is the level of IGF-1, which is induced by GH, has a longer half life, and maintains a more constant serum concentration over time. Normal levels of IGF-1 are age and sex dependent, so results must be interpreted in this context. While elevation of IGF-1 relative to appropriately matched control levels is highly suggestive of GH hypersecretion, the definitive test remains the oral glucose tolerance test. In this test, baseline glucose and GH levels are measured just prior to administration of a 75 g oral glucose load to a fasting patient. Growth hormone and glucose levels are then assayed at 30 minute intervals for the next 150–180 minutes. The oral glucose load should result in suppression of GH levels to <1 ng/mL by the end of the test, and failure to suppress to this level definitively diagnoses GH hypersecretion. Monitoring glucose levels during the same test can diagnose impaired glucose tolerance, which is said to be present if the glucose level remains elevated above 140 mg/dL at the conclusion of the test.

Surgical resection is the treatment of choice for GH-secreting adenomas because of the significant improvement in morbidity and survival that results from rapid and durable reduction of GH and normalization of IGF-1 levels. Transphenoidal resection results in normalization of IGF-1 levels in 75–95% of patients with microadenomas and 40–68% of patients with macroadenomas. Medical management with somatostatin receptor ligands (octreotide, lanreotide), GH receptor agonists (pegvisomant), or dopamine agonists (cabergoline) can normalize IGF-1 levels in 60–90% of patients but are costly and are unlikely to achieve definitive cure, requiring life-long administration [2]. Medical management strategies are useful for preoperative reduction in tumor size, for up-front or postoperative control in patients with tumors not amenable to gross total resection, in patients without symptoms of mass effect awaiting definitive treatment, in patients with surgical contraindications, or in preparation for or as an adjunct to radiation therapy or radiosurgery [1, 2].

Case description 2

History: A 36-year-old female was referred by her dermatologist. She had been followed for several years for acne that had been poorly controlled with standard medical management. Over the past year she had noticed the appearance of purple abdominal striae and multiple ecchymoses on her arms and legs. When she reported these findings to her dermatologist she was referred to the neuroendocrine clinic for evaluation. She stated that she was generally healthy except for depression and anxiety, which caused difficulty sleeping. On detailed questioning she reported an increased appetite over the past 6 months with 15–20 pounds of unintentional weight gain. She had also had irregular menstrual cycles over a similar time period, which she attributed to stress and to her depression. She had no acute complaints. Her medications included duloxetine 60 mg QD for her depression and anxiety. Her medical and surgical histories were otherwise unremarkable. She drank 2–3 beers per day and smoked 2 packs of cigarettes per week. She had never been pregnant.

Examination: She was a 36-year-old woman in no distress. She was 163 cm tall and weighed 79.5 kg (BMI 30). She had normal visual fields and acuity. Her cranial nerves were intact. She had 4/5 deltoid strength bilaterally with some muscle atrophy but had no other neurologic deficits. Her face was rounded, and she had mild hirsutism and prominent supraclavicular fat deposits. Her abdominal exam was remarkable for the presence of red stria. The remainder of her physical exam was unremarkable and was notable for the absence of galactorrhea and acral enlargement.

Radiology: Non-enhanced magnetic resonance imaging demonstrated a normal sellar region with a pituitary gland of normal size and configuration. With gadolinium contrast, there was a 3 mm area of abnormal intensity to the right of midline within the anterior pituitary gland. No other lesions were seen (Figure 55.1).

Laboratory evaluation: Laboratory tests were obtained as shown in Table 55.2. Normal values are indicated in parentheses.

Diagnosis: Cushing's disease – pituitary microadenoma.

Discussion: Cushing's syndrome (CS) is the clinical manifestation of cortisol excess, and Cushing's disease (CD) specifically describes cortisol excess caused by an ACTH-secreting pituitary adenoma. There are several clinical hallmarks of CS. First is progressive obesity, including generalized weight gain, truncal obesity, and fat deposits in the face ("moon face") and dorsal cervical and supraclavicular regions ("buffalo hump"). Next are dermatologic manifestations, including acne, skin hyperpigmentation, abdominal striae, easy bruis-

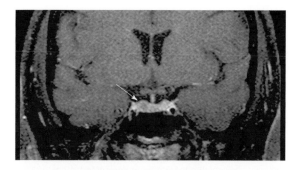

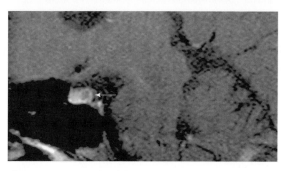

Figure 55.1. Coronal gadolinium-enhanced magnetic resonance image of the sella. The arrow indicates a small area of decreased enhancement that suggests a possible pituitary microadenoma.

ability, skin atrophy, and frequent fungal infections [3]. Third are signs of androgen excess, including hirsutism, virilization, oily skin, and irregular menstruation in women. Other systemic symptoms, including diastolic hypertension, osteopenia, and proximal muscle wasting are observed. Finally, psychiatric symptoms including anxiety, depression, and emotional lability are frequently seen in patients with CS [3]. Like acromegaly, the many systemic effects of CS lead to increased mortality, which may be as high as 4–5-fold that of the general population.

Hypercortisolemia can result from unregulated production of cortisol by the adrenal glands or through a normal adrenal response to central or ectopic elevations of ACTH. The case above represents an example of the challenges associated with diagnosing CS and identifying the source of cortisol excess. The first step is to identify elevated cortisol levels. In this patient, the 00:00 and 07:00 random cortisol levels were at the high end of normal, and the 24-hour urine free cortisol was mildly elevated. While this suggests cortisol excess, it leaves open the possibility of hypercortisolism associated with other medical conditions (termed "pseudo-Cushing's"), including physical or emotional stress, infection, depression, or alcoholism, all of which are suggested by her history. Her failure to

Table 55.2. Laboratory test result for patient in case description 2.

CBC, BMP:	WBC 13 K/µL (3 K/µL)	LH: 6 mU/mL (<12 mU/mL)	
Urine β		GH: 1.2 ng/mL (0–3 ng/mL)	
Prolactin:	3 ng/µL (2 ng/µL)	IGF-1: 201 ng/mL (117–329 ng/mL)	
TSH:	4.000 µU/mL (0.500 µU/mL)	Total cortisol, 07:00: 25 µcg/dL (3.4–26.9 mcg/dL)	
Free T4:	1.2 ng/dL (0.7 ng/dL)	Total cortisol, 00:00: 5 mcg/dL (<5 mcg/dL)	
FSH:	6 mU/mL (1 mU/mL)	ACTH: 50 pg/mL (8–20 pg/mL)	

24-hour urine free cortisol (UFC): 65 mcg/24h (<45 mcg/24h).
Low-dose dexamethasone (1mg) suppression test: 3.2 mcg/dL (<1.8 mcg/dL).
High-dose dexamethasone (8mg) suppression test: 4.2 mcg/dL (<1 mcg/dL).

Corticotropin Releasing Hormone (CRH) stimulation test							
	15 minutes before CRH (t_{-15})	5 minutes before CRH (t_{-5})	CRH Dose (t_0)	15 minutes after CRH (t_{15})	30 minutes After CRH (t_{30})	45 minutes After CRH (t_{45})	60 minutes After CRH (t_{60})
Cortisol (mcg/dL) [% over baseline]	25 [0%]	26 [4%]	25 [0%]	24 [−4%]	30 [20%]	31 [24%]	28 [12%]
ACTH (pg/mL) [% over baseline]	52 [2%]	50 [−2%]	51 [0%]	66 [29%]	72 [41%]	70 [37%]	63 [24%]

Inferior petrosal sinus sampling (IPSS)						
ACTH (pg/mL)						
		Petrosal Sinus				
				ACTH Ratio		
	Peripheral	Right	Left	R/P	L/P	R/L
CRH (−10 min)	37	212	36	5.7	0.97	5.9
CRH (−5 min)	41	451	43	11.0	1.0	10.5
CRH (+2 min)	34	1214	44	35.7	1.3	27.6
CRH (+5 min)	63	2855	92	45.3	1.5	31.0
CRH (+10 min)	80	90	112	1.1	1.4	0.8
CRH (+15 min)	82	152	136	1.9	1.7	1.1

adequately suppress on the low-dose dexamethasone suppression test, however, makes a definitive diagnosis of true hypercortisolemia [4]. This patient's MRI suggests a potential microadenoma; however, even a normal pituitary MRI does not rule out an occult pituitary lesion. The next step is therefore to use physiologic testing to determine if the excess cortisol is being produced *de novo* from an adrenal lesion or represents a normal adrenal response to abnormally elevated ACTH. In this patient, the laboratory finding of elevated serum ACTH narrows the differential to a pituitary or an ectopic source of ACTH. The high-dose dexamethasone suppression test is used to make this distinction, because pituitary adenomas producing ACTH will generally be suppressed with high doses of dexamethasone while ectopic sources will not. Cortisol levels <1 mcg/dL reflect normal physiology or a pituitary source, levels >5 mcg/dL suggest an ectopic source, and levels from 1–5 mcg/dL are suggestive of a pituitary etiology but are considered equivocal [4, 5].

This patient demonstrated an equivocal response, which argues toward a pituitary source but is not definitive. In this circumstance additional testing is required. The cortrosyn releasing hormone (CRH) stimulation test measures serum ACTH and cortisol levels in response to intravenous administration of 100 mcg of ovoid CRH. ACTH-secreting pituitary adenomas will respond to CRH stimulation by increasing ACTH and cortisol production, while ectopic (and adrenal) sources will demonstrate no response. The patient is considered to respond if ACTH increases to 35–50% over baseline by 30 minutes or if cortisol increases to 20–50% over baseline by 60 minutes. In this patient the maximum ACTH increase was 41% over baseline (at 30 minutes) and the maximum cortisol increase was 24% (at 45 minutes). These findings also suggest a pituitary source, but the values are borderline. The final, definitive test involves CRH stimulation followed by direct sampling of ACTH levels in blood collected from the bilateral inferior petrosal sinuses (IPS), the central cerebral venous structures into which the pituitary vascular plexus drains. Comparing the IPS ACTH levels to those of ACTH in the peripheral venous system is used to compute a central-to-peripheral ACTH gradient. A gradient value greater than 2-fold before stimulation or greater than 3-fold within 10 minutes after stimulation is consistent with a pituitary etiology for the hypercortisolemia [4, 5]. This patient demonstrates a baseline right IPS:peripheral ratio of 5.7:1 at baseline and 45.3:1 at 5 minutes. This is diagnostic for a pituitary etiology of CS or CD. Of note, these findings do not necessarily localize the lesion to the right side of the pituitary gland.

The treatment of CD involves surgical resection of the pituitary adenoma, because removal of the lesion and rapid normalization of the serum cortisol improves survival in these patients. In patients with occult microadenomas, surgery often involves a transsphenoidal approach and surgical exploration of the entire gland. If abnormal-appearing tissue is identified it is resected and sent to pathology for definitive identification of the adenoma. When an ACTH-secreting tumor is identified and completely removed, 85–90% of patients will achieve sustained remission. If no grossly abnormal tissue is apparent, hemihypophysectomy (guided by the IPS data) may be considered. If no adenoma is identified on final pathology and/or if cortisol levels fail to normalize postoperatively, early surgical re-exploration and possibly, complete hypophysectomy may be required. Such patients will experience panhypopituitarism and will require lifelong hormone supplementation, but they will gain the survival benefits associated with control of their hypercortisolemia [6].

References

1. **A. Ben-Shlomo, S. Melmed**. Acromegaly. *Endocrinol Metab Clin N Amer* 2008; **37**: 101–22.

2. **S. Melmed, A. Colao, A. Barkan** et al. The pituitary Society and the European Neuroendocrine Association. Guidelines for acromegaly management: an update. *J Clin Endocrinol Metab* 2009; **95**: 1509–17.

3. **J. Newell-Price, X. Bertagna, A. B. Grossman** et al. Cushing's syndrome. *Lancet* 2006; **367**: 1605–17.

4. **B. M. Biller, A. B. Grossman, P. M. Stewart** et al. Treatment of adrenocorticotropin-dependent Cushing's syndrome: a consensus statement. *J Clin Endocrinol Metab* 2008; **93**: 2454–62.

5. **L. K. Nieman, B. M. Biller, J. W. Findling** et al. The diagnosis of Cushing's syndrome: An Endocrine Society Clinical Practice Guideline. *J Clin Endocrinol Metab* 2008; **93**: 1526–40.

6. **M. B. Elamin, M. H. Murad, R. Mullan** et al. Accuracy of diagnostic tests for Cushing's syndrome: a systematic review and metaanalyses. *J Clin Endocrinol Metab* 2008; **93**: 1553–1562.

Neuroendocrine surgery

Acromegaly and gigantism

D. John Doyle

An excess of growth hormone (GH) from a pituitary adenoma can result in gigantism and acromegaly; neurosurgical intervention is often required. Airway management is a prime consideration in the anesthetic management of these patients [1–3].

Case description

A 36-year-old female weighed 115 kg and was 218.5 cm tall. She was scheduled for a transsphenoidal resection of the pituitary adenoma that had caused her gigantism. She also had obvious acromegalic features. The upper airway evaluation showed a large protruding tongue with grade IV Mallampati score. Due to the anticipated difficult airway management, awake fiberoptic intubation was performed after local anesthetic topicalization of the upper airway. The fiberoptic laryngoscopy proceeded with difficulty given the pronounced macroglossia and redundant tissue surrounding the glottis. Several hypertensive episodes were treated with labetolol. After securing the upper airway, the patient had general anesthesia and an uneventful surgery.

Discussion

The term "acromegaly" comes from the Greek words for "extremities" (acro) and "enlargement" (megaly). Giants have been known from biblical times. The acromegalic patient suffers from an excess of GH, usually from a pituitary adenoma derived from somatotroph cells. If the condition occurs prior to closure of the epiphyseal growth plates, gigantism may occur. Once the growth plates have fused in adolescence, the patient may take on acromegalic features.

The goals of treatment are to normalize GH production while avoiding adverse effects on other pituitary functions (adrenocorticotropic hormone, follicle stimulating hormone, luteinizing hormone, prolactin, thyroid stimulating hormone, etc.), to relieve pressure on nerves and other structures exerted by the tumor,

and to reverse the symptoms of acromegaly. Treatment options include surgical removal of the tumor, drug therapy (bromocriptine, octreotide), and radiation to the pituitary. If the tumor has not invaded surrounding brain tissue, surgical removal of the tumor, often via a transsphenoidal approach, is usually the first choice. Radiation therapy is usually reserved for patients who have tumor remaining after surgery. Drug therapy can be useful in nonpituitary causes of acromegaly as well as to shrink large tumors before surgery.

From the viewpoint of airway management in the acromegalic patient, several concerns exist: (1) the tongue may be very enlarged; (2) redundant folds of tissue may be present in the oropharynx; (3) the epiglottis is often enlarged; and (4) laryngeal stenosis occurs more frequently compared with the general population. These factors may make laryngoscopy and intubation considerably more difficult and also increase the likelihood of airway obstruction during anesthetic induction and recovery. Acromegalic patients are also prone to obstructive sleep apnea. In the case of gigantism, several additional potential problems should also be considered: (1) possible need for an extra long operating table; (2) possible need for an extra large laryngoscope; (3) endotracheal tubes may need to be placed deeper than usual; and (4) an extra large face mask may be needed as in our case.

A number of decades ago, if direct laryngoscopy or blind intubation was unsuccessful, tracheotomy was occasionally required to manage the airway in these patients. However, the development of the fiberscope has greatly reduced the need for this. Still, it should be emphasized that acromegalic patients can be a great airway challenge. In a study by Schmitt *et al.* the authors found that laryngoscopy was difficult (grade III view) in over one quarter (26%) of acromegalic patients [3]. Consequently, special attention should be paid to the availability of alternative airway management techniques, such as the use of airway adjuncts, fiberoptic intubation, video laryngoscopy, etc. Awake intubation may be needed in some cases [4, 5].

References

1. **S. Z. Hassan, G. J. Matz, A. M. Lawrence** *et al.* Laryngeal stenosis in acromegaly: a possible cause of airway difficulties associated with anesthesia. *Anesth Analg* 1976; **55**: 57–60.

2. **J. P. Southwick, J. Katz**. Unusual airway difficulties in the acromegalic patient – indications for tracheostomy. *Anesthesiology* 1979; **51**: 72–3.

3. **H. Schmitt, M. Buchfelder, M. Radespiel-Troger** *et al.* Difficult intubation in acromegalic patients: incidence and predictability. *Anesthesiology* 2000; **93**: 110–14.

4. **P. A. Seidman, W. A. Kofke, R. Policare** *et al.* Anaesthetic complications of acromegaly. *Br J Anaesth* 2000; **84**: 179–82.

5. **E. C. Nemergut, Z. Zuo**. Airway management in patients with pituitary disease: a review of 746 patients. *J Neurosurg Anesthesiol* 2006; **18**: 73–7.

Neuroendocrine surgery

Perioperative diabetes insipidus

Juan P. Cata and Ehab Farag

Sodium disturbances are common in patients presenting with neurologic disease. However, postoperative development of sodium dysregulation may be seen after transphenoidal surgery.

Case description

A 45-year-old male with a 1-year history of right temporal anopsia and impotence underwent a successful transphenoidal resection of a 21 mm (in maximal diameter) suprasellar mass (meningioma) under general anesthesia. Intraoperative management was unremarkable with an estimated blood loss of 125 mL. After surgery and successful extubation of the trachea, the neurologic exam was unremarkable and visual fields were grossly intact. He was then transferred to the postanesthesia recovery unit and 8 hours later transferred to the general medical ward. On postoperative day 1, he started complaining of thirst, his urinary output increased to 300 mL/hour and reached a total volume of 7.8 liters on postoperative day 1. A laboratory analysis was remarkable for urinary specific gravity of 1.000 and serum glucose of 161 g/dL. Due to the clinical suspicion of central diabetes insipidus (DI), he was treated conservatively with liberal access to oral intake of water and intravenous fluids. On postoperative day 2, he developed signs of dehydration and was hypernatremic, therefore 0.1 mg of oral desmopressin was given after which his urinary output decreased to 90 mL/hour and the urinary specific gravity increased to 1.010. On postoperative day 3, he was asymptomatic, the serum sodium level was 138 mEq/L and serum osmolality was 300 mOsm/kg. The urinary output remained stable. He was discharged on postoperative day 4.

Discussion

Disorders of sodium after transphenoidal surgery occur due to the irritation or destruction of the pituitary stalk [1]. The two main disorders are: (1) syndrome of inappropriate antidiuretic hormone secretion, and (2) central DI. The first is caused by inappropriate secretion of vasopressin and the second, by the lack of release of the hormone. It is necessary to differentiate central DI (caused by insufficient production of vasopressin) from nephrogenic DI, which is caused by an impaired response of the kidneys to vasopressin. In both, there is a failure to concentrate urine [2].

Perioperative central DI is a common finding in patients undergoing pituitary surgery. Preoperative DI can be part of a panhypopituitarism syndrome in patients with large pituitary prolactinomas or non-prolactinomas [3]. However, central DI develops most commonly in the postoperative setting. The incidence of transient postoperative central DI ranges from 5% to 80% of those undergoing pituitary surgery [3–5]. However, fewer patients develop permanent central DI [3]. A third form of postoperative central DI called "triphasic" has also been described. The first phase is characterized by thirst and polyuria and is present within 24 to 72 hours after surgery. The second phase develops 7–10 days after surgery and is characterized by antidiuresis. Two to 3 weeks after surgery, polyuria returns and marks the onset of the third phase. Predictive factors of central DI after pituitary surgery are resection of a Rathke's cleft cyst and intraoperative cerebrospinal fluid leak. However, conflicting results exist between the incidence of central DI and pituitary adenoma size [5].

The clinical manifestation of central DI ranges from mild thirst to significant polyuria, polydipsia, dehydration and, if severe, hypotension. Commonly, the onset of signs and symptoms of DI starts on postoperative day 1 to 2 and may last for 1 or 2 weeks. A urine output >250 mL/hour for 2 consecutive hours is a clinical indicator of DI. However, DI is diagnosed when *all* the following criteria are met: polyuria of >2.5 L, a day with concomitant polydipsia, serum Na >140 mmol/L, spontaneous urine specific gravity <1.005, and glycemia <180 mg/dL [4].

The clinical management of patients with central DI after pituitary surgery is initially conservative. Most patients undergoing pituitary surgery are awake and cooperative after surgery, which facilitates the treatment of central DI. Monitoring of daily weights, fluid balance, and the oral intake of water are fundamental during the initial management of these patients. The use of exogenous vasopressin is indicated in patients with significant urinary output and hypernatremia. Vasopressin can be administered intravenously, intranasally, subcutaneously, and orally. Several authors recommend a daily oral dose of 0.1 mg of desmopressin as the first choice. Serum sodium has to be followed during vasopressin administration because the excessive retention of free water can lead to hyponatremia. See Case 83 for further discussion of sodium abnormalities in the neurosurgical population.

References

1. **I. Ciric, A. Ragin, C. Baumgartner** *et al.* Complications of transsphenoidal surgery: results of a national survey, review of the literature, and personal experience. *Neurosurgery* 1997; **40**: 225–36.

2. **G. L. Robertson**. Diabetes insipidus. *Endocrinol Metab Clin North Am* 1995; **24**: 549–72.

3. **N. Fatemi, J. R. Dusick, C. Mattozo** *et al.* Pituitary hormonal loss and recovery after transsphenoidal adenoma removal. *Neurosurgery* 2008; **63**: 709–18.

4. **R. A. Kristof, M. Rother, G. Neuloh** *et al.* Incidence, clinical manifestations, and course of water and electrolyte metabolism disturbances following transsphenoidal pituitary adenoma surgery: a prospective observational study. *J Neurosurg* 2009; **111**: 555–62.

5. **D. G. Sigounas, J. L. Sharpless, D. M. Cheng** *et al.* Predictors and incidence of central diabetes insipidus after endoscopic pituitary surgery. *Neurosurgery* 2008; **62**: 71–8.

Pediatric neuroanesthesia

Craniotomy

William Bingaman and Marco Maurtua

Pediatric surgical patients present special anesthetic challenges including induction without intravenous (IV) access, a higher incidence of airway complications (laryngospasm and bronchospasm), and a greater incidence of hemodynamic instability due to surgical blood loss [1].

Brain tumors are the second most common cause of cancer in pediatric patients [2]. Between 5 and 60% of these central nervous system tumors are infratentorial and include medulloblastoma, low-grade cerebellar astrocytoma, ependymoma, glioma, and low-grade brainstem astrocytoma. Supratentorial tumors are the second most common location and include low-grade astrocytoma, malignant and mixed glioma, ependymoma, ganglioglioma, oligodendroglioma, choroid plexus tumor, and meningioma [3].

Case description

An 8-year-old child (120 cm tall and 24.6 kg) presented with partial complex seizures characterized by staring spells accompanied by oral and manual automatisms. These persisted despite adequate trials of three different anticonvulsant medications. Preoperative evaluation (magnetic resonance imaging) demonstrated a non-enhancing heterogeneous lesion in the mesial aspect of the right temporal lobe consistent with low-grade glial neoplasm. Right tailored temporal lobectomy was scheduled to obtain tissue for diagnosis, resect the lesion, and eliminate the seizures.

After the preoperative evaluation the patient was premedicated with 10 mg oral midazolam. Once in the operating room standard ASA monitors were applied and an inhalation induction with sevoflurane took place. Intravenous access was secured followed by tracheal intubation. A radial arterial line was also placed prior to cranial fixation with the three-point head holder. Prior to fixating the head, the patient was given a bolus of intravenous propofol to blunt the hypertensive response elicited by head pinning.

Maintenance of anesthesia was achieved with isoflurane 0.6%, remifentanil infusion at 0.1 mcg/kg/min and nitrous oxide 70%. Muscle relaxation was obtained with intermittent rocuronium administration that in this case was more frequent secondary to the hepatic enzyme induction produced by anticonvulsant medications, which were further available in the operating room if needed. During the skin closure, fentanyl 25 mcg was administered to provide analgesia in the immediate postoperative period. The surgical procedure was performed without complications with 200 mL estimated blood loss. A neurologic assessment was performed after extubation and it showed no neurologic deficits. Subsequently the patient was transported to the pediatric intensive care unit where his recovery was satisfactory. The pathology was ganglioglioma.

Discussion

Preoperative assessment

In elective cases the nothing by mouth (or Nil Per Os) guideline currently followed is the "2–4-6–8" rule, which indicates that clear fluid intake is allowed 2 hours before surgery, breast milk 4 hours before surgery, formula 6 hours before surgery, and solid food 8 hours before surgery [4].

A complete history should be performed focusing on the past medical history, family history, and past experiences with anesthesia if applicable. Co-morbid conditions should be accounted for including maternal complications during pregnancy, delivery and history of prematurity and its complications. A system-based review including screening for cardiac, pulmonary, renal, hepatic, and neurologic disease should be performed. The past surgical and anesthetic history of the patient is relevant to identify prior anesthetic complications such as difficulties with airway management, previous anesthetic drug reactions, and the type of surgical procedures performed in the past. Family history of complications with anesthesia is aimed at identification of diseases and conditions that can be transmitted genetically such as malignant hyperthermia, Duchenne's muscular dystrophy, etc. to prevent patient exposure to triggering agents and depolarizing muscle relaxants. Allergies should be identified and medications reviewed; precautions should be instituted for conditions such as latex allergy. Anticonvulsant medications should be continued and administered the day of surgery to prevent intraoperative and postoperative seizures.

During the patient's clinical assessment, one should start with the patient's airway examination, including Mallampati score, thyromental distance, degree of cervical spine extension, presence of craniofacial abnormalities such as craniosynostosis or syndromes such as Crouzon's, Pierre Robin, Goldenhar, etc. that generally are accompanied by micrognathia, an independent predictive factor for difficult ventilation and/or intubation. The clinical assessment should continue by examining the patient's pulmonary status, especially in patients with generalized seizures or mental retardation to diagnose preoperatively the presence of pulmonary aspiration. The clinician should be alert to signs of dehydration, especially if the patient had a history of intermittent nausea and vomiting due to increased intracranial pressure (ICP). A thorough physical examination should follow. A neurologic examination should include documentation of abnormal neurologic development, presence of cognitive delay, level of alertness and orientation. A motor and sensory exam should also be performed. Any signs or symptoms of raised ICP need to be documented and discussed with the surgical team. In newborns the presence of lethargy or irritability may indicate an increase in ICP.

Cell blood counts may be altered due to the use of carbamazepine or valproic acid. Electrolyte abnormalities due to vomiting secondary to increased ICP may be found and should be corrected prior to the surgical procedure. In pediatric patients the head is larger in proportion to the body surface area compared with the adult patient. This is an important fact that leads to a greater blood loss and third spacing losses that can make the pediatric patient hemodynamically unstable intraoperatively. Close monitoring of blood loss and coagulation parameters during surgery is crucial to avoid potentially serious complications. Therefore blood should be available before starting a craniotomy in newborns and infants.

Premedication: Prior to bringing the patient to the operating room, patients older than 1 year of age should be premedicated with oral midazolam (0.5 mg/kg) or nasal midazolam (0.1 to 0.2 mg/kg). If increased ICP is present or suspected, premedication should be avoided to prevent a further increase in ICP due to sedation and hypercarbia.

Intraoperative management

Induction of anesthesia: Inhalation induction can be performed in the child without IV access and who does not have clinical signs of increased ICP. If increased ICP is present and the patient has been vomiting, an intravenous line should be placed and volume replacement initiated to treat dehydration. Clinical signs of hypovolemia, such as decrease in skin turgor, sunken fontanelles, crying without tears, low urine output, and lethargy, imply a decrease in intravascular volume that should be corrected prior to induction of anesthesia.

Placement of invasive monitors should take place after induction of anesthesia, including an arterial line to monitor acute changes in blood pressure due to blood loss or bradycardia seen after stimulation of the dura or other central nervous system structures and also to accurately determine $PaCO_2$ levels. Bladder catheterization is mandatory to monitor urine output that is frequently increased due to the administration of hyperosmotic therapy. Intravenous access can be accomplished with the placement of two large-bore peripheral IVs. If peripheral IV access cannot be achieved, placement of a central venous line should be performed. Finally, if the procedure will increase the risk for air embolism, a precordial Doppler ultrasound should be utilized for early detection of air embolism especially in surgeries involving brain venous sinuses.

Maintenance of anesthesia can be achieved by the administration of inhalation anesthetics, such as sevoflurane, isoflurane, and desflurane. It is important to remember that these agents produce dose-dependent cerebral vasodilation that is noticeable during surgery and a decrease in cerebral metabolic rate ($CMRO_2$) producing an uncoupling effect. Nitrous oxide can be used during pediatric neurosurgical procedures, however avoidance of this agent is indicated within 1 month after a previous craniotomy since pneumocephalus may have not yet been resolved. Nitrous oxide is also contraindicated in patients with pneumothorax, or after trauma of the chest and should be used cautiously or completely avoided in those procedures where there is an increased risk for air embolism. Similarly to the described fluorinated inhalation anesthetics, nitrous oxide produces a dose-dependent cerebral vasodilation, but the difference is that it increases $CMRO_2$.

Narcotic infusions in conjunction with inhalation anesthetics are currently used in pediatric patients for neuroanesthesia maintenance. Remifentanil is a narcotic approximately 100 times more potent than morphine. It is useful in neuroanesthesia because of its short context-sensitive half life due to its unique metabolism by nonspecific plasma and tissue esterases. It has been proven to be an ideal drug in pediatric neuroanesthesia, allowing for a faster wake up and reliable postoperative neurologic exam. Remifentanil's side effects include bradycardia, hypotension, and decreased cardiac output. A general recommendation is to avoid remifentanil boluses and if given as an infusion the starting dose should be low and may be increased only if the hemodynamic parameters are stable. Chest rigidity can also be seen as a complication of any intravenous narcotic and should be considered if increased inspiratory pressures are suddenly detected and a right main-stem intubation has been ruled out. Other narcotic infusions are also used in pediatric neuroanesthesiology, such as fentanyl infusions. Due to its high lipid solubility, fentanyl is stored in adipose tissue; the longer the infusion is delivered the higher the plasma concentration will get and the greater the time required for the patient to return to therapeutic plasma levels. Therefore, it is imperative to stop the fentanyl infusion at least 1 hour before emergence from anesthesia so a thorough immediate postoperative neurologic examination is achievable. A common advantage of all narcotic infusions is that they potentiate inhalation anesthetics, decreasing their requirement and allowing a decrease in their plasma concentration. In a prospective randomized clinical trial performed in our institution, we showed that an infusion of remifentanil at 0.13 mcg/kg/min adds 50% minimum alveolar concentration in adult patients when combined with 0.6% isoflurane [5]. This decrease in inhalation anesthetic requirements leads to a decreased cerebral vasodilation, that as we mentioned is dose dependent, offering the neurosurgeon a more relaxed, less edematous surgical field.

Keeping the patient immobilized during the surgical procedure is essential because of the risk of head dislodgement from the head holder, injury to the brain from patient movement during the surgical procedure, and cervical spine injury from body motion with a fixed cranium. Nondepolarizing muscle relaxants should be used in pediatric patients undergoing elective procedures to avoid hyperkalemic responses seen in children with undiagnosed myopathies after the administration of succinylcholine. Patients taking antiepileptic medications have an increased activity of the cytochrome P450 system, which produces rapid metabolism of muscle relaxant drugs and decreases their usual half life. Therefore close monitoring of muscle relaxation with a muscle twitch monitor should be routine. Neurosurgeons are often concerned with brain swelling during surgery. Useful techniques to combat this include hyperventilation therapy, hyperosmotic therapy, head elevation, and reduction of inhaled anesthetics. Hyperventilation can be performed in children to decrease brain volume by producing central nervous system vasoconstriction. One needs to be cognizant about the theoretical risk of producing cerebral ischemia at $PaCO_2$ levels below 25 mmHg. Hyperosmolar therapy is useful to reduce cerebral swelling. Mannitol can be administered in a dose of 0.25–1.0 g/kg body weight. Mannitol has a biphasic effect after its intravenous administration; first there is an increase in intravascular volume due to a transient increase in intravascular osmotic effect that drives fluids from the interstitial space to the intravascular space, followed by a second effect of osmotic diuresis producing a decrease in intravascular volume by increasing urine output.

Conclusion

Approaching the care of a child with a central nervous system lesion requires a systematic approach that takes into consideration the principles of both pediatric anesthesiology and neuroanesthesiology.

References

1. **G. Olson, B. Hallen.** Laryngospasm during anaesthesia. A computer aided incidence study in 136 929 patients. *Acta Anaesthesiol Scand* 1984: **28**: 567–75.

2. **M. D. Walker.** Diagnosis and treatment of brain tumors. *Pediatr Clin North Am* 1976; **23**: 131–46.

3.   **I. F. Pollack**. Brain tumors in children. *N Engl J Med* 1994; **331**: 1500–7.

4.   **L. R. Ferrari, F. M. Rooney, M. A. Rockoff**. Preoperative fasting practices inn pediatrics. *Anesthesiology* 1999; **90**: 978–80.

5.   **M. A. Maurtua, A. Deogaonkar, M. H. Bakri** *et al*. Dosing of remifentanil to prevent movement during craniotomy in the absence of neuromuscular blockade. *J Neurosurg Anesthesiol* 2008; **20**: 221–5.

Pediatric neuroanesthesia

Ventriculoperitoneal shunt

Ruairi Moulding and Peter Stiles

Hydrocephalus is a common childhood disorder that may present with a spectrum of symptoms from nonspecific nausea and fatigue to life-threatening intracranial hypertension. Timely surgical correction is mandatory in emergent cases in order to reduce intracranial pressure (ICP) and decrease any secondary injury, which may result from interstitial cerebral edema.

A ventriculoperitoneal (VP) shunt – a series of catheters with a unidirectional valve to divert cerebrospinal fluid (CSF) from the brain by draining it into the peritoneum – may be implanted from birth onwards as a definitive surgical correction for hydrocephalus. Shunt failure, however, is common. A large cohort study demonstrated that 81% of shunt patients experience at least one episode of blockage in the first 12 years following implantation. Further, as many as 40% of those will fail within 1 year of revision [1]. Once a shunt has failed the subsequent revision also has a reduced survival time.

Case description

A 15-month-old female with a history significant for stenosis of the aqueduct of Sylvius, epilepsy, and VP shunt placement as an infant, presented to the emergency department for evaluation. She was obtunded and had a 1-day history of lethargy, nausea, and vomiting. Although she had walked unaided since the age of 14 months, she had difficulty taking more than two steps. Her mother also noted that disinterest and frequent crying developed over a 1-week interval. Physical examination revealed an obtunded 15-month-old female with large head and bulging fontanelle. Pupils were equal and reactive to light. Brain computed tomography (CT) showed dilated ventricles (Figure 59.1) when compared with previous images, but a shunt series of plain films failed to reveal localizable abnormality. Laboratory values were unremarkable. The patient's temperature was 37.0 °C. Lumbar

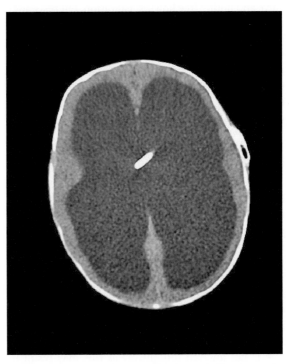

Figure 59.1. Computed tomography of severely dilated ventricles in an infant, with compressed and thinned cerebral hemispheres at the periphery. The tip of the ventricular shunt is evident, inserted via a left frontal approach.

puncture was not performed given likely increased ICP and resulting risk of herniation. She was diagnosed with recurrent hydrocephalus due to shunt malfunction at an unknown location along the apparatus and possible shunt infection. The patient required immediate surgical revision of her VP shunt.

Although the patient was lethargic on presentation, every effort was made not to further stimulate the child. An intravenous catheter was placed and fluids given. In view of the patient's history of vomiting and her altered mental state, no sedation was given and a modified rapid sequence induction with fentanyl, propofol, and rocuronium was performed. Fentanyl was used to obtund the laryngeal reflex in order to avoid increased ICP. Endotracheal intubation via direct laryngoscopy was confirmed and general anesthesia was maintained with intravenous anesthesia and intermittent opioids. A loading dose of phenytoin for seizure prophylaxis was administered at 18 mg/kg [2]. A Foley catheter was placed to monitor urine output. Intraoperative CSF sample yielded no white cells. The surgical team localized the VP shunt obstruction to the peritoneal portion by accessing the apparatus' valve and noting free flowing aspiration, but resistance to injection. The case was without complication and took 2 hours to complete with minimal blood loss and uneventful emergence. The patient was transferred to the pediatric intensive care unit for overnight observation then transferred to the general pediatric ward the following day. The patient recovered neurologically, regaining the ability to walk after 2 days.

Discussion

Any child with increased ICP presents a variety of concerns for the anesthesiology team. First, the patient is drowsy and has been vomiting. This mandates a rapid sequence induction together with attention to any electrolyte abnormalities and dehydration. Second, a patient with increased ICP requires a high degree of vigilance as any further increase in ICP and therefore reduction in cerebral perfusion pressure (CPP) may cause irreparable damage. Third, if the shunt revision is successful, the anesthesiology and surgical teams must maintain excellent communication to ensure that ICP is not lowered too quickly as this may result in further intracranial pathology. Finally, the VP shunt patient population is at risk for seizures and proper prophylaxis must be administered.

Hydrocephalus is the accumulation of cerebrospinal fluid (CSF) within the brain. It may be acquired or congenital, communicating or noncommunicating. Communicating hydrocephalus means that CSF can still flow between ventricles but flow is blocked as it exits the ventricles. Noncommunicating hydrocephalus, such as in the above patient with aqueductal stenosis, is also known as obstructive hydrocephalus. This occurs when the flow of CSF is blocked along one of the interconnecting passages between the ventricles. The aqueduct of Sylvius, also called the aqueduct of the midbrain, is a canal that communicates between the third and fourth ventricles.

Hydrocephalus can present as a neurosurgical emergency requiring quick action to reduce the pressure. Although medical management may alleviate some increases in ICP, definitive treatment is surgical. In the above scenario, the patient exhibited an insidious progression of symptoms. However, the presence of nausea and vomiting is a concerning symptom and warrants closer scrutiny as it may be a sign of acute decompensation. Surgical management will depend on the cause of the ICP elevation. If there is no evidence of an infectious etiology, then a simple mechanical obstruction is likely and the shunt does not need to be externalized.

Elevation of ICP can result in catastrophic consequences for neural tissue and may result in poor outcomes for patients if prompt interventions are not instituted. Normal values for ICP are age dependent, although no consensus exists. Elevations in ICP can be chronic or acute depending on etiology. Occasionally a chronically elevated ICP can change rapidly to life-threatening acute intracranial hypertension. In any patient with elevated ICP, it is important to control any further increase to reduce the risk of secondary damage from interstitial cerebral edema as well as stopping the progression from uncontrolled intracranial hypertension to a herniation syndrome and death.

Control of ICP requires avoidance of hypercarbia, hypoxemia, acidemia, hyperthermia, cerebral edema, coughing, airway obstruction, obstruction to the venous drainage of the head, and high metabolic demand states such as seizures. Medical interventions that reduce ICP include head elevation to facilitate venous drainage, hyperventilation (after intubation), and hyperosmolar therapy. These measures may need to be employed in patients prior to definitive surgery.

Cerebral perfusion pressure (CPP) is the pressure gradient driving cerebral blood flow. Cerebral perfusion pressure is derived from mean arterial pressure (MAP) minus ICP:

$$CPP = MAP - ICP$$

If central venous pressure (CVP) is higher than ICP then it directly affects CPP. Reduction in CPP decreases the supply of metabolic substrate and oxygen to the brain, potentially resulting in ischemic damage. It is therefore especially important to maintain a MAP appropriate to adequate CPP in the setting of increased ICP. Mean arterial pressure may be increased using intravenous fluid resuscitation or vasopressors. It is worth noting that excess intravenous fluid may be detrimental, potentially causing

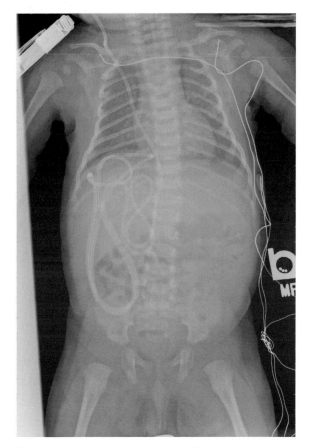

Figure 59.2. X-ray of infant with blocked VP shunt showing the pathway from the neck, over the right hemithorax, with redundant tubing in the abdomen. No evidence of kinking or tube disruption is evident.

tissue edema. Therefore, extreme care should always be taken when instituting intravenous fluids in any patients with raised ICP.

Ventriculoperitoneal shunts can fail to perform their intended function for a variety of reasons. The most common etiology of shunt failure in first-time revisions is obstruction, accounting for 66.7% of all instances [3]. Ventriculoperitoneal shunt blockage may be caused by occlusion of the ventricular catheter with choroid plexus, blood, or even brain tissue. Alternatively, the peritoneal catheter may be occluded by clot or scar tissue. Finally, the unidirectional valve, responsible for regulating flow, may malfunction and obstruct CSF drainage (Figure 59.2). Other, less common causes of shunt failure include infection (19%), loculated ventricles (7.7%), and overdrainage (5.7%) [3].

Patients undergoing emergent correction of acute hydrocephalus require a high degree of vigilance. Invasive intra-arterial blood pressure measurement is often unnecessary unless the patient is unstable or has significant co-morbidities. The use of central venous catheters is rarely indicated. Duration of surgery may be difficult to judge, therefore it is prudent to assume all such patients will need urinary catheters and attention to positioning.

Increased ICP can lead to nausea and vomiting. If a patient presents with profuse vomiting, he or she may display changes in biochemistry and suffer dehydration. These fluid and electrolyte abnormalities may need to be corrected perioperatively. Nausea and vomiting also exposes the patient to risk of aspiration during induction of anesthesia and therefore mandates a rapid securing of the patient's airway with an endotracheal tube [4].

Although perioperative anticonvulsants are not always indicated, elevated ICP predisposes to seizures and the associated increase in cerebral metabolic demand may be catastrophic. Additionally, if a patient is already on seizure prophylaxis they may have subtherapeutic plasma levels due to the nausea and vomiting and therefore further intravenous dosing may be required. It should be noted that some anticonvulsant medications are hepatic enzyme inducers, meaning that the metabolism and clearance of some anesthetic drugs is increased. Perioperative antibiotics may be indicated as prophylaxis. Occasionally the surgeon may ask for antibiotics to be withheld until a CSF sample has been taken for analysis if an infectious etiology of shunt failure is suspected.

Some patients with indwelling VP shunts may present for non-neurologic abdominal surgery, for example, appendectomy. There is no consensus on what measures should be taken in these instances although case series suggest that if an abdominal surgical site is infected then the VP shunt apparatus may need to be externalized temporarily until that local infection has cleared. These case series suggest VP shunts may fail if subjected to infectious assaults [5].

The hydrocephalus exhibited by patients requiring VP shunts may be part of a syndrome or disease process and a thorough history and physical examination may elicit signs and symptoms of other organ dysfunction.

Hydrocephalus is a common childhood disorder and surgical correction utilizes a shunt system to divert excess CSF out of the brain. If the drainage system obstructs then the patient may suffer from recurrence of their hydrocephalus with accompanying symptoms and signs. If timely surgical intervention is not undertaken, intracranial hypertension can lead to more serious consequences such as herniation syndrome and death. The obtunded child with acute hydrocephalus requires careful preoperative assessment and monitoring in order to formulate an appropriate anesthetic plan to avoid further rises in ICP.

References

1. **C. Sainte-Rose, J. H. Piatt, D. Renier** *et al.* Mechanical complications in shunts. *Pediatr Neurosurg* 1991; **17**: 2–9.

2. **P. Marik, K. Chen, J. Varon** *et al.* Management of increased intracranial pressure: a review for clinicians. *J Emerg Med* 1999; **17**: 711–19.

3. **S. Tuli, J. Drake, J. Lawless** *et al.* Risk factors for repeated cerebrospinal shunt failures in pediatric patients with hydrocephalus. *J Neurosurg* 2000; **92**: 31–8.

4. **R. K. Hamid, P. Newfield**. Pediatric neuroanesthesia. Hydrocephalus. *Anesthesiol Clin North America* 2001; **19**: 207–18.

5. **G. Li, S. Dutta**. Perioperative management of ventriculoperitoneal shunts during abdominal surgery. *Surg Neurol* 2008; **70**: 492–5.

Pediatric neuroanesthesia

Craniosynostosis repair

Vera Borzova and Julie Niezgoda

Craniosynostosis is a common multifactorial congenital anomaly affecting approximately 1 in 2000 births. It is the result of premature fusion of cranial sutures with the development of skull deformity that may negatively affect future brain development. Surgical procedures for craniofacial malformations are one of the most challenging cases in pediatric anesthesia. The difficulties arise in part due to the well recognized and frequently unavoidable complications of this type of surgery. Major considerations with regard to the management of these patients are (1) patient size: early surgical correction of craniosynostosis is recommended to avoid development of intracranial hypertension due to restricted skull growth and to potentially improve neurocognitive function of the brain; (2) management of the airway in patients with mid-facial hypoplasia; (3) extensive blood loss that coincides with the time of the physiologic nadir of the hematocrit in the newborn; (4) potential for development of coagulopathy related to massive blood transfusion; (5) risk of venous air embolism; (6) prolonged surgery and hypothermia; and (7) possibility of raised intracranial pressure when more than one suture is involved, or in the older child.

Case description

A 3-month-old male who had an uncomplicated term delivery presented for repair of craniosynostosis. His past medical history was significant for Crouzon syndrome (see Table 60.1). Magnetic resonance imaging (MRI) of the brain revealed fusion of the coronal sutures and mid-face hypoplasia. Preoperative laboratory evaluation was remarkable for a hematocrit of 30%.

Premedication was avoided and a peripheral intravenous catheter was started because of the young age, presence of mid-facial hypoplasia, and concern regarding potential problems with ventilation and intubation. The infant received glycopyrrolate

as an antisialagogue and sympathomimetic effect in the event of bradycardia with airway manipulation. Propofol was titrated to maintain spontaneous respiration during induction. The airway was secured nasally with the assistance of a flexible fiberoptic bronchoscope. In addition to standard ASA monitors, an arterial line and central line were placed to assist with blood pressure monitoring as well as fluid and electrolyte management.

Typed and crossed packed red blood cells were present in the operating room at the start of the skin incision. Anesthesia was maintained with isoflurane, remifentanil and vecuronium infusion. Estimated blood loss was equal to 50% of the total blood volume and the infant was transfused to maintain a hematocrit >27%. Upon completion of the surgery the infant was warm and hemodynamically stable. The trachea was left intubated due to concern about fluid shifts and airway edema in the presence of difficult airway. He was transferred to pediatric intensive care for recovery where he was extubated successfully a few hours later.

Discussion

Craniosynostosis is a congenital deformity of the skull related to premature closure of one or more cranial sutures. Craniosynostosis can be a primary anomaly (80%) or can be associated with a syndrome, most commonly Apert, Crouzon, and Pfeiffer. Isolated craniosynostosis typically affects only one suture, usually sagittal, which is also called scaphocephaly. Syndromic craniosynostosis often affects two or more sutures and can have other congenital anomalies, most noticeably mid-facial hypoplasia and obstructive sleep apnea, as in patients with Apert and Crouzon syndromes. Despite some uncertainty about the impact of early correction of craniosynostosis on future brain growth and cognitive development, it is current practice to perform surgery in early infancy.

Table 60.1. Most common syndromes associated with craniosynostosis.

Syndrome	Airway	Cerebral	Cardiac	Musculoskeletal
Apert	Maxillary hypoplasia, narrow palate, +/− cleft palate, difficult airway	Craniosynostosis, hydrocephalus	CHD	syndactyly
Crouzon	Maxillary hypoplasia with inverted, V-shaped palate, large tongue, difficult airway	Craniosynostosis, shallow orbits with proptosis		
Pfeiffer	Choanal atresia, laryngo-, tracheo-, and bronchomalacia	Craniosynostosis, hydrocephalus, Arnold–Chiari malformation		Syndactyly, broad thumbs and toes

CHD, Congenital heart disease.

In addition to routine preoperative evaluation including history and physical examination with particular attention to airway and any other associated anomalies, laboratory evaluation includes hematocrit, platelet count, coagulation profile and type/cross for packed red blood cells equal to one estimated blood volume. The potential need for postoperative mechanical ventilation, intensive care unit admission and blood transfusion should be discussed with parents.

Intraoperative monitoring should include standard ASA monitors along with arterial line for precise blood pressure monitoring and frequent blood sampling. Intravenous access sufficient for rapid blood and fluid replacement is mandatory. Blood should be checked and available prior to skin incision. Two large-bore intravenous catheters (22–20 gauge in the infant) are often adequate but central venous access may be desired if large volume blood loss is anticipated as in a multi-suture correction or the risk of venous air embolism is high. Routine use of precordial Doppler is recommended for early detection of air emboli. A bladder catheter will allow monitoring of sufficient urine output.

Most infants with primary craniosynostosis are healthy and their airway can be secured with direct laryngoscopy in an anesthetized state after inhalation induction. However, all necessary equipment to deal with the difficult airway should be immediately available especially in an infant with syndromic craniosynostosis. Spontaneous ventilation should be maintained whenever there is a concern about the likelihood of successful ventilation or intubation until the airway is secured. Meticulous attention should be paid to the endotracheal tube during positioning of the patient for surgery. Occasionally nasal or oral endotracheal tubes may be sutured or wired to avoid displacement during extreme neck manipulation. In the patient with a tracheotomy, the stoma is intubated with an armored tube and sutured in place.

The small size of infants presenting for craniosynostosis repair translates into low absolute blood volumes, such that a small amount of blood loss can result in significant hemodynamic compromise. Cardiac arrests were described due to sudden massive blood loss from sinus or extradural venous tears. Slow blood loss from bone edges and scalp incisions is often difficult to quantify secondary to a significant portion being absorbed into surgical drapes, gowns, and the plastic reservoir that is used to drain irrigation and blood from the surgical field. Because evaluation of blood loss is difficult intraoperatively, the anesthesiologist must pay meticulous attention to the monitoring of intravascular status via the arterial pressure, central venous pressure, urine output, as well as serial determination of acid-base status, hematocrit, platelet count and coagulation profile. The anesthesiologist and the surgeon need to be in ongoing communication.

Probably the most challenging part of the anesthetic management of craniosynostosis repair is the significant blood loss and frequent rate of blood product transfusion [1]. Various attempts have been made to reduce the need for allogenic blood including preoperative administration of erythropoietin and iron, autologous blood donations, acute normovolemic hemodilution, intraoperative and postoperative blood salvaging, use of less invasive surgical procedures, and combinations of the above. To date there is no "ideal" technique that can guarantee freedom of allogenic blood transfusion. Different techniques can, however, play a role in decreasing and in some patients eliminating the need for blood transfusion.

Local infiltration of the skin with epinephrine is used by surgeons to decrease blood loss. However, most of the blood loss is from the periosteum and bone. Human recombinant erythropoietin given at a dose of 600 U/kg subcutaneously for 3 consecutive weeks in combination with supplemental iron significantly increased preoperative hematocrit from a mean of 24% to a mean of 38% in 41 infants with a mean age of 5.7 months [2]. The same authors showed that combination of erythropoietin with intraoperative use of cell saver resulted in lower transfusion rates (5% vs 100% control) and less amount of blood transfused than in the control group (0.05 pediatric units vs 1.74 pediatric units). In both groups hypervolemic hemodilution using an additional 30–50 mL/kg of colloid or crystalloid solution was used as needed [2]. Although cell saver appears to be an attractive option, its use does not completely eliminate the need for transfusion, since the transfusion is often started early in the procedure to maintain hemodynamic stability, before salvaged blood is available. It can, however, decrease use of allogenic blood postoperatively.

Preoperative autologous blood donation has been described but has been considered to be impractical especially in children less than 3 years of age due to smaller blood volumes and intolerance to repeated vascular access for the donation process. Acute normovolemic hemodilution is another technique where whole blood is exchanged for an equal amount of colloid or crystalloid solution to maintain normovolemia. As a result the volume of blood lost during the surgery stays the same but the amount of red blood cell mass lost is less due to a lower hematocrit of the blood [3]. This technique may be beneficial in infants with rare blood types.

Induced hypotension was proposed as a means to decrease intraoperative blood loss. It has not gained acceptance for craniosynostosis repair. Reasons cited include compromised cerebral perfusion especially in the presence of elevated intracranial pressure, lowering mean arterial and central venous pressure increases the risk for air emboli and the potential for added hemodynamic instability during rapid blood loss [4]. There are no guidelines that specifically address blood transfusion practice in children.

The American Society of Anesthesiologists Task Force on Blood Component Therapy excluded infants and children in their practice guidelines in 1996. The British Committee for Standards in Hematology Transfusion [5] recommended the following for neonates and older children:

- Cytomegalovirus-negative blood should be used during first year of life.
- All components should be leukocyte reduced.
- A screen filter should be used for transfusion of all blood components.
- Old packed red blood cells (greater than 2–3 weeks) should be avoided whenever possible.

The amount of blood given will depend on the clinical circumstances (estimated blood loss, presence of hemodynamic instability despite maintenance of euvolemia with crystalloid or colloid solution, extent of the surgery, presence of lactic acidosis as a marker of compromised tissue perfusion). One can calculate the amount of blood to be transfused using desired, actual hemoglobin (Hb) and patient's weight: Hb desired (g/dL) – Hb actual (g/dL) × weight (kg) × 3. Since postoperative oozing is common and can lead to significant blood loss, one may consider transfusing the whole unit to which the patient has been exposed in anticipation of postoperative blood loss in order to minimize exposure to additional units.

A more practical option is to have 20 mL/kg aliquots separated in order to extend the expiration time from 4 to 24 hours after it has been spiked. Hyperkalemic cardiac arrest was described in infants who received large amounts of blood rapidly due to high concentration of potassium in stored blood. Calcium homeostasis has to be maintained especially when large volumes of citrate-containing blood products are given. Acquired coagulopathy is rarely a problem unless blood loss has reached greater than 1.5 times or more of the estimated blood volume. Platelets, fresh frozen plasma, and cryoprecipitate may be necessary in the presence of microvascular bleeding or when laboratory studies confirm coagulopathy due to component deficiency. Keep in mind that activated partial thromboplastin time is often prolonged in the first 6 months of age at baseline.

Venous air embolism has been reported during craniofacial surgery. A high index of suspicion should be maintained particularly during any phase of acute blood loss with reduction in central venous pressure. Hydration and keeping up with ongoing blood loss is critical to limit the gradient between the surgical field and the right atrium. Although transesophageal echocardiography is the most sensitive monitor for detection of emboli, its use is limited in small infants. As previously stated, the precordial Doppler, continuous monitoring of end-tidal CO_2 and nitrogen, central venous and arterial pressure waveforms may be useful in detecting significant venous air emboli.

Children with complex craniosynostosis have a higher incidence of increased intracranial pressure than those with simple craniosynostosis. Cranial vault reconstruction increases intracranial capacity and reduces intracranial pressure. Techniques to decrease elevated intracranial pressure intraoperatively include hyperventilation to $PaCO_2$ of 25–30 mmHg, cerebral dehydration with mannitol 0.25–1 g/kg and furosemide 0.5–1 mg/kg, dexamethasone 0.5 mg/kg, reverse Trendelenburg position to improve venous drainage, avoidance of extreme flexion or extension of the neck and occasionally placement of subarachnoid drain.

Maintaining normothermia is very important during surgery. Large surface-to-weight ratio, increased metabolic rate, lack of significant body fat for insulation as well as large surface area of the head that is exposed to heat loss, coupled with the need for infusion of large volumes of intravenous fluids and blood products, place infants at risk for hypothermia. Techniques for maintaining the patient's temperature include prewarming the operating room, warming fluids, and using convective air warmers.

Conclusion

Craniosynostosis repair presents a number of challenges to the anesthesiologist: (1) small size of the patients; (2) significant and often unavoidable blood loss; (3) need for intraoperative transfusion of blood products; (4) risk of venous air emboli, especially during hypotensive episodes; (4) tendency to develop hypothermia; and (5) associated anomalies including airway problems and obstructive sleep apnea. All of these potential complications call for careful preoperative and intraoperative planning, meticulous attention to intravascular volume status and hemodynamic stability as well as maintenance of normothermia. Anticipation of the above difficulties along with the treatment plan should be discussed with the surgeon and any anesthesia provider participating in the management of the patient.

References

1. G. Tuncbilek, I. Vargel, A. Erdem et al. Blood loss and transfusion rates during repair of craniofacial deformities. J Craniofac Surg 2005; 16: 59–62.

2. K. Krajewski, R. Ashley, N. Pung et al. Successful blood conservation during craniosynostotic correction with dual therapy using procrit and cell saver. J Craniofac Surg 2008; 19: 101–5.

3. C. Di Rocco, G. Tamburrini, D. Pietrini. Blood sparing in craniosynostosis surgery. Semin Pediatr Neurol 2004; 11: 278–87.

4. J. Koh, H. Gries. Perioperative management of pediatric patients with craniosynostosis. Anesthesiol Clin 2007; 25: 465–81.

5. B. E. Gibson, A. Todd, I. Roberts. Transfusion guidelines for neonates and older children. Br J Haematol 2004; 12: 433–53.

Pediatric neuroanesthesia

Scoliosis

George N. Youssef

Scoliosis is a complex deformity of the spine with lateral curvature and rotation of the thoracolumbar vertebrae leading to rib cage deformity. There are different causes for scoliosis (Table 61.1). Adolescent idiopathic scoliosis (AIS) is the commonest form of scoliosis and it affects 1–3% of children aged 10–16 years [1].

Measuring Cobb's angle has been the gold standard for quantification of the severity of scoliosis. A diagnosis is made when the curvature is 10% or more. There is a female predominance when considering curves >30 degrees, with some authors estimating the female to male ratio to be 8:1. Clinicians and patients base their treatment decisions on the risk of curve progression. For curves <50 degrees at skeletal maturity progression usually ceases. For curves >60 degrees progression is common and can compromise pulmonary function; curves >90 degrees are usually associated with significant reduction in pulmonary function.

The goals for surgical treatment are to prevent progression, improve alignment and balance, and to avoid negative outcomes of the natural history of the disease without introducing iatrogenic complications.

Case description

A 16-year-old female presented for posterior spinal instrumentation and fusion from T4–L2. She had a history of idiopathic scoliosis that started when she was 11 years old. The scoliosis curve was estimated at 60 degrees – she was otherwise healthy and extremely scared of needles. She was 56 kg with a hematocrit of 40; the patient fainted during the blood draw for the preoperative blood work.

Risks, benefits, and alternatives of the anesthetic together with the personnel involved were discussed with the patient and her family. The plan for induction of anesthesia included invasive monitors, blood conservation, neurophysiologic monitoring with the possibility of performing a "wake up test." The possibility of postoperative facial swelling and the remote chance

Table 61.1. Etiologic classification of scoliosis.

Idiopathic	Infantile: less than 4 years Juvenile: 4–10 years Adolescent: older than 10 years until skeletal maturity
Congenital	Failure of formation, e.g., hemivertebrae Failure of segmentation Mixed
Neuromuscular	Cerebral palsy Muscular dystrophy Myelomeningocele Spinal muscular atrophy Friedreich's ataxia Charcot Marie Tooth disease
Vertebral disease	Tumor Infection or metabolic bone disease
Spinal cord disease	Tumor Syringomyelia
Disease associated	Neurofibromatosis Marfan syndrome Connective tissue disorder, e.g., Ehlers–Danlos syndrome

of postoperative mechanical ventilation were also discussed. The patient was premedicated with 20 mg oral midazolam 30 minutes before the surgery.

After the application of ASA standard monitors in the operating room inhalational induction of anesthesia using nitrous oxide/oxygen and sevoflurane was performed. Two large-bore peripheral intravenous lines were started and 2 mcg/kg of fentanyl + 0.5 mg/kg of rocuronium were given to facilitate intubation. After the endotracheal tube was secured, a nasogastric tube was placed and taped to the nose, an esophageal temperature probe/stethoscope was inserted and a soft bite block was placed. An arterial line was placed and isovolemic hemodilution was started where two units of blood were obtained from the arterial line and replaced with 5% albumin at a ratio of 1:1.

Meanwhile, the neurophysiology technician worked on the placement of the monitoring leads/

needles and the operating room nurse catheterized the patient's bladder. The surgical team was then called to the operating room to help with positioning the patient on the surgical table. After proper positioning a forced air warming blanket was placed on the lower body before the patient was draped for surgery. Baseline somatosensory evoked potentials (SSEPs) and motor evoked potentials (MEPs) were obtained and anesthetic was maintained with <0.5 minimum alveolar concentration (MAC) of isoflurane with 50% nitrous oxide in oxygen; a remifentanil infusion was titrated to keep mean arterial pressure between 60–75 mmHg.

During the procedure periodic inspection of the positioning of the patient's face and arms was performed; blood work including arterial blood gases, electrolytes, hemoglobin, hematocrit, and lactate were obtained. Lactated Ringer's solution was used for fluid maintenance and replacement in addition to periodic cell saver blood. The patient continued to be hemodynamically stable despite the continuous ooze of blood throughout the procedure. By the time all the pedicle screws and rods were placed and the surgeon was ready for spine distraction, the hematocrit was 20 and the mean arterial pressure (MAP) was 59 mmHg. We transfused the patient with her own blood in addition to cell saver blood, both of which brought the MAP to 75 mmHg and the hematocrit to 26.

Somatosensory evoked potentials and MEPs were intact throughout the procedure. Before wound closure, two epidural catheters were placed by the surgeon for postoperative pain management. The patient was given 20 mcg/kg of hydromorphone IV with preparation for wake up and other anesthetics were tapered off. After the dressing was applied, the patient was turned to supine position on the hospital bed. On waking up the patient was asked to wiggle her toes and bend her legs before the endotracheal tube was pulled out and epidural catheters were loaded with 0.2 mL/kg of 0.2% ropivacaine with epinephrine 1:200 000 divided over the two catheters.

Discussion

The most common form of scoliosis encountered is adolescent idiopathic scoliosis followed by neuromuscular scoliosis and their management can be quite different (Table 61.2). Despite being healthy otherwise, AIS patients pose a number of different challenges to the anesthesiologist in all stages of their manage-

ment. Psychological preparation of the patients and their families is of the utmost importance, as well as thorough preoperative teaching and assurance to alleviate their anxiety. It is crucial to assess the developmental level of each patient and to individualize the anesthetic plan according to each patient's needs. Preoperative sedation with oral midazolam was chosen with our case as was inhalational induction given the patient's high anxiety level and her needle phobia. For more mature patients, intravenous induction would be preferred. Isovolemic hemodilution was performed in addition to cell salvage to help avoid allogenic blood transfusion. The option of preoperative blood donation should be considered and discussed with the patient before scheduling the surgery, although this is fraught with its own set of problems.

Great care has to be given to patient positioning by the surgical and anesthesia teams. Care has to be given to the positions of the arms which are normally flexed at the elbow and parallel with the head to avoid injury to the brachial plexus. All the pressure points have to be well padded. The abdomen has to be free to avoid increased intra-abdominal pressure, which can lead to increased surgical bleeding. Eyes have to be clear with no compression from the padding to avoid increased intraocular pressure leading to postoperative visual loss. Visual loss after spine surgery is a rare but devastating complication with incidence of 0.28% after surgery for scoliosis repair. Pediatric patients are at increased risk for development of nonischemic optic neuropathy with hypertension being a risk factor [2]. Slight head-up reverse Trendelenburg position is usually helpful to decrease facial edema by the end of the procedure and might decrease the chances of optic neuropathy.

The main determinant of anesthetic maintenance choice is compatibility with neurophysiologic monitoring. Usually both SSEPs and MEPs are monitored. The plan has to be agreed upon by the anesthesiologist and the neurophysiologist. We chose low-dose isoflurane/nitrous oxide plus remifentanil infusion. Remifentanil is the easiest narcotic to titrate and provides the fastest wake up in the event a wake up test is needed. However, there are many anesthetic alternatives. Propofol is shown to better preserve cortical SSEP and provide a deeper level of hypnosis compared with low-dose isoflurane/N_2O or low-dose isoflurane alone but with the risk of delayed emergence. Sevoflurane produces a faster decrease and recovery of SSEP amplitude as well as a better conscious state

Table 61.2. Clinical consideration for anesthetic management of idiopathic versus neuromuscular scoliosis.

	Idiopathic	Neuromuscular
General health	Usually healthy	Usually associated with other disease states and malnutrition
Heart	Usually normal	
Lungs	Usually normal – unless severe curvature	Possible cardiomyopathy or cor pulmonale
		Possible severe restrictive lung disease
Preoperative testing	CBC, coagulation studies, Blood type and cross match	As idiopathic + Comprehensive metabolic panel + albumin, CXR, EKG, echocardiography, PFT if patient is cooperative
	PFT only if severe curve or Reactive airway disease	
Induction	Usually intravenous + propofol occasionally inhalation if scared of needles	Usually inhalational unless risk of MH
Lines/invasive monitoring	Usually 2 PIVs + arterial line	Central venous access +arterial line +PIV
Neurophysiologic monitoring	SSEP+MEP	SSEP+MEP unless seizure disorder
Anesthetic maintenance	Narcotic infusion + propofol infusion or low-dose inhalational agent	Narcotic infusion + low-dose inhalational agent or TIVA with dexmedetomidine or ketamine if associated with cardiomyopathy or risk of MH
Estimated blood loss (EBL)	Less EBL per segment	Higher EBL
	Blood conservation techniques more successful	Allogenic blood usually needed
		Aminocaproic acid shown to decrease EBL
Number of segments to be fused	Usually less than 12	Commonly thoracic and lumbar vertebrae into the pelvic
Emergence	Usually extubated by the end	Higher possibility of post operative mechanical ventilation
ICU stay	Short, usually one night	Longer, usually a few days
Postoperative pain management	IV PCA or PCEA	Narcotic infusion or epidural infusion
Risk of infection	Minimal	Higher rate of infection

ICU, intensive care unit; CBC, complete blood count; PFT, pulmonary function tests; PIV, peripheral intravenous line; SSEP, somatosensory evoked potential; MEP, motor evoked potential; IV PCA, intravenous patient controlled analgesia; PCEA, patient controlled epidural analgesia; CXR, chest X-ray; EKG, electrocardiogram; MH, malignant hyperthermia; TIVA, total intravenous anesthesia.

on emergence than propofol. The use of dexmedetomidine infusion was shown to reduce propofol infusion requirements with potential to facilitate faster awakening compared with propofol alone [3]. Muscle relaxants are either avoided completely or an infusion is titrated to keep two twitches on the train-of-four monitor – this will have the benefit of decreasing the background noise and might improve the quality of the SSEP.

At the time of spine distraction care has to be given to optimize the patient's hemodynamics and oxygen carrying capacity to prevent ischemia to the cord. Some clinicians try to keep the MAP above 90 mmHg during this critical part of the procedure.

Epidural analgesia was chosen because it was proven to provide better analgesia and allows for quicker return to consumption of solid food with fewer side effects [4]. Other options include: (1) intrathecal morphine, which provides excellent pain control but is limited to <24 hours; (2) intravenous narcotic infusion, which is associated with increased sedation, respiratory depression, delayed return of bowel function, and increased risk of nausea and vomiting; (3) intravenous patient controlled analgesia provides good pain control during the day with fewer side effects but with increased pain whenever the patient drifts to sleep; and (4) intravenous patient-controlled analgesia with a basal narcotic infusion provides better pain control but with increased side effects.

Despite modern technology, scoliosis still carries a small but grave risk of mortality and morbidity. The key for an uneventful anesthetic is proper planning and knowledge of potential complications in order to avoid them.

References

1. **J. A. Janicki, B. Alman.** Scoliosis: review of diagnosis and treatment. *Paediatr Child Health* 2007; **12**: 771–6.

2. **C. G. Patil, E. M. Lad, S. P. Lad** *et al.* Visual loss after spine surgery. *Spine* 2008; **33**: 1491–6.

3. **N. E. Ngwenyama, J. Anderson, D. G. Hoernschemeyer** *et al.* Effects of dexmedetomidine on propofol and remifentanil infusion rates during total intravenous anesthesia for spine surgery in adolescents. *Paediatr Anaesth* 2008; **18**: 1190–5.

4. **T. A. Milbrandt, M. Singhal, C. Minter** *et al.* A comparison of three methods of pain control for posterior spinal fusions in adolescent idiopathic scoliosis. *Spine* 2009; **34**: 1499–503.

Pediatric neuroanesthesia

Hemispherectomy for treatment of intractable epilepsy in an infant with congenital antithrombin III deficiency

Rami Karroum and Alina Bodas

Perinatal cerebral artery occlusion is responsible for ischemic cerebral infarction and can lead to brain cavitation and gliosis. The etiology of perinatal ischemic accidents remains uncertain in most cases. Only in a minority of cases can a causative factor be identified, but one cause is congenital antithrombin III (ATIII) deficiency. The territory of the middle cerebral artery is most frequently involved and epilepsy can be an associated co-morbidity. Most of these epilepsy cases can be managed medically, but 6–7% are refractory [1]. Patients who are refractory to medical management can be candidates for surgical treatment such as anatomical or functional hemispherectomy.

Case description

The patient was a 10-month-old, 7.5 kg male who was born at 36 weeks gestation. Shortly after birth he was noted to have a left-sided hemiparesis. Magnetic resonance imaging of the brain showed a large right middle cerebral artery infarction. A work-up revealed congenital ATIII deficiency. The patient subsequently developed seizures refractory to medical treatment and presented for a right functional hemispherectomy.

The primary concerns of the anesthesiology team were (1) perioperative management of congenital ATIII deficiency including the administration of pooled ATIII from human plasma (thrombate III); (2) the risk of using invasive hemodynamic monitors in the setting of increased risk of thromboembolic events secondary to congenital ATIII deficiency; and (3) complications associated with hemispherectomy, especially the increased risk of bleeding.

Following his perinatal thrombotic event, anticoagulation therapy was initiated and consisted of 8 mg subcutaneous enoxaparin, injected twice daily. Twenty-four hours prior to surgery, enoxaparin was held. A baseline ATIII activity was found to be at 50%

of normal and the patient received 400 IU thrombate III. Antithrombin III activity drawn 20 minutes after the treatment was 136%. Our target range of ATIII activity in the perioperative period was set to be between 80–120% of normal. Given the risk of blood loss and large volume shifts that can occur during functional hemispherectomy, we decided that invasive hemodynamic monitors were necessary during the operation. Prior to the start of surgery, an ATIII level was drawn.

After inhalational induction, two peripheral intravenous lines were secured and the trachea was intubated. Anesthesia was maintained using balanced technique of isoflurane in oxygen and nitrous oxide combined with remifentanil infusion. Rocuronium was used to provide muscle relaxation. A left arterial catheter was placed. A double lumen right internal jugular central venous catheter was placed using ultrasound guidance. Both lines were frequently flushed intraoperatively and all lumens remained patent intraoperatively.

We closely monitored for signs and symptoms of thromboembolism including limb or face discoloration, swelling, or change in temperature of extremities.

Antithrombin III level drawn in the immediate perioperative period was at 86% activity. In consultation with the hematologist, we gave a dose of thrombate III, 125 units over 20 minutes. There were no complications associated with infusion. The operation was otherwise uneventful; there was no major bleeding or thrombotic event. The trachea was extubated successfully in the operating room and the patient subsequently transferred to the pediatric intensive care unit for further management.

Postoperatively, ATIII levels were checked twice daily and infusions of thrombate III were dosed accordingly. The patient's arterial catheter was removed a few hours after the end of the surgery because blood could no longer be aspirated from the catheter. There was no sign of thromboembolism in the left upper extremity. The central venous catheter remained in place until postoperative day 5. By the time of removal both lumens had clotted. An ultrasound of the upper extremity did not reveal any evidence of thrombosis. On postoperative day 6, thrombate III infusion was stopped and ATIII levels followed. Once the levels dropped to the 80% range, enoxaparin subcutaneous injection was restarted at a dose of 1 mg/kg twice daily. The patient did not suffer any thrombotic or hemorrhagic events throughout his hospital stay.

Discussion

Early surgery for intractable epilepsy is recommended as it has been shown to improve functional outcomes. Anatomic hemispherectomy consists of the resection of the frontal, parietal and occipital cortices, complete temporal lobectomy and insular resection. Perioperative complications associated with this procedure include significant changes in systemic and pulmonary vascular resistance, arrhythmias, cardiac arrest, neurogenic pulmonary edema, seizures, cerebral edema, massive blood loss, and coagulopathy. Modification of this procedure led to introduction of functional hemispherectomy. This procedure leaves the anterior frontal and posterior occipital lobes intact while a temporal lobectomy and central resection are performed. The remaining cortex is completely disconnected by resecting the corpus callosum. In this manner, the frontal and occipital lobes remain, but are functionally disconnected from the brain. This procedure is associated with reduced hemorrhage and other complications. Patients undergoing hemispherectomy are usually on chronic anticonvulsant therapy. This leads to hepatic enzyme induction and consequently opioids and muscle relaxants are more rapidly metabolized [2]. Thus, more frequent or larger dosing of these medications is often required.

Antithrombin III is a serine protease inhibitor that plays an important role in modulating coagulation by inhibiting factor IIa (thrombin), factor Xa and to a lesser extent factors IX, XI, XII (Figure 62.1). Antithrombin III is produced by the liver and has normal plasma concentrations of 112–140 mcg/mL (equivalent to approximately 100 IU/dL of ATIII activity) with a half life of 2–3 days [3]. Congenital ATIII deficiency is the most clinically important of the inherited thrombophilias resulting in thrombosis in the majority of those affected. The challenge in managing these patients is preventing potentially life-threatening thrombosis, while minimizing the equally significant risk of hemorrhage associated with long-term anticoagulation.

Patients with congenital ATIII deficiency have around 50% normal levels of antithrombin activity. Interestingly, childhood is a period that carries the lowest thrombotic risk. Increasing age and presence of hypercoagulable states such as pregnancy, surgery, or immobility raise the risk of thrombosis markedly. Even rarer is the instance of arterial thrombotic events, with venous thrombotic events being much more prevalent. Our patient represents a very rare case in that one of his thrombotic events that he developed in the perinatal period was arterial in origin. While primary prophylaxis with anticoagulant therapy is generally not recommended in asymptomatic ATIII deficiency [4], our patient required low molecular weight heparin therapy perioperatively given his serious thromboembolic complications. In addition, our patient received thrombate III in the pre-, intra-, and postoperative periods. Despite the absence of a randomized controlled trial to prove benefit to this treatment and despite the inherent risk associated with the use of pooled plasma products, its use has been considered appropriate in patients undergoing procedures with a high risk of venous thromboembolic events. Antithrombin III could be continued for few days until it is safe to administer therapeutic doses of anticoagulants. Side effects of ATIII include: hypersensitivity, dizziness, chest tightness, dyspnea, or nausea. The risk of viral transmission such as human immunodeficiency virus, hepatitis C virus, hepatitis B virus, or other infectious agents is very rare.

Potency of thrombate III is expressed in international units (units) as tested against activity of the World Health Organization reference standard. One unit is approximately equivalent to the amount of ATIII (mg) in 1 mL of pooled human plasma from healthy donors. The initial loading dose of thrombate III is calculated by the following equation:

$$\text{Initial dose (units)} = [(\text{Goal ATIII level \%} - \text{baseline ATIII level \%}) \times \text{body weight (kg)}] / 1.4.$$

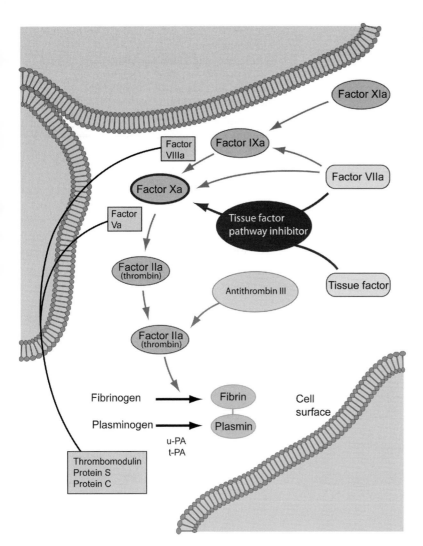

Figure 62.1. The anticoagulant action of antithrombin III.

The formula is based on the expected incremental in vivo increase of antithrombin III concentrations above baseline values of 1.4% for each unit/kg administered. Thrombate III is given as an infusion over 10–20 minutes. Strict aseptic technique is recommended during reconstitution since the drug contains no preservative. It should be diluted with sterile water and used within 3 hours after reconstitution. The maintenance dosage is calculated by determining the preinfusion (trough) and peak postinfusion ATIII concentrations. Additional doses of ATIII are administered at appropriate intervals (e.g., every 24 hours) until peak and trough concentrations are maintained within the therapeutic range of 80–120% of normal. Therapy with thrombate III is usually continued for 2–8 days following thromboembolism or surgical or obstetric procedures, depending on the clinical situation. It is not known whether supraphysiologic concentrations (e.g., 150–200% of normal) increase bleeding risk in patients with congenital ATIII deficiency [5].

Care of these patients not only requires an integrated team approach with close collaboration among the anesthesiologist, hematologist, surgeon, and intensivist, but an acute sense of vigilance in monitoring for signs of thromboembolic events – particularly in relation to foreign material such as indwelling catheters. Invasive venous and arterial catheters were used safely in this patient and were only kept in place for as long as absolutely necessary.

References

1. **P. Uvebrant**. Hemiplegic cerebral palsy. Aetiology and outcome. *Acta Paediatr Scand Suppl* 1988; **345**: 1–100.

2. **S. G. Soriano, L. J. Sullivan, K. Venkatakrishnan** *et al.* Pharmacokinetics and pharmacodynamics of vecuronium in children receiving phenytoin or carbamazepine for chronic anticonvulsant therapy. *Br J Anaesth* 2001; **86**: 223–9.

3. **P. S. Maclean, R. C. Tait**. Hereditary and acquired antithrombin deficiency. *Drugs* 2007; **67**: 1429–40.

4. **Haemostasis and Thrombosis Task Force, British Committee for Standards in Haematology.** Investigation and management of heritable thrombophilia. *Br J Haematol* 2001; **114**: 512–28.

5. **Talecris Biotherapeutics.** *Thrombate® III (antithrombin III) injection prescribing information.* Research Triangle Park, NC; 2006.

Neurosurgical procedures for pediatric patients with cardiac malformations

Stephen J. Kimatian, Kenneth Saliba and Erin S. Williams

In the USA, approximately 30 000 infants are born annually with congenital heart disease (CHD) and currently there are an estimated 750 000–1 000 000 children and adults with CHD who may present for noncardiac surgery [1, 2]. With advances in medical and surgical care, patients are surviving complex cardiac palliative procedures and living well beyond adolescence into adulthood. This underscores important issues regarding the safe and proper anesthetic management of the CHD patient having noncardiac surgery. Since the presence of CHD increases the risk for noncardiac surgery, the anesthesiologist must understand the pathophysiology of the cardiac lesion and how their anesthetic management affects the patient's cardiovascular system.

In order to minimize complications, the anesthesiologist must tailor their anesthetic management according to the age of the patient, type of lesion, extent of corrective procedure, and presence of other congenital anomalies [3].

Case description

The patient was a 7-year-old female with a history of hypoplastic left heart syndrome (HLHS) who was status post Fontan completion operation 3 years ago and who presented for resection of a right temporal lobe mass. She was premedicated with oral midazolam 0.5 mg/kg in the preoperative suite and then brought to the operating room, where she underwent an uneventful inhalation induction. Two large-bore peripheral intravenous catheters were placed, as well as an arterial line. General anesthesia was maintained with isoflurane and fentanyl, with neuromuscular blockade achieved with rocuronium.

The primary concerns of the anesthesiology team included the avoidance of increased pulmonary vascular resistance (PVR), the maintenance of adequate systemic oxygenation, the avoidance of increased intracranial pressure, and the maintenance of adequate

cerebral perfusion pressure. Pulmonary vascular resistance is critical after a Fontan procedure, as blood flows directly from the right atrium to the pulmonary arteries – increased PVR can lead to cyanosis.

After removal of the bone flap the surgeon stated that the dura was tight, so the anesthesiologist hyperventilated the patient to an end-tidal CO_2 of 32. The surgery proceeded uneventfully and the tumor was resected. The patient remained hemodynamically stable throughout the case and the trachea was extubated in the operating room at the end of the procedure.

Discussion

When managing a CHD patient for noncardiac surgery it is imperative to address the specific anatomy and physiology following any palliative procedures. Also, one must appreciate the presence of intracardiac or systemic-to-pulmonary artery shunts as well as how manipulations of PVR and systemic vascular resistance (SVR) affect these shunts. Lastly, the presence of dysrhythmias, polycythemia, and hyperviscosity should be identified, along with the observance of subacute bacterial endocarditis (SBE) prophylaxis [4]. In this case, the patient had undergone a total cavopulmonary anastamosis following the Fontan procedure, without significant residual shunt. Thus, no further surgical intervention was required and arterial saturations were typically 94–98%.

Preoperative management

The history and physical examination are extremely important in evaluating a patient with CHD. During the physical examination, the clinician should assess the airway, heart, lungs, and extremities. The extremities can be assessed for ease of vascular access and the presence of adequate pulses, clubbing, or edema. It is imperative that the patient be euvolemic with adequate peripheral perfusion and hydration prior to the induction of general anesthesia. This can also be assessed by evaluating the patient on physical examination. Signs such as tachycardia, low blood pressure, decreased skin turgor, dry mucous membranes, and decreased capillary refill all indicate dehydration and hypovolemia; therefore intravenous access should be obtained and the patient adequately resuscitated before proceeding with induction. If possible, the intake of clear liquids should be encouraged up to 2 hours before the planned institution of general anesthesia in the post Fontan population to optimize intravascular volume status [5].

Evaluation of the most recent electrocardiogram, echocardiogram, and cardiac catheterization is paramount. Ideally, the patient would have had a cardiologist consultation within the prior 6 months, or as part of their preoperative evaluation [6].

The presence of a fenestration in the Fontan conduit also carries the risk for paradoxical embolism; therefore, strict bubble precautions must be adhered to throughout the perioperative infusion of intravenous fluids or medications.

The history and physical examination is essential in determining the presence of congestive heart failure. Krane developed 10 rules that can help the anesthesiologist when examining a child with CHD. These include:

1. You cannot auscultate a crying child.
2. Examine the heart first.
3. Most systolic murmurs will be benign.
4. All pan-systolic murmurs are pathological.
5. All diastolic murmurs are pathological.
6. All murmurs that radiate are pathological.
7. The louder the murmur the smaller the shunt.
8. The softer the murmur the larger the shunt, the sicker the child.
9. Children develop biventricular failure.
10. Obtain blood pressure readings in upper and lower extremities [7].

It is also important for the anesthesiologist to understand how to manage preload, PVR, SVR, heart rate, and contractility in patients with CHD.

For example, in patients with tetralogy of Fallot, it is imperative to maintain preload while decreasing heart rate and contractility. Pulmonary vascular resistance should also be decreased to minimize right to left shunting while SVR remains increased. If the anesthesiologist is presented with a patient that has undergone a Fontan, the physiologic goals for this

Table 63.1. Effect of intracardiac shunts on intravenous and inhalation induction.

Shunt type	Intravenous induction	Inhalation induction
Left to right	Slower	Faster or unchanged
Right to left	Faster	Slower

patient would include maintaining preload and avoiding anything that could increase the PVR in order to maximize pulmonary circulation. Systemic vascular resistance should be maintained and no changes are warranted with heart rate and contractility [3].

Since patients with CHD will possibly have undergone multiple surgeries, they can have a great deal of preoperative anxiety. Therefore, premedication can be administered unless the patient is hemodynamically unstable, symptomatic from mass effect, or lethargic. Typically, midazolam is given either orally, intranasally, or intravenously.

Intraoperative management

The presence of intracardiac shunts can affect the speed of induction. The anesthesiologist should be knowledgeable of these changes (see Table 63.1). For example, a patient with left-to-right shunt will have a quicker inhalation induction because there is more blood passing through the lungs and thereby more blood being delivered to the brain, thus leading to unconsciousness sooner. Patients with right-to-left shunts have slower inhalation inductions because blood is diverted away from the lungs [3]. With right-to-left shunts, however, intravenous induction agents bypass the lungs and go directly to the systemic circulation – this makes the possibility of overdose much higher. Thus, the clinician must appropriately adjust his or her dosages.

Once induction is underway, the anesthesiologist must vigilantly prevent any increases in intracranial pressure. This can be done by maintaining an adequate depth of anesthesia during laryngoscopy, as well as during the most stimulating portions of the planned operative procedure, such as skull pin placement, and dural reflection, as well as the remainder of the surgical procedure. During the maintenance phase of anesthesia, volatile anesthetics along with intermediate acting neuromuscular blockers, such as rocuronium, and fentanyl are acceptable. Oxygen and air mixtures would be optimal since nitrous oxide can cause expansion of venous air emboli, which could lead to acute increases in PVR and catastrophic cardiovascular collapse. In addition, patients with Fontan anatomy will often have a fenestration between the venous and arterial systems at the level of the atrial baffle setting the stage for right-to-left shunting in the presence of increased PVR and emboli to the arterial circulation. Monitors such as capnography and precordial Doppler are vital in diagnosing a venous air embolism. The transesophageal echocardiogram is the most sensitive monitor for detection of air emboli, but its availability, size, and encroachment near the surgical field, plus the requisite expertise, may limit its feasibility.

Patients with Fontan circulation are dependent upon central venous pressure for pulmonary blood flow. Blood must flow passively through the lungs to fill the heart, making the management of pulmonary blood flow an important aspect of care for these patients. It is imperative that preload, oxygenation, and ventilation be maintained to avoid catastrophic elevations in PVR. Other etiologies of increased PVR such as stress, hypothermia, acidosis, and atelectasis must be avoided.

Given the need to maintain adequate cerebral oxygenation, cerebral perfusion, and to avoid intracranial hypertension, an arterial line must supplement standard ASA monitors, and will allow real-time measurement of blood pressure, as well as providing the ability to follow PaO_2, $PaCO_2$, and electrolytes. End-tidal CO_2 to $PaCO_2$ differences can also be followed as measurement of relative pulmonary dead space and an indirect indicator of West Lung Zone 1 and pulmonary blood flow.

With regard to SBE or infective endocarditis prophylaxis, the American Heart Association has guidelines regarding the administration of appropriate antimicrobial therapy to susceptible patients. Subacute bacterial endocarditis can develop after noncardiac surgery in any mucosal penetrating procedure that permits bacteria to seed on prosthetic endocardium [3]. The previous guidelines recommended routine SBE prophylaxis for all patients at risk undergoing dental, gastrointestinal, or genitourinary procedures; however, this is no longer the case. Prophylaxis is now recommended only for patients considered at highest risk of acquiring SBE, such as:

1. Patients with prosthetic heart valves or with prosthetic material used in valve repair.

2. History of previous endocarditis.
3. Specific CHD (unrepaired cyanotic CHD, completely repaired CHD with prosthetic material during the past 6 months, repaired CHD with residual defect).
4. Cardiac transplant patients with cardiac valvular disease (American Heart Association: www.heart.org/HEARTORG/).

Postoperative management

In patients status post Fontan procedures, spontaneous ventilation allows for better pulmonary blood flow than does positive-pressure ventilation. Thus, if the operation has been otherwise uneventful and the patient is hemodynamically stable and normothermic, extubation of the trachea in the operating room should be considered. Reversal of neuromuscular blockade must first take place. Postoperative pain management can include carefully titrated opioids such as fentanyl, hydromorphone, or morphine with special care to avoid respiratory compromise that can result in hypercarbia, hypoxia, atelectasis, and increased PVR. Early postoperative emergence and extubation will also facilitate postoperative neurologic examination.

References

1. **R. R. Clancy**. Neuroprotection in infant heart surgery. *Clin Perinatol* 2008; **35**: 809–21.

2. **R. Sumpelmann, W. Osthaus**. The pediatric cardiac patient presenting for non-cardiac surgery. *Curr Opin Anaesthesiol* 2007; **20**: 216–20.

3. **R. Mohindra, D. Beebe, K. Belani**. Anesthetic management of patients with congenital heart disease presenting for non-cardiac surgery. *Ann Card Anaesth* 2002; **5**: 15–24.

4. **M. Cannesson, M. Earing, V. Collange** et al. Anesthesia for noncardiac surgery in adults with congenital heart disease. *Anesthesiology* 2009; **111**: 432–40.

5. **C. D. McCLain, F. X. McGowan, P. G. Kovatsis**. Laparoscopic surgery in a patient with fontan physiology. *Anesth Analg* 2006; **103**: 856–8.

6. **L. Diaz, S. Hall**. Anesthesia for non-cardiac surgery and magnetic resonance imaging. In **Andropoulos D. B., Stayer S. A., Russell I. A.**, eds. *Anesthesia for Congenital Heart Disease*. Malden, MA: Blackwell Futura, 2005; 427–52.

7. **E. Krane**. Anesthesia in children with congenital heart disease. *Pediatric Anesthesia and Pain Management*; 2–15. Available from http://pedsanesthesia.stanford.edu/downloads/guideline-chd.pdf.

Neuroprotection during pediatric cardiac anesthesia

Stephen J. Kimatian, Erin S. Williams and Kenneth Saliba

In the USA, approximately 30 000 infants are born annually with congenital heart disease (CHD) [1]. Of these 30 000 infants, about 11 000 will require some form of surgical correction [1]. Such procedures place these infants at risk for morbidity and mortality associated with cardiac surgery. However, with advances in medicine and surgical technique patients are surviving these intricate procedures, leading us to focus our attention toward issues such as optimizing the neurologic outcomes of patients who have undergone congenital heart surgery [1].

The overall incidence of neurologic injury associated with cardiac surgery in children is 2–25% [2]. These insults can stem from preoperative brain anomalies, perioperative hypoxemia and low cardiac output states, as well as sequelae from cardiopulmonary bypass and deep hypothermic circulatory arrest. It has also been found that approximately half of school-aged survivors of infant heart surgery receive some sort of special education assistance [1]. In a study of 171 children after repair of d-transposition of the great arteries (d-TGA), these children had more developmental delay, speech problems, learning disorders, and attention problems than controls at the same age [3]. With such prevalence and such an effect on psychosocial development, it is important that anesthesiologists monitor and protect the pediatric neurologic system.

Case description

The patient was a 3-day-old neonate with a history significant for hypoplastic left heart syndrome. The patient was born at 37 weeks gestation and was currently on a prostaglandin infusion to maintain patency of the ductus arteriosis. As expected in a patient with complete mixing of oxygenated and deoxygenated blood in a single ventricle, pulse oximetry showed saturations in the low to mid 80s.

The patient was scheduled for a Norwood procedure. The Norwood procedure would result in the creation of a single "neo aorta" to provide systemic blood flow, with pulmonary blood flow from a surgically created shunt between the systemic and pulmonary arterial systems (Blalock Taussig Shunt). Such extensive reconstruction of the aortic arch requires a period of low flow or no flow while on cardiac bypass, placing the child at significant risk for neurologic injury.

In addition to standard ASA monitors, intraoperative monitoring included an arterial line, central venous line, and near infrared spectroscopy (NIRS). The patient was induced intravenously with ketamine 2 mg/kg, pancuronium 0.1 mg/kg and fentanyl 2 mcg/kg. The focus of the anesthesiology team was maintaining a balance between pulmonary and systemic blood flow (Qp:Qs) that would ensure adequate cardiac output and oxygen content such that end organ perfusion and oxygenation was maintained. This child's single ventricle morphology resulted in blood flowing to the lungs or body proportional to the relative resistance of the two respective systems. Maintaining homeostasis would require active manipulation of pulmonary, systemic, and cerebral vascular resistance. The surgery was approximately 5 hours in duration requiring 40 minutes of deep hypothermic circulatory arrest (DHCA) during which time the patient was cooled to 18 °C and cerebral perfusion was maintained via selected perfusion of the innominate artery. The patient remained stable throughout the case and the trachea was extubated 3 hours after surgery without any gross neurologic sequelae.

Discussion

When considering the etiology of negative neurologic outcomes after cardiac bypass surgery, the adult literature cites primarily embolic causes, while the pediatric literature cites a number of different possibilities [2]. The neurologic sequelae in infants who have undergone cardiac surgery include seizures, stroke, and choreoathetosis [1]. During DHCA the pediatric patient endures a planned period of low, or no, cerebral blood flow. This insult causes changes very similar to the changes seen in hypoxic ischemic encephalopathy [1].

In the past, it was thought that infants who underwent cardiac surgery had normal brains and that any injury that occurred was simply secondary to surgery. However, magnetic resonance imaging of the brains of neonates with CHD has shown a significant incidence of anatomical components that appear premature compared with term neonates without CHD. In a study by Williams et al., preoperative magnetic resonance imaging showed white matter injury in >15% of neonates and cerebral atrophy changes in one-third of children with CHD [3]. Additionally, there are increased amounts of periventricular leukomalacia, also known as white matter neuropathology, as well as microcephaly, hypotonia, and delayed brain maturation [3].

Cerebral injury after cardiac surgery continues to be a significant source of morbidity, and there are numerous pharmacologic and nonpharmacologic modalities that have been implemented to prevent such injury. During the course of cardiac bypass surgery involving DHCA, the patient is actively cooled via the cardiopulmonary bypass (CPB) circuit to a core temperature of 18 °C prior to the initiation of the low- or no-flow period. Once the repair is complete, the patient is slowly rewarmed prior to being weaned from CPB. Various techniques have been employed to minimize or modify the period of DHCA as prolonged DHCA with no flow (>30 minutes) has been associated with a higher incidence of neurologic complications [3]. One method is regional low-flow perfusion. This allows the brain and upper body to be perfused via a GoreTex graft connected to the innominate artery. The graft allows for CPB blood flow to the right common carotid and right vertebral artery to directly perfuse the right side of the brain. Assuming an intact circle of Willis, the left side of the brain is also indirectly perfused. Animal studies have shown better neurologic outcomes and less apoptosis in piglets exposed to regional low-flow perfusion compared with those subjected to DHCA [3]. Other perfusion methods that may lead to better neurologic outcome include intermittent cerebral perfusion and low-flow CBP.

Hematocrit while on bypass affects the oxygen carrying capacity to end organs as well as the viscosity and flow dynamics in capillary beds. Recent studies have suggested that higher hematocrits in the range of 25–30 result in better neurologic outcomes than the hematocrits in the low to mid 20s that had been traditionally used [4].

Neurologic monitoring should be used during surgery for congenital cardiac lesions, however, it is important to note that many of these modalities represent indirect measurements of neurologic function or cerebral oxygen status and are not without limitations. The electroencephalogram (EEG), by providing a measure of cerebral electrical activity, can provide an indirect measure of cerebral metabolic oxygen demand as well as display characteristic changes in the presence of cerebral hypoxia. Inducing an isoelectric EEG via thermal or pharmacologic intervention prior to the initiation of DHCA or low flow can provide assurance that cerebral oxygen demand is at its lowest prior to the anticipated insult. Using intraoperative EEG does require dedicated personnel with expertise to place the electrodes and interpret the waveforms during the surgery. Intraoperative monitoring is further complicated by many sources of artifact not seen in normal EEGs including distortion by anesthetics, electrical surgical equipment, CPB and patient temperature [3]. Austin et al. found that EEG changes were associated with only 5% of adverse neurologic outcomes and that aberrant readings did not consistently correlate with negative postoperative outcomes [5]. For these reasons the routine use of EEG in pediatric cardiac surgery was not recommended. Processed EEG, such as the BIS monitor, has been studied as a means of judging depth of anesthesia but has not been shown to correlate with cerebral injury in children.

Near infrared spectroscopy is a noninvasive method for monitoring cerebral oxygenation. It uses light at wavelengths 700–1000 micrometers in a manner similar to pulse oximetry, but without a discernible pulse to distinguish arterial from venous flow, NIRS provides an indication of regional tissue saturation. A monitor that emits near infrared light is placed on the forehead of the patient, which penetrates an approximately 10 mL banana-shaped region of tissue in the frontal cortex. The only Food and Drug Administration-approved instrument for measuring cerebral oxygen saturation specifically uses the term regional saturation index (rSO_2i). In order to interpret the rSO_2i, it is assumed that 75% of cerebral blood volume is venous while the remaining 25% is arterial. For pediatric patients there are pediatric-specific probes (4–40 kg), which account for anatomical differences such as a thinner skull and smaller radius of curvature. The rSO_2i value indicates a relative ratio of oxyhemoglobin to total hemoglobin that results in a numerical score reported as a raw score of 15–95. These values are not considered actual percent saturation of oxygen but rather a relative value from baseline. This means that proper interpretation of the NIRS readings requires a baseline measurement at the start of the case, preferably prior to the induction of anesthesia. Adult studies have suggested that decreases of >20% from baseline could be associated with neurologic injury [3].

Although it is difficult to make direct application of animal studies to humans, there may be some relevance to low rSO_2i and cell dysfunction, cell death, and subsequently negative neurologic outcome. Piglet models that used NIRS with different variables showed that the nadir of rSO_2i occurred earlier with lower hematocrits and higher temperatures. In addition, lower rSO_2i readings were seen with the use of alpha-stat pH management when compared with pH-stat management. It has been suggested that this difference seen with pH-stat management results from better cerebral blood flow and more effective cooling of the brain [3]. Near infrared spectroscopy has also been shown to be effective in detecting cerebral desaturation with superior vena cava occlusion in a piglet model. Extrapolation of these studies to the neonatal population has been suggested for superior vena cava cannulation for bypass, which can result in partial occlusion [3].

One study of 26 infants and children undergoing bypass and DHCA found that the three patients with low rSO_2i had acute postoperative neurologic events, which included seizures in one and prolonged coma in the other two patients [2]. With such findings, it appears that NIRS may be beneficial in identifying potential neurologic injury. There are, however, limitations to NIRS such as the small area that is assessed for cerebral desaturation, the variation in rSO_2i preoperatively (depending on the cardiac anatomy), and the need for more prospective outcome studies.

The transcranial Doppler allows real time assessment of cerebral blood flow velocity and emboli during cardiac surgery. The most common blood vessel evaluated is the middle cerebral artery. Typically, a 2 MHz probe is placed above the zygoma and anterior to the tragus of the ear. This position allows visualization of the bifurcation of the middle and anterior cerebral artery in which there is antegrade (toward the transducer with the middle cerebral artery) and retrograde flow (away from transducer with the anterior cerebral artery) [2]. The anterior fontanelle is an alternative site that can be used in infants [2]. In addition to showing flow velocity and emboli, case reports have also shown that transcranial Doppler can detect cerebral steal in the presence of systemic to pulmonary shunts [6].

Transcranial Doppler has several technical and logistic issues that must be considered. Placement of the probe can be technically difficult and maintaining probe position in the operative environment can be challenging. In addition, artifact can also produce false "hits" and requires a trained eye to distinguish emboli from artifact. It is also important to remember that cerebral blood flow velocity depends upon the size of the cerebral vasculature, and cerebral blood flow is affected by cerebral vascular resistance. Thus, the clinician must consider anesthetic and physiologic changes that affect cerebral vascular resistance when interpreting changes in flow velocity. While this can be a very useful tool, the technical difficulties coupled with the expertise required for accurate interpretation makes regular use impractical in many institutions. As the technology improves, it has the potential of being a useful adjunct for neurologic monitoring in the future.

Conclusion

With so many patients surviving very complex congenital heart surgeries, the anesthesiologist should lead the way in preventing, assessing, and treating neurologic injury in order to obtain the highest quality of life possible for these children. While intraoperative neurologic monitoring for pediatric cardiac surgery is still a relatively new science, it shows a great deal of promise for future application in minimizing cerebral injury and optimizing neurodevelopmental outcome.

References

1. **R. R. Clancy**. Neuroprotection in infant heart surgery. *Clin Perinatol* 2008; **35**: 809–21.

2. **D. B. Andropoulos, S. A. Stayer, L. K. Diaz** et al. Neurologic monitoring for congenital heart surgery. *Anesth Analg* 2004; **99**: 1365–75.

3. **G. D. Williams, C. Ramamoorthy**. Brain monitoring and protection during pediatric cardiac surgery. *Semin Cardiothorac Vasc Anesth* 2007; **11**: 23–33.

4. **S. J. Kimatian, K. J. Saliba, X. Soler** *et al.* The influence of neurophysiologic monitoring on the management of pediatric cardiopulmonary bypass. *ASAIO* 2008; **54**: 467–9.

5. **E. H. Austin 3rd, H. L. Edmonds Jr, S. M. Auden** *et al.* Benefit of neurophysiologic monitoring for pediatric cardiac surgery. *J Thorac Cardiovasc Surg* 1997; **114**: 707–15, 717; discussion 715–16.

6. **S. J. Kimatian, J. L. Myers, S. K. Johnson** *et al.* Transcranial Doppler-revealed retrograde cerebral artery flow during Norwood operation. *ASAIO* 2006; **52**: 608–10.

65 Pregnant patient with aneurysm

Karen K. Wilkins and Alexandra S. Bullough

Approximately 1–2% of pregnant women undergo nonobstetric surgery during their pregnancy. The challenge in these cases is that the anesthesia care provider must take into consideration both mother and fetus. Neurosurgery during pregnancy is rare and as a result there are few evidence-based recommendations in the literature to provide guidance. Concerns are often raised about the perinatal implications of anesthetic exposure. An understanding of maternal physiology and a multidisciplinary approach are imperative to ensure a successful outcome.

Case description

A 37-year-old G9 P6, ASA 3, Jehovah's Witness female with multiple hematologic co-morbidities presented at 18 weeks gestation with a 1-year history of perioral and periocular twitching, memory lapses and a recent sensory loss and painful paresthesias affecting the right side of her body. Magnetic resonance angiography demonstrated a 7-mm saccular aneurysm involving the anterior communicating artery. Her co-morbidities included von Willebrand's disease type I, alpha thalassemia trait and antiphospholipid antibody syndrome. After a multidisciplinary discussion involving neurosurgery, obstetrics, and hematology it was decided to proceed with intracranial aneurysm clipping via craniotomy at 18 weeks gestation.

Primary concerns for the anesthesiology team were (1) risk of significant blood loss given her multiple hematologic dyscrasias and Jehovah's Witness status; (2) maintenance of hemodynamic stability – hypotension would be detrimental to placental perfusion and perioperative hypertension risks aneurysm rupture; (3) maternal aspiration; and (4) fetal survival and wellbeing.

On the day of surgery, Humate-P was administered preoperatively per hematology recommendations. Humate-P (lyophilized concentrate of Factor VIII and von Willebrand's Factor) is given perioper-atively to patients with von Willebrand's disease to promote platelet aggregation and adhesion to damaged vascular endothelium. Fetal heart tones were confirmed by the obstetricians. A private discussion between the anesthesiologist and patient regarding blood replacement therapy also took place. The patient agreed to receive a transfusion of packed red blood cells if more than one unit was required to maintain maternal and fetal safety. She also agreed to cell saver blood replacement if the system maintained continuity with her circulation. The patient had a 16 g peripheral intravenous catheter and a radial arterial line placed preoperatively.

A smooth intravenous rapid sequence induction with cricoid pressure was performed using lidocaine, fentanyl, propofol, and succinylcholine. After anesthetic induction, a subclavian central line was placed for potential administration of vasopressors or fluid resuscitation. Esmolol was utilized during cranial pin placement. Hemodynamic stability was achieved throughout the case using phenylephrine and remifentanil infusions. The patient received two units of packed red blood cells due to increasing phenylephrine requirements and a hematocrit of 17 prior to manipulation of the aneurysm. The remainder of the case proceeded without incident and the trachea was extubated postoperatively. In the recovery room, the fetal heart tones were confirmed to be in the 150s. Her postoperative course was uneventful and she was transferred out of the intensive care unit on postoperative day 2 and discharged home on day 5 without neurologic sequelae.

Discussion

Intracranial aneurysms have an estimated rupture rate of approximately 20 in 100 000 pregnancies with most cases occurring between the 30th week of pregnancy and 6 weeks postpartum [1–3]. An increase in aneurysm rupture risk is most likely due to the

Table 65.1. Physiologic changes in pregnancy.

System	Physiologic changes	Comments
Cardiovascular	↑ Cardiac output ↑ Blood volume ↑ Resting heart rate ↓ Systemic vascular resistance ↓ Blood pressure (second trimester) Dilutional anemia Aortocaval compression after 16–20 weeks ↑ Risk of thromboembolic disease	Maintain systolic blood pressure >100 mmHg Left uterine displacement after 16–20 weeks
Pulmonary	↑ Respiratory rate ↑ Tidal volume ↑ Minute ventilation ↓ Functional residual capacity Respiratory alkalosis Mucosal engorgement/edema Potentially difficult airway	Preoxygenation Optimal "sniffing position" or ramping Alternative intubation plan (intubating laryngeal mask airway, Glidescope, fiberoptic scope)
Gastrointestinal	↓ Gastric motility ↓ Esophageal sphincter tone	Nonparticulate antacid Rapid sequence induction
Central nervous system	↓ Minimum alveolar concentration ↓ Local anesthetic requirements	

changes that occur in cardiac physiology during pregnancy (Table 65.1), which comprise a 50% increase in cardiac output and blood volume expansion as well as a hormonal softening of vascular connective tissue [1, 3]. Maternal mortality associated with a ruptured aneurysm is approximately 35% [1, 2, 4].

In this case, in addition to the usual concerns of a neurosurgical patient undergoing aneurysm clipping such as intraoperative aneurysmal rupture and central nervous system ischemic episodes, the parturient has issues that are specific and unique to pregnancy. Concerns are often raised about the perinatal implications of anesthetic exposure. In general, propofol, morphine, local anesthetics, muscle relaxants, and inhalational agents are considered safe in pregnancy. Antiseizure medications known to be teratogenic include carbamazepine, phenytoin, and valproic acid and should be avoided in pregnant neurosurgical patients. It is recommended that elective nonobstetric surgery in the pregnant patient be performed during the second trimester. Surgery during the first trimester, the time of organogenesis and rapid growth, is associated with an increased risk of teratogenesis and intrauterine fetal demise. Surgery performed in the third trimester is associated with an increased risk of premature labor. In this patient, the obstetricians and neurosurgeons agreed that 18 weeks gestation was an optimal time to perform maternal surgery.

Vascular neurosurgery may be associated with rapid blood loss and hemodynamic instability, thus large-bore intravenous access and invasive monitoring are warranted. In addition to the typical invasive lines and monitors utilized for neurosurgery, one must consider fetal monitoring for pregnant patients. Fetal viability is generally accepted to be 24 weeks gestation. Prior to 24 weeks gestation, fetal monitoring is typically limited to a pre/postoperative assessment of heart tones. After 24 weeks, severe changes in baseline fetal heart tones may be predictive of neonatal mortality and loss of fetal heart rate variability may be associated with hypoxia, sedative medications, and fetal sleep. Beyond 24 weeks, the decision to monitor fetal heart tones intraoperatively is both institution- and case-dependent. If a decision is made to monitor fetal heart tones intraoperatively, it is recommended to establish a preoperative management plan after a patient, surgery, anesthesiology, and neonatology consensus has been reached on how to respond to unfavorable changes in fetal heart tones and whether a Cesarean section is desired or even feasible. If severe fetal bradycardia is detected the anesthesiologist must ensure adequate maternal blood pressure, ventilation, and oxygenation.

Special attention is required during induction of anesthesia in a pregnant patient. A rapid sequence induction with cricoid pressure is recommended from 16 weeks gestation and left uterine displacement is required after 16–20 weeks gestation to avoid aorto-caval compression [3]. Due to generalized mucosal and vascular engorgement as well as potential airway edema, intubation may prove to be more challenging in the pregnant patient. It is advisable to have a smaller diameter endotracheal tube available and be prepared for a potentially difficult airway. When considering respiratory physiologic changes in pregnancy, pregnant women have a decreased functional residual capacity and increased oxygen consumption and will desaturate rapidly during periods of hypoventilation or apnea, such as seen during anesthetic induction. Preoxygenation is therefore of critical importance.

Hemodynamically, aneurysm clipping in a pregnant patient carries two major risks – hypertension and hypotension. All patients are at particular risk of hypertension and subsequent aneurysm rupture during direct laryngoscopy, placement of the head in pins, incision, and during removal of the bone flap. The hypertensive response may be attenuated with esmolol (potential for transient fetal bradycardia), labetolol, lidocaine, nitroglycerin or nitroprusside (long-term use is associated with fetal cyanide toxicity). Hypotension in the pregnant patient (systolic BP <100 mmHg) causes a decrease in uteroplacental blood flow and fetal wellbeing. Contrary to past teaching, phenylephrine is now considered the vasopressor of choice for pregnant patients due to evidence that it improves neonatal acid-base status [5].

In this case, hemodynamic stability was achieved using a multimodal approach. An adequate depth of anesthesia was assured prior to endotracheal intubation through the use of fentanyl, lidocaine, and propofol. Postinduction hypotension due to the administration of Humate-P was treated with phenylephrine. The hypertensive response to cranial pin placement was anticipated and preemptively treated with esmolol boluses. Hemodynamic stability was maintained throughout this case with carefully titrated phenylephrine and remifentanil infusions.

Acceptable methods that assist with reducing maternal intracranial pressure include: slight head-up position, decreased tidal volumes, avoidance of bucking on the endotracheal tube, and moderate hyperventilation (PaCO$_2$ 28–30 mmHg). The normal parturient PaCO$_2$ is 30–32 mmHg (respiratory alkalosis) due to increased ventilation during pregnancy. Intraoperatively, it is important to avoid severe hyperventilation (PaCO$_2$ <28 mmHg) to prevent a leftward shift of the maternal oxyhemoglobin dissociation curve impairing transfer of oxygen across the placenta [6]. In this case, the patient's PaCO$_2$ was kept between 30–34 mmHg. Mannitol administration in the parturient to decrease intracranial pressure is controversial. Intravenous mannitol use may result in fetal accumulation leading to fetal hyperosmolality, decreased fetal lung fluid production and urinary blood flow, decreased plasma Na+ concentration, and fetal dehydration. However, mannitol doses of 0.25–0.5 g/kg have been reported in some cases without ill effects [1]. This patient received 0.3 g/kg of mannitol.

Conclusion

In conclusion, neurosurgery in a pregnant patient is rare and requires a thorough understanding of the physiologic changes of pregnancy and the associated concomitant anesthetic risks to both mother and fetus. A multidisciplinary approach is essential to optimize outcomes for both mother and fetus.

References

1. **L. P. Wang**, **M. J. Paech**. Neuroanesthesia for the pregnant woman. *Anesth Analg* 2008; **107**: 193–200.

2. **R. Qaiser**, **P. Black**. Neurosurgery in pregnancy. *Semin Neurol* 2007; **27**: 476–81.

3. **D. H. Chestnut**, **L. S. Polley**, **L. C. Tsen** *et al.* *Chestnut's Obstetric Anesthesia: Principles and Practice.* Philadelphia, PA: Mosby Elsevier Press, 2009.

4. **A. M. Bader**, **D. Acker**. Neurologic and muscular disease. In **Datta S.**, ed. *Anesthetic and Obstetric Management of High-risk Pregnancy.* New York, NY: Springer-Verlag, 2004; 133–42.

5. **D. W. Cooper**, **M. Carpenter**, **P. Mowbray** *et al.* Fetal and maternal effects of phenylephrine and ephedrine during spinal anesthesia for caesarean delivery. *Anesthesiology* 2002; **97**: 1582–90.

6. **K. M. Kuczkowski**. Nonobstetric surgery during pregnancy: what are the risks of anesthesia? *Obstet Gynecol Surv* 2004; **59**: 52–6.

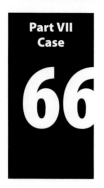
Anesthetic management of pregnant patients with brain tumors

Alaa A. Abd-Elsayed and Ehab Farag

Physiologic changes during pregnancy may result in the development or growth of nervous system tumors. Such cases at the interface of neuroanesthesia and obstetric anesthesia pose unique challenges.

Case description

A 36-year-old female presented at 36 weeks gestation with headache, nausea, and vomiting. The patient also reported that she experienced seizures at her 34th week of gestation and was prescribed lorazepam as a treatment. Computed tomography (CT) scan of the head revealed the presence of a mass in the left frontal lobe measuring 5 × 4 cm. Given the signs of intracranial hypertension, a decision was made to perform urgent concomitant Cesarean section and craniotomy to save both the mother and the fetus. Standard monitors were applied; large-bore intravenous access and an arterial line were also placed. Back-up emergency airway equipment was prepared in the event of difficult endotracheal intubation. A rapid sequence induction was performed uneventfully using fentanyl, propofol, and rocuronium and anesthetic maintenance was achieved using desflurane and remifentanil. The Cesarean section was performed and the baby was delivered with normal Apgar scores. Craniotomy then proceeded. After resection of the tumor, pathological examination of the mass revealed anaplastic glioma. The estimated blood loss during surgery was 100 mL; the patient received a total of 1800 mL intravenous fluids during surgery.

Discussion

Brain tumors tend to become larger during pregnancy due to fluid retention, increased blood volume, and hormonal changes. Therefore they may be diagnosed earlier than in the nonparturient. There are currently no guidelines for the management of intracranial tumors in the pregnant woman. A possible algorithm to follow is shown in Figure 66.1 [1].

Medical management

Corticosteroids are often used to reduce cerebral edema. These are safe in pregnancy and have the additional advantage of promoting fetal lung maturity.

First and early second trimesters

During this time, the fetus is remote from viability and, as the hemodynamic changes in the pregnant woman have not peaked, the risks of intraoperative hemorrhage are not so significant. If the patient is stable, gestational advancement may be permitted into the early second trimester, where surgical management of the tumor can be undertaken. Furthermore, radiotherapy, radiosurgery and image-guided surgery during gestation beyond the first trimester may also be options. If the patient is unstable, urgent neurosurgery is indicated.

Late second and third trimesters

Maternal intravascular volume peaks at the end of the second trimester and tumor resection risks significant hemorrhage: delay of surgery until term is preferred. In stable patients, gestational advancement can be permitted, with close observation of the mother and fetus. In a patient with worsening symptoms, radiotherapy may be an option to delaying surgery. In an unstable patient with impending herniation, delivery of the baby by Cesarean section under general anesthesia, followed immediately by surgical decompression, may be necessary.

Term gestation

At term, delivery can be expedited. In a stable patient, induction of vaginal delivery is an option. A shortened second stage can be achieved with epidural anesthesia; although it should be used with care if intracranial pressure is elevated. Most authors advocate Cesarean section only for accepted obstetric and fetal indications, as this procedure does not seem to provide any

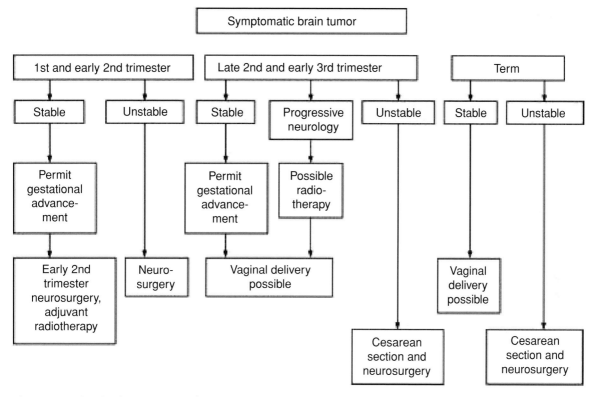

Figure 66.1. Algorithm for management of brain tumors in the pregnant woman.

definitive advantage over vaginal delivery in protecting from increased intracranial pressure. In the unstable patient, as above, Cesarean section under general anesthesia, followed immediately by surgical decompression, is advised.

If an asymptomatic patient is discovered to have a brain tumor during pregnancy, options include a "watch and wait" approach in the face of possible acute worsening or initiating the above measures. Mannitol and hypocapnia were avoided in our case to prevent fetal dehydration and cerebral ischemia/hypoxia, respectively. Perioperative vigilance for pulmonary embolism is essential due to the combined risk of hypercoagulable state/thromboembolism from pregnancy, craniotomy, and brain tumor.

Previous reports suggest that general anesthesia is safe to use in parturients with intracranial tumors. Tracheal intubation is very important as it allows maternal hyperventilation thereby controlling raised intracranial pressure. Patients should be premedicated with a nonparticulate antacid and ranitidine to protect against the sequelae of vomiting and aspiration.

Propofol was used in our case without producing any serious side effects. It is still controversial if it is safe to use propofol in such cases or not. We chose desflurane because of its rapid onset and titratibility. Although sevoflurane is one of the most prevalent volatile anesthetics, there are no data regarding neuronal structure or neurocognitive function after sevoflurane administration in humans or animals. However, sevoflurane can lead to electroencephalographic abnormalities and seizures.

Remifentanil was used in our case without any adverse neonatal effects. This can be explained by the fact that it has a unique metabolism by plasma and tissue esterases and a context-sensitive half life of 3–4 min, independent of the duration of infusion [2]. Opioid properties of remifentanil allow both control of the intraoperative stress response and a more rapid recovery than with other commonly used opioids. Because of its metabolism and short duration of action, remifentanil can be considered to be safe and effective for general anesthesia for emergency Cesarean section in patients with neurologic risk factors.

Clinically relevant concentrations of remifentanil induce rapid, persistent increases in N-methyl-D-aspartate (NMDA) responses. A NMDA-receptor blockade during a critical stage in brain development leads to depression of neuronal activity, which initiates the apoptotic cell death cascade in immature neurons [3]. So, remifentanil potentially prevents this process and has a neuroprotective effect in the fetal brain.

Nitrous oxide was not used in our case. There are no human trials examining the effects of nitrous oxide in young children on neuronal structure and neurocognitive performance, but nitrous oxide is known to inhibit methionine synthase. Case studies in neonates after exposure to nitrous oxide in utero during the third trimester of pregnancy or during Cesarean delivery indicated at least transient neurologic sequelae [4].

Oxytocin and tocolytics were not used in our case although oxytocin has been used in patients with intracranial tumors without any adverse effects. Although osmotic diuresis with mannitol is routinely used to decrease brain bulk and intracranial pressure, we did not use them in our case as mannitol has been shown to cross the placenta, and it may accumulate in the fetus, leading to changes in fetal osmolality, volume and the concentrations of various electrolytes.

Dexamethasone was used in our case to decrease cerebral edema. Its acute use may be safe for the fetus but chronic use of corticosteroids may result in fetal adrenal suppression and fetal hypo-adrenalism, particularly during the third trimester. It is believed that the administration of high-dose steroids for at least 24–48 hours would facilitate fetal lung development for premature delivery of the fetus. Our patient received lorazepam for the treatment of her seizures; eclampsia must also be investigated with any presentation of seizures in the parturient.

Mechanisms of anesthesia-induced neurotoxicity and selectivity of anesthesia-induced neurodegeneration are actively being investigated. It has been suggested that anesthesia-induced gamma-aminobutyric acid type A (GABA-A) receptor activation and NMDA-receptor blockade during a critical stage in brain development lead to depression of neuronal activity, which initiates the apoptotic cell death cascade in immature neurons [5]. Several adjuvants, such as estradiol, pilocarpine, melatonin, and dexmedetomidine, have been identified in animal studies to ameliorate anesthesia induced neurodegeneration [3]. Repeated evidence for clinical doses of isoflurane leading to a dramatic increase in neuronal apoptotic cell death in animal models raises serious concerns for anesthesia practice. The neurodegenerative effects of etomidate, desflurane, and sevoflurane have yet to be closely studied, whereas there is evidence from one study that the rarely used anesthetic, xenon, in clinical doses does not have neurodegenerative effects and may be neuroprotective [6].

Conclusion

Management of brain tumors in pregnant women is mainly reliant on case reports and inherited wisdom. Therefore, close communication among the neurosurgeon, neuroanesthesiologist, obstetrician, and patient is of paramount importance.

References

1. K. S. Tewari, F. Cappuccini, T. Asrat et al. Obstetric emergencies precipitated by malignant brain tumors. Am J Obstet Gynecol 2000; 182: 1215–21.

2. T. Loop, H. J. Priebe. Recovery after anesthesia with remifentanil combined with propofol, desflurane, or sevoflurane for otorhinolaryngeal surgery. Anesth Analg 2000; 91: 123–9.

3. V. Jevtovic-Todorovic. General anesthetics and the developing brain: friends or foes? J Neurosurg Anesthesiol 2005; 17: 204–6.

4. K. Eishima. The effects of obstetric conditions on neonatal behaviour in Japanese infants. Early Hum Dev 1992; 28: 253–63.

5. T. Gerstner, S. Demirakca, T. Demiracka et al. Psychomotorische Entwicklung nach neonataler Phenobarbitaltherapie. Monatsschr Kinderheilkd 2005; 153: 1174–81.

6. A. Fredriksson, T. Archer, H. Alm et al. Neurofunctional deficits and potentiated apoptosis by neonatal NMDA antagonist administration. Behav Brain Res 2004; 153: 367–76.

Neurologic sequelae in other patient populations. Pregnancy

Eclamptic seizures

Negmeldeen F. Mamoun

Eclampsia refers to the occurrence of one or more generalized convulsions and/or coma in the setting of preeclampsia, and in the absence of other neurologic conditions. It occurs with an incidence of 5 cases per 10 000 live births in developed countries. It usually develops after 20 weeks of gestation and just over one-third of cases occur at term, usually developing intra-partum or within 48 hours of delivery.

Case description

The patient was a 23-year-old G4 P1 female who was 33 weeks pregnant with a history of poor prenatal care and preeclampsia during previous pregnancies. She presented with worsening headaches, generalized edema, and blood pressure of 195/115 mmHg. The patient was given a loading dose of 6 g magnesium sulfate ($MgSO_4$), followed by infusion of 2 g/hour for prophylaxis of imminent eclampsia. Blood pressure was managed with labetalol infusion of 1 mg/min, in addition to intermittent doses of hydralazine. Blood tests revealed mild anemia, normal electrolytes and creatinine, platelet count of 95 000/μL, partial thromboplastin time (PTT) of 36, International Normalized Ratio (INR) of 1.3, and elevated transaminases. The plan was to manage the patient expectantly, but she was given betamethasone to promote fetal lung maturity in case preterm labor occurred.

The patient had a brief episode of generalized tonic-clonic convulsions a few hours later; she was given supplemental O_2, placed in left uterine displacement position, and given a bolus of 2 g $MgSO_4$. This episode was associated with fetal bradycardia that lasted for a few minutes, but loss of beat-to-beat variability persisted, which along with poorly controlled blood pressure, urged the obstetrician to proceed with Cesarean section.

The anesthesiologist favored spinal over general anesthesia despite mild coagulopathy; however, while positioning the patient on the OR table, she had a second episode of generalized convulsions. Rapid sequence induction with cricoid pressure was performed using thiopental and succinylcholine, which terminated the seizure within seconds. The trachea was intubated with the aid of a Glidescope (video laryngoscopy), after a failed first attempt of intubation using direct laryngoscopy. Anesthesia was maintained with 0.5 minimum alveolar concentration (MAC) of isoflurane and a low birth weight baby was delivered with Apgar scores of 7 and 9 at 1 and 5 minutes respectively.

The patient had a brief episode of subtle facial and limb twitches about 20 minutes after induction, raising concerns that she might be experiencing another episode of eclamptic seizures. Due to the recurrent nature of her convulsive episodes, continuous electroencephalogram (EEG) monitoring was urgently requested. Emergence was associated with another episode of generalized convulsions, which was evident both clinically and on EEG (Figure 67.1a–d). This episode was quickly controlled by ventilating the patient with 2 MAC of isoflurane until isoelectric silence was achieved. Propofol infusion was then started, aiming to replace isoflurane while maintaining isoelectric silence.

The patient was transported to the intensive care unit on a propofol infusion; multiple fluid boluses and intermittent phenylephrine infusion were used to support her blood pressure. The propofol infusion was discontinued 24 hours later, with no evidence of seizure activity, and the trachea was extubated a few hours thereafter with no problems. $MgSO_4$ infusion was discontinued 48 hours postpartum due to clinical improvement. The patient did not have any more convulsive episodes and was not maintained on any long-term antiseizure medication.

Discussion

The exact cause of seizures in eclampsia is not known. Two hypotheses have been proposed: (1) cerebral

(a)

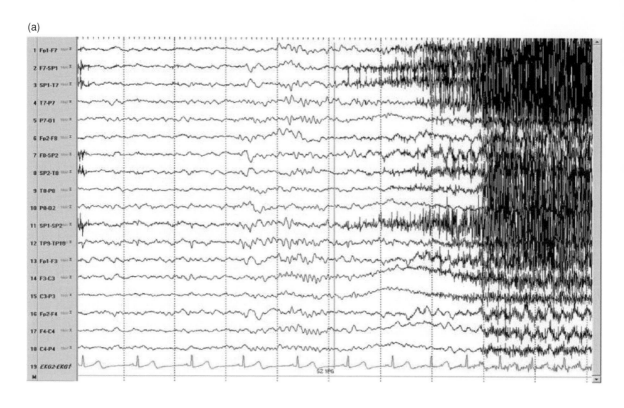

(b)

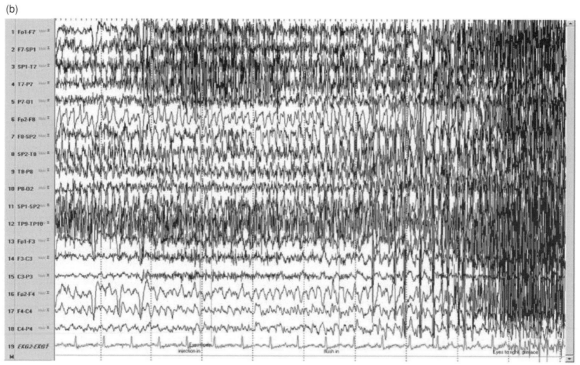

Figure 67.1a–d. Progression of an eclamptic seizure during emergence.

(c)

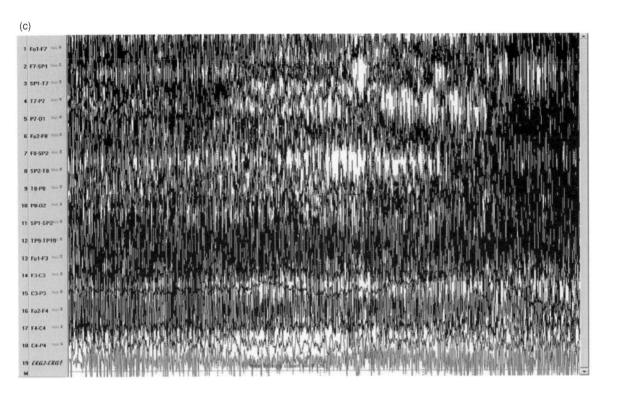

(d)

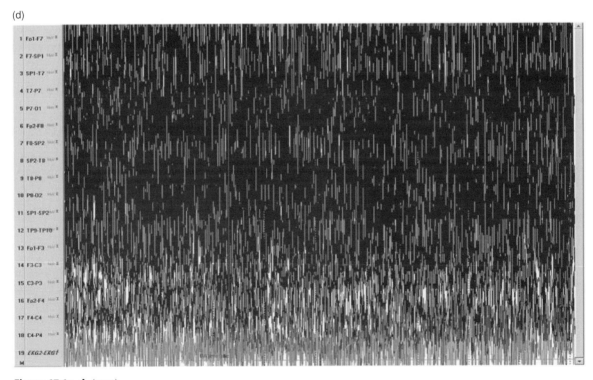

Figure 67.1a–d. *(cont.)*

overregulation in response to high blood pressure results in vasospasm of cerebral arteries, localized ischemia, and intracellular edema; (2) loss of autoregulation of cerebral blood flow in response to high blood pressure results in hyperperfusion, and vasogenic edema.

Eclampsia is a clinical diagnosis, presenting with generalized tonic-clonic convulsions that are usually self-limiting, lasting <3–4 minutes (average of 60–75 seconds), but may be recurrent. Premonitory symptoms include persistent frontal or occipital headache, blurred vision, photophobia, altered mental status, right upper quadrant or epigastric pain. Maternal complications include abruptio placentae, disseminated intravascular coagulopathy, acute renal failure, liver rupture, intracerebral hemorrhage, cardiorespiratory arrest, aspiration pneumonitis, and acute pulmonary edema.

Eclamptic seizures are usually associated with fetal bradycardia, but may also be associated with compensatory fetal tachycardia and loss of beat-to-beat variability, or transient late decelerations. This does not necessitate emergent delivery; stabilizing the mother can help the fetus recover from the effects of maternal hypoxia and hypercarbia. If the fetal heart rate tracing remains non-reassuring for more than 10–15 minutes despite maternal and fetal resuscitative efforts, emergent delivery should be considered. Continuous maternal–fetal monitoring is indicated intrapartum to identify worsening hypertension, deteriorating hepatic, renal, cardiopulmonary, or hematologic function, and uteroplacental insufficiency.

Eclamptic seizures are clinically and electroencephalographically indistinguishable from other generalized tonic-clonic seizures. Other etiologies are particularly important in pregnant women with atypical eclampsia, such as patients who seize before 20 weeks of gestation, or patients with focal neurologic deficits. Differential diagnosis includes:

- Stroke.
- Hypertensive encephalopathy.
- Infection (meningitis, encephalitis).
- Idiopathic epilepsy.
- Cerebral vasculitis.
- Space-occupying lesions (brain tumor, abscess).
- Metabolic disorders (hypoglycemia, hyponatremia).
- Use of illicit drugs (methamphetamine, cocaine).
- Reversible posterior leukoencephalopathy syndrome (RPLS).

In addition to the management principles that apply to other seizures with different etiologies such as prevention of hypoxia, trauma, and recurrent seizures, management of eclamptic seizures includes control of severe hypertension if present, and evaluation for prompt delivery.

General principles

Maintenance of airway patency and prevention of aspiration should be the first priority. Supplemental O_2 should be administered, and the patient should be placed in a left uterine displacement position to improve uteroplacental perfusion. A bed with raised, padded side rails provides protection from trauma.

Treatment of hypertension

Antihypertensive therapy is recommended for sustained diastolic blood pressures ≥ 110 mmHg or systolic blood pressures ≥ 160 mmHg to prevent maternal complications. Although clinical trials have not adequately addressed the question of how aggressively to lower a preeclamptic patient's blood pressure, experts consider systolic blood pressure of 140–160 mmHg and diastolic blood pressure of 90–110 mmHg to be a reasonable goal; their rationale is to avoid potential reduction in either uteroplacental blood flow or cerebral perfusion pressure [1].

The most frequently used antihypertensives are labetalol and hydralazine; labetalol is preferred because it is associated with less maternal hypotension. Nifedipine, nicardipine, α methyl dopa, and diazoxide are less frequently used. It is not recommended to use calcium channel blockers and $MgSO_4$ concurrently due to their synergistic depressive effects on cardiac function.

Treatment of convulsions

Noneclamptic status epilepticus is traditionally treated with four main categories of drugs: benzodiazepines, phenytoin, barbiturates, and propofol. Benzodiazepines are considered the first-line treatment because they control seizures quickly, with lorazepam as the first-line drug. Lorazepam is more effective than diazepam in termination of seizures, and has a duration of action of 4–6 hours compared with 20–30 minutes after a single dose of diazepam [2]. Phenytoin or fosphenytoin are usually used as an adjunct to a benzodiazepine; they are effective in preventing recurrence for extended periods of time. Propofol, barbiturates (pentobarbital and thiopental), and continuous infusion of midazolam are usually reserved for refractory status epilepticus. General anesthesia with isoflurane or other inhalational agents may be temporarily effective in stopping seizures, but is used only in extreme circumstances due to logistical problems.

In eclamptic seizures, obstetricians usually favor $MgSO_4$ as the drug of choice, whereas neurologists tend to favor other traditional anticonvulsants such as lorazepam. There is strong evidence that $MgSO_4$ is more effective than other anticonvulsants in reducing the risk of recurrent seizures in eclamptic women. $MgSO_4$ halves the risk of eclampsia, and probably reduces the risk of maternal mortality [3]. The American College of Obstetricians and Gynecologists recommends its use in women with severe preeclampsia, and the World Health Organization, the Federation Internationale de Gynecologie et d'Obstetrique, the International Society for the Study of Hypertension in Pregnancy advocate its use in the prevention and treatment of eclampsia.

The mechanism of action of $MgSO_4$ as an anticonvulsant is not clearly understood. It is likely multifactorial including both vascular and neurologic mechanisms such as vasodilatation of the cerebral vasculature, inhibition of platelet aggregation, prevention of calcium ion entry into ischemic cells, or its role as a N-methyl-D-aspartate receptor antagonist [4].

A recommended loading dose of 4–6 g $MgSO_4$ is given intravenously, usually followed by a maintenance infusion of 2 g/hour. The maintenance dose should be adjusted in renal insufficiency, and is given only if a patellar reflex is present, respiratory rate >12/min, and average urine output of >25 mL/hour. Recurrent seizures occurring in patients on maintenance $MgSO_4$ therapy can be treated with an additional bolus of 2 g $MgSO_4$. If two such boluses do not control seizures, other medications should be used such as lorazepam or diazepam.

Eclamptic seizures are typically self limiting, and EEG monitoring is usually not required for management, but due to our patient's recurrent convulsive episodes despite therapy, there were concerns that she might be at a higher risk of developing cerebral hemorrhage, which is the major cause of maternal mortality in this patient population. Continuous EEG monitoring was not done solely for diagnostic purposes, but mainly to ensure that the patient was not having recurrent subclinical seizures postpartum.

Anticonvulsants are usually administered for 24–48 hours postpartum. The optimal duration of therapy has not been determined, but therapy is usually discontinued in women who are clearly improving clinically as evidenced by absence of symptoms (no headache, visual disturbances, or epigastric pain), and signs (sustained blood pressure <150/100 mmHg, or spontaneous diuresis >100 ml/hour for >2 hours) [5].

Delivery

The definitive treatment of eclampsia is delivery, which reduces the risk of maternal morbidity and mortality. Maternal end-organ damage and nonreassuring tests of fetal wellbeing are indications for delivery at any gestational age. Antenatal corticosteroids (betamethasone) should be administered to women less than 34 weeks of gestation to promote fetal lung maturity.

General anesthesia in parturients is typically maintained with <1 MAC of inhalational agents due to decreased anesthetic requirements during pregnancy. This relatively lower concentration of isoflurane was probably not enough to suppress one of our patient's recurrent seizures; its clinical presentation with subtle twitches may be due to residual muscle relaxation. Prolongation of neuromuscular blockade is expected in patients receiving $MgSO_4$ therapy, which potentiates the effect of both depolarizing and nondepolarizing muscle relaxants.

Neuraxial anesthesia (spinal, epidural, or combined spinal epidural) is the anesthetic technique of choice in patients with severe preeclampsia in the absence of coagulopathy. Hypotension is a major concern with neuraxial anesthesia, as those patients usually have depleted intravascular volume despite total body fluid overload. Major concerns with general anesthesia include: (1) increased risk of difficult intubation secondary to airway edema; difficult intubation should be anticipated, and equipment for management of a difficult airway including emergent cricothyroidotomy should be readily available; (2) exacerbation of a poorly controlled blood pressure with intubation; (3) increased risk of aspiration; aspiration prophylaxis (bicitra and metoclopramide) should be administered, and the airway is managed either awake or after rapid sequence induction.

Conclusion

In conclusion, eclampsia is associated with increased risk of maternal and fetal morbidity and mortality. Aggressive attempts should be made to control seizures and hypertension. $MgSO_4$ is considered the drug of choice for prevention and treatment of eclampsia.

References

1. **B. M. Sibai**. Diagnosis, prevention, and management of eclampsia. *Obstet Gynecol* 2005; **105**: 402–10.

2. **K. Prasad, P. R. Krishnan, K. Al-Roomi** *et al.* Anticonvulsant therapy for status epilepticus. *Br J Clin Pharmacol* 2007; **63**: 640–7.

3. **D. Altman, G. Carroli, L. Duley** *et al.* Do women with preeclampsia, and their babies, benefit from magnesium sulphate? The Magpie Trial: a randomised placebo-controlled trial. *Lancet* 2002; **359**: 1877–90.

4. **A. G. Euser, M. J. Cipolla**. Magnesium sulfate for the treatment of eclampsia: a brief review. *Stroke* 2009; **40**: 1169–75.

5. **C. M. Isler, P. S. Barrilleaux, B. K. Rinehart** *et al.* Postpartum seizure prophylaxis: using maternal clinical parameters to guide therapy. *Obstet Gynecol* 2003; **101**: 66–9.

68

Postpartum headache

Alexandra S. Bullough

Headache is a common complaint in the postpartum period. Most cases of postpartum headache (PPH) are attributed to dural puncture, migraine, pneumo-cephalus, or nonspecific causes, but all differential diagnoses need to be considered [1, 2].

Spontaneous internal carotid artery dissection (ICAD) is a rare cause of PPH. An arterial dissection involves an intimal layer tear and the resulting intra-mural hematoma may compress and distort the lumen resulting in local stenosis or thrombosis. The conse-quent hypoperfusion or subsequent distal emboliza-tion may lead to an ischemic stroke which is already a recognized risk in the puerperium [3].

Case description

A healthy 36-year-old G3 P1 female with no known history of vascular disease or connective tissue disor-der was admitted at full term in spontaneous labor. A lumbar labor epidural catheter was placed without complications. Five hours after successful neuraxial analgesia the patient delivered a healthy 3.8 kg infant with only 20 minutes of expulsive effort. The epidu-ral catheter was removed with the tip intact and the woman was discharged home the next day.

Four days postpartum the woman contacted the obstetric triage desk by telephone complaining of a persistent frontal headache radiating to the back of her neck with increased pain on the left side. There was no definite postural component to the headache and the patient did not complain of fever, photopho-bia, nausea, or any other focal neurologic symptoms. As she had received epidural analgesia, she was reas-sured and told to increase her oral fluid uptake, remain supine, take regular simple analgesia and drink caf-feinated beverages for a suspected postdural puncture headache.

On postpartum day 8, the woman presented to obstetric triage with a severe global headache. Both anesthesiology and neurology teams were consulted. There was no postural component to the headache and a postdural puncture headache was dismissed as a diagnosis.

Neurologic examination was normal. The patient underwent magnetic resonance imaging (MRI) to exclude venous sinus thrombosis. The MRI revealed normal sinuses and no evidence of an intracranial mass, hemorrhage, or dural enhancement. However, an absent flow void pattern was noted in the left internal carotid artery. The MRI report also com-mented upon the presence of abnormal bilateral ver-tebral arteries, which was suggestive of fibromus-cular dysplasia but not conclusive without further investigations.

Further investigation of the left internal carotid artery with magnetic resonance angiography (MRA) revealed a narrowing of the left carotid artery 2 cm distal to the bifurcation, consistent with a left ICAD. Follow-up MRI scanning revealed a healing but not total resolution of left internal artery integrity. The patient was commenced on anticoagulation ther-apy comprising low molecular weight heparin and coumadin. While on anticoagulation therapy, the patient complained of right-sided visual blurring and right-hand numbness that resolved spontaneously after 5 minutes. She remained in the hospital for a fur-ther 3 days during which time her headache localized to the occipital region and radiated to her neck.

Coumadin therapy was continued for 8 months until the left ICAD resolved, whereupon a long-term aspirin regimen was prescribed. An unpleasant com-plication of her dissection was the subsequent devel-opment of frequent complex migrainous headaches, which persisted for several days and involved right-hand and leg numbness as well as occasional visual disturbances. The patient was placed on divalproex sodium which did provide some migraine pain relief.

Discussion

Pregnancy and puerperium increase the risk for focal ischemic cerebrovascular events. The hypercoaguable state in pregnancy and the immediate puerperium most certainly contributes to this risk. Some 60–80% of ischemic strokes occurring in pregnancy and puerperium are believed to be due to arterial occlusions and approximately 40% of these occlusions occur up to a month later in the postpartum period [3].

Spontaneous ICAD is a rare cause of postpartum headache; the mean age of patients with ICAD is 40–46 years [4]. In most cases no specific etiology is found, but ICAD has been associated with minor trauma to the head or neck, as well as connective tissue disorders such as Ehlers–Danlos syndrome or Marfan's syndrome. Other trigger factors may include: "headbanging," prolonged telephone usage, chiropractic manipulations, whiplash, childbirth, and even turning one's head to the same side during breastfeeding. In most cases no specific etiology is found. An arterial intimal wall tear may also be associated with straining and Valsalva maneuver during vaginal delivery. It is unclear whether the association between puerperium and arterial dissection is causative or coincidental [3].

Extracranial ICAD usually presents as a headache, cervical pain, Horner's syndrome, or pulsatile tinnitus without cerebral ischemia. An ICAD headache is typically ipsilateral and hemicranial [5]. In this case the patient initially complained of a frontal headache, which is usually associated with a dural puncture. All parturients who receive neuraxial labor anesthesia and who later complain of a headache are usually treated for postdural puncture headache, but this represents only one possible diagnosis for postpartum headache (Table 68.1). In this instance, postdural puncture headache was discounted early as there was no postural element associated with the headache or any history of traumatic epidural placement.

The neurology team wanted to exclude venous sinus thrombosis and therefore rapidly requested MRI, MRA, and magnetic resonance venography (MRV) investigations. Magnetic resonance imaging can visualize morphological details, while MRA and MRV reflect intraluminal blood flow [5]. Duplex ultrasonography may also be used to detect extracranial ICAD, but use is limited in intracranial internal carotid involvement and high cervical occlusions. A skilled operator is paramount for ultrasound investigation of ICAD.

Table 68.1. Differential diagnoses of postpartum headache.

Causes	Description of headache
Postdural puncture	Fronto-occipital, throbbing in nature, postural-relieved when supine
Nonspecific coincidental headache	
Migraine	Generalized or unilateral throbbing pain, visual disturbances, nausea and vomiting, photophobia, may last minutes or days
Preeclampsia/eclampsia	Hypertension, proteinuria, seizure
Pregnancy-induced hypertension	Throbbing, visual disturbances
Pneumocephalus after epidural	Frontal, worsening headache, dull and persistent
Meningitis	Sudden onset, severe and persistent +/− fever, stiff neck, nausea and vomiting, behavioral changes, altered level of consciousness
Cerebral vein thrombosis	Intermittent, diffuse and "pounding," other signs may include papilledema, intracranial hypertension, focal neurologic deficits, seizures, and altered level of consciousness
Nontraumatic intracranial hemorrhage	
Intracerebral	Severe headache
Subdural	Mild to severe, localized or generalized
Subarachnoid	"Worst headache of my life," all intracranial bleeds may be associated with nausea, vomiting, neurologic sequelae and loss of consciousness
Cervicocephalic arterial dissection	Variable presentation, mild to severe pain, ipsilateral or bilateral, transient ischemic attack, stroke, Horner's syndrome, visual disturbance due to ophthalmic artery occlusion
Cerebral vasculitis	Constant headache +/− transient ischemic attack, tinnitus, visual disturbance
Reversible cerebral vasoconstriction	"Thunderclap" headache +/− confusion, visual disturbances, seizures
Cerebral tumor	No unique characteristics, headache depends on location and size of tumor

Initial MRI findings reported that the left internal carotid artery lacked a normal flow-void pattern throughout the petrous and cavernous portion on the left side which could represent thrombosis or dissection. On a subsequent MRA an abnormality was noted to begin after the level of carotid bifurcation and extend up to the cavernous segment.

Usual angiographic findings of extracranial ICAD include a string sign, double lumen, as well as irregular and tapered stenosis, which usually begins 2–3 cm above the bifurcation as occurred in this case and extends to the base of the skull [4].

Fortunately MRV images demonstrated no evidence of dural venous sinus thrombosis. A final follow-up MRI scan 8 months later showed a persistent asymmetrical small left internal carotid artery, unchanged since the previous studies several months earlier.

Treatment usually comprises immediate anticoagulation to prevent cerebral ischemia which is usually delayed yet may appear up to 1 month later. A study by Lucas *et al.* [6] proposes that most cerebral ischemic events after ICAD are embolic rather than hemorrhagic in origin. The optimal guideline duration of anticoagulant therapy is yet to be established but 3–6 months has been recommended. Duration is usually determined by the recanalization of the artery as demonstrated on MRI or duplex follow-up [4].

Surgical intervention in ICAD is only required when anticoagulant therapy does not prevent progressive cerebral ischemic events.

Medication was later prescribed to assist with management of debilitating migraines. Divalproex sodium is teratogenic and should not be prescribed for women of child-bearing age. The patient stated she wanted no further children. Teratogenic effects are severe and include anencephaly and spina bifida.

Conclusion

In conclusion, postpartum headache caused by ICAD is a rare yet treatable condition with a favorable prognosis when recognized. Noninvasive MRI scanning is the investigation of choice due to high sensitivity and specificity in detecting an ICAD. Therapy comprises anticoagulation until recanalization of the internal carotid artery is achieved followed by an antiplatelet regimen, the duration of which is determined by the patient risk profile. Complications such as ICAD serve as a reminder to consider a broad differential for the evaluation of postpartum headache, as catastrophic neurologic sequelae may occur [2].

References

1. **J. Waidelich, A. S. Bullough, J. M. Mhyre.** Internal carotid artery dissection: an unusual cause of postpartum headache. *Int J Obstet Anesth* 2008; **17**: 61–5.

2. **G. A. Mashour, L. H. Schwamm, L. Leffert.** Intracranial subdural hematomas and cerebral herniation after labor epidural with no evidence of dural puncture. *Anesthesiology* 2006; **104**: 610–12.

3. **A. P. Gasecki, H. Kwiecinski, P. A. Lyrer** *et al.* Dissections after childbirth. *J Neurol* 1999; **246**: 712–15.

4. **J. Bogousslavy, P. A. Despland, F. Regli.** Spontaneous carotid dissection with acute stroke. *Arch Neurol* 1987; **44**: 137–40.

5. **M. Zetterling, C. Carlström, P. Konrad.** Internal carotid artery dissection *Acta Neurol Scand* 2000; **101**: 1–7.

6. **C. Lucas, T. Moulin, D. Deplanque** *et al.* Stroke patterns of internal carotid artery dissection in 40 patients. *Stroke* 1998; **29**: 2646–8.

69

Increased intracranial pressure with acute liver failure

Ryen D. Fons and Paul Picton

Acute liver failure (ALF) is a rare clinical syndrome characterized by coagulopathy and hepatic encephalopathy. There are multiple etiologies, the clinical course is variable, and the mortality rate is high. Despite recent advances in the development of hepatic assist devices, the only therapy with proven survival benefit is liver transplantation. According to the US ALF Study Group database, approximately 45% of adult patients with ALF recover with medical treatment alone, 25% receive liver transplantation, and the remaining 30% die without liver transplantation [1]. Multisystem organ failure secondary to sepsis and cerebral herniation secondary to increased intracranial pressure (ICP) are the leading causes of death. The decision to place an ICP monitor to facilitate goal-directed management of intracranial hypertension remains controversial.

Case description

The patient was a 36-year-old female with newly diagnosed depression who ingested approximately >100 tablets (500 mg each) of acetaminophen in a suicide attempt. She presented to a local hospital later that evening with severe nausea, vomiting, and abdominal pain. There was no other significant past medical history. Laboratory evaluation revealed aspartate aminotransferase (AST) of 218 IU/L, alanine aminotransferase (ALT) of 288 IU/L, International Normalized Ratio (INR) of 1.6, and creatinine of 1.7 mg/dL. Oral N-acetylcysteine and vitamin K were administered. Over the next 24 hours, her AST increased to 2078 IU/L, ALT to 1979 IU/L, with an INR of 2.6, prothrombin time (PT) 31.5, total bilirubin of 2.9 and creatinine of 1.5. She developed lethargy and personality changes consistent with grade 2 hepatic encephalopathy (Table 69.1) and was transferred to a tertiary care center for intensive care management and liver transplant evaluation.

One day after patient transfer (third day post acetaminophen ingestion), her AST was 6120, ALT 6233, INR 3.7, total bilirubin 4.8, creatinine 3.2, and platelets of 64 K/mm^3. Her mental status deteriorated to somnolence and profound disorientation (grade 3 hepatic encephalopathy) and the patient was listed as United Network for Organ Sharing (UNOS) status IA. An ICP monitor was not placed in this patient due to the risk of intracranial hemorrhage.

The patient underwent orthotopic liver transplantation (OLT) 4 days following initial acetaminophen overdose. Intraoperatively she received 2 units packed red blood cells, 7 units fresh frozen plasma (FFP), and 10 units of platelets. She remained in the intensive care unit for 5 days and was discharged home on postoperative day 13 without neurologic complications.

Discussion

Acute liver failure is a syndrome defined as the development of coagulopathy (INR ≥1.5) and hepatic encephalopathy within 26 weeks of the onset of jaundice in a patient without a prior history of liver disease. Acute liver failure is further subdivided based on the jaundice-to-encephalopathy interval with hyperacute liver failure occurring ≤7 days, ALF between 8 and 28 days, and subacute liver failure between 28 days and 26 weeks (Table 69.2). While the overall mortality of ALF without liver transplantation is >50%, the rate of spontaneous recovery from acute liver failure is inversely proportional to the length of the jaundice-to-encephalopathy interval. The rate of spontaneous recovery is 80–90% for hyperacute liver failure, 50–60% for acute liver failure, and 15–20% for subacute liver failure (Table 69.2).

Common causes of acute liver failure

Drug-induced hepatotoxicity remains the leading cause of ALF in the USA with acetaminophen overdose constituting approximately 50% of all cases [1]. Other medications commonly implicated include isoniazid, sulfonamides, phenytoin, disulfiram,

Table 69.1. West Haven criteria for grading of hepatic encephalopathy and rate of spontaneous recovery of hepatic function.

Grade	Signs and symptoms	Rate of spontaneous recovery
Grade 0	No signs or symptoms	
Grade 1	Trivial lack of awareness Euphoria or anxiety Decreased attention span Impaired performance of addition	65–70%
Grade 2	Lethargy or apathy Minimal disorientation to time or place Subtle personality change Inappropriate behavior Impaired performance of subtraction	
Grade 3	Somnolence, but responsive to verbal stimuli Confusion Gross disorientation	40–50%
Grade 4	Coma (unresponsive to verbal or noxious stimuli)	<20%

Table 69.2. Acute liver failure classification.

Acute liver failure subcategory	Onset of jaundice to encephalopathy	Spontaneous survival %	Incidence of clinically significant cerebral edema	Common causes
Hyperacute	0–7 days	80–90%	24%	Acetaminophen overdose, hepatitis A, hepatic ischemia
Acute	8–28 days	50–60%	23%	Hepatitis B, drug reaction
Subacute	28 days to 26 weeks	15–20%	9%	Drug reaction, indeterminate

troglitazone, propylthiouracil, bromfenac, and herbal supplements [1]. Common viral causes include hepatitis A and B, while infrequent viral causes include hepatitis C and E, cytomegalovirus, herpes-simplex virus and Epstein–Barr virus. Other less frequent causes include autoimmune hepatitis, "shock liver" (ischemic hepatitis), acute Wilson's disease, acute Budd–Chiari syndrome, lymphoma, and acute fatty liver of pregnancy. In approximately 15% of adult patients, the cause remains indeterminate.

Neurologic manifestations of acute liver failure: encephalopathy, cerebral edema, and increased intracranial pressure

By definition, ALF requires the presence of hepatic encephalopathy. The prognosis for spontaneous recovery of liver function decreases with increasing severity of encephalopathy (Table 69.1). The exact etiology of hepatic encephalopathy remains unclear, but increased levels of toxins (ammonia, mercaptans, serotonin, c-aminobutyric acid, endogenous benzodiazepines, and tryptophan), altered neurotransmitter levels, glutamatergic receptor activation and changes in GABAergic tone have been proposed [2]. In contrast to chronic liver failure where encephalopathy is common but cerebral edema is rare, ALF is often accompanied by cerebral edema, especially when acetaminophen overdose is the cause (26% of patients). The mechanism of cerebral edema is multifactorial and includes increased blood flow from disruption of cerebral autoregulation, astrocyte swelling, and inflammation. Because the cranium is noncompliant, dramatic increases in ICP may result from small increases in brain volume once compensatory mechanisms have been exhausted. Normal ICP is <15 mmHg for adults. An ICP >20 mmHg is defined as intracranial hypertension. Prolonged increases of ICP >40 mmHg and/or cerebral perfusion pressure <40 mmHg for

>2 hours are associated with cerebral herniation and poor prognosis for neurologic recovery following liver transplantation [3].

Coagulopathy

In addition to hepatic encephalopathy, ALF is defined by the presence of coagulopathy. The coagulopathy of ALF is multifactorial, including impaired synthesis of clotting factors and fibrinogen, increased peripheral consumption, and thrombocytopenia. Correction of elevated INR, thrombocytopenia, hypofibrinogenemia, or specific clotting factors is not routinely recommended due to the low rate (~10%) of spontaneous and clinically significant hemorrhage in patients diagnosed with ALF [3]. Additionally, correction of coagulopathy may mask the signs of spontaneous recovery and lead to unnecessary liver transplantation. Empiric administration of vitamin K is recommended for all patients with ALF. If clinically significant bleeding develops or an invasive procedure (e.g., ICP monitor) is planned, correction of INR to ~1.5, platelet count of >50 000/mm³, and fibrinogen to >100 mg/dL is recommended [3]. If FFP does not correct the INR or the patient is unable to tolerate the volume load, recombinant factor VIIa (40 mcg/kg) may be considered immediately prior to the planned procedure [4]. Additionally, isovolumetric plasmapheresis may also be effective [5].

Intracranial pressure monitor placement

In the presence of coagulopathy associated with ALF, placement of an ICP monitor to facilitate goal-directed management of intracranial hypertension remains controversial. The US Acute Liver Failure Study Group currently does not recommend routine placement of ICP monitors in all patients with ALF since survival at 30 days was similar in patients with and without ICP monitoring who underwent OLT [3]. However, they do recommend considering an ICP monitor for all patients with grade 3 or 4 hepatic encephalopathy for whom OLT is planned [3].

Four types of ICP monitors are used in clinical practice: epidural, subdural bolt, intraparenchymal, and intraventricular. Ventriculostomy additionally allows for removal of cerebrospinal fluid to treat increased ICP. The rate of hemorrhagic complications from placement of an ICP monitor is approximately 10% in ALF despite reversal of coagulopathy [4]. The

risk of intracranial hemorrhage varies depending on the site of monitor placement (epidural 4%, subdural 20%, and intraparenchymal/intraventricular 22%). The risk of fatal hemorrhage for the various monitoring choices is 1%, 5%, and 4%, respectively [5]. The US ALF Study Group does not recommend intraventricular ICP monitor placement due to the high risk of hemorrhagic complications [3]. In general, epidural catheters have the lowest complication rate, but tend to overestimate ICP. Subdural bolts are currently the most commonly placed device in the USA for ICP management in patients diagnosed with ALF [4].

Conclusion

In conclusion, ALF is rare but carries a high mortality. The leading cause within the USA is acetaminophen overdose. The associated encephalopathy seen with patients diagnosed with ALF is commonly caused by cerebral edema. The combination of coagulopathy, increased ICP, and grade 3 or 4 hepatic encephalopathy presents a difficult and controversial dilemma for the critical care physician. While placement of an ICP monitor to facilitate goal-directed management of intracranial hypertension may insure that cerebral perfusion is preserved, the risks of intracranial hemorrhage (~10%) from ICP monitor placement and blood product administration must be considered. This is especially true given the lack of definitive evidence of a benefit in patient mortality.

References

1. W. M. Lee, R. H. Squires Jr., S. L. Nyberg et al. Acute liver failure: Summary of a workshop. *Hepatology* 2008; **47**: 1401–15.

2. J. G. O'Grady. Acute liver failure. *Postgrad Med J* 2005; **81**: 148–54.

3. R. T. Stravitz, A. H. Kramer, T. Davern et al. Intensive care of patients with acute liver failure: recommendations of the U.S. Acute Liver Failure Study Group. *Crit Care Med* 2007; **35**: 2498–508.

4. J. Vaquero, R. J. Fontana, A. M. Larson et al. Complications and use of intracranial pressure monitoring in patients with acute liver failure and severe encephalopathy. *Liver Transpl* 2005; **11**: 1581–9.

5. R. T. Stravitz. Critical management decisions in patients with acute liver failure. *Chest* 2008; **134**: 1092–102.

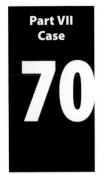

70 Permissive hypertension in a patient with von Willebrand's disease and a preexisting ventriculoperitoneal shunt

Miguel Cruz, Maged Guirguis and Wolf H. Stapelfeldt

Hypertension is not usually considered acceptable in patients with abnormal coagulation, including von Willebrand's disease. The present case describes a situation in which significant permissive hypertension may have *prevented* an otherwise likely adverse outcome.

Case description

A 56-year-old male reporting a remote history of stroke with residual left-sided weakness, prior radiation therapy of a pontine brain tumor, a seizure disorder, ventriculoperitoneal (VP) shunt, and history of von Willebrand's disease underwent robot-assisted laparoscopic radical prostatectomy for prostate cancer. A previous laparoscopic cholecystectomy performed elsewhere had been complicated by significant postoperative bleeding, requiring surgical drainage as well as multiple blood product transfusions. Prophylactic pretreatment with intravenous desmopressin was completed 1 hour before the current surgery. After placement of routine monitors, general anesthesia was induced and invasive blood pressure monitoring initiated via a radial arterial catheter. The patient was placed into a steep Trendelenburg position. Immediately following CO_2 insufflation into the peritoneal cavity, a dramatic and refractory blood pressure rise was noted with mean pressure exceeding 130 mmHg despite adequate analgesia (including supplemental doses of 0.8 mg hydromorphone) and sufficient anesthetic depth based on end-tidal anesthetic concentration (Figure 70.1, arrow 1), suggesting some underlying cause other than inadequate anesthesia. Because of the team's concern about increased risk of cerebral hemorrhage the possibility was considered to abort the surgical procedure. Release of the intra-abdominal insufflation pressure caused mean arterial pressure (MAP) to rapidly normalize into the 80–90 mmHg range (Figure 70.1, arrow 2). Based on this

observation it was reasoned that the patient's blood pressure increase might have represented a compensatory response to the increased intracranial pressure occurring during abdominal inflation, conceivably brought about by a malfunctioning valve of the VP shunt, transmitting increased abdominal pressure to the cerebrospinal fluid (CSF) and brain. A lateral skull X-ray was performed to rule out the possibility of pressurized gas having passed into the cerebral ventricles along such a conceivable path. In the absence of any evidence (Figure 70.2) the team resolved to cautiously proceed with the prostatectomy while having cerebral blood flow continuously monitored by transcranial Doppler. Immediately upon renewed inflation of the peritoneal cavity, the patient's systemic blood pressure again rose precipitously (Figure 70.1, arrow 3). Doppler measurements confirmed that cerebral blood flow was adequately maintained under these conditions with mean velocities ranging between 34–46 cm/second (Figure 70.3). The decision was made to complete the surgical procedure while keeping peritoneal insufflation pressure at a minimally acceptable level (around 8 mmHg) (Figure 70.1, arrow 4). For the balance of the case the patient's mean arterial blood pressure remained within the 80–100 mmHg range. Transfusion of platelets became necessary to control excessive and persistent bleeding from the prostate bed. After completion of surgery the patient was permitted to awaken from anesthesia and to be tracheally extubated after exhibiting the ability to sustain head lift and follow commands. There was no evidence for any adverse event or new neurologic deficit resulting from either cerebral ischemia or hemorrhage, which might conceivably have occurred during the above episodes. After the patient's return to the operating room that same evening to undergo an exploratory laparotomy for continued postoperative intra-abdominal hemorrhage from the resection site, the patient was ultimately discharged from the hospital without further complication.

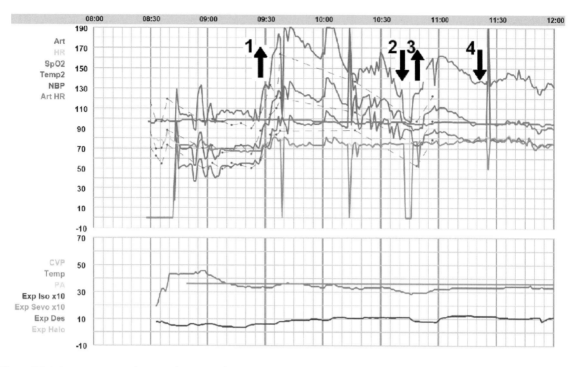

Figure 70.1. Intraoperative vital signs, with arrows indicating changes in intra-abdominal pressure caused by inflation (up) and deflation (down).

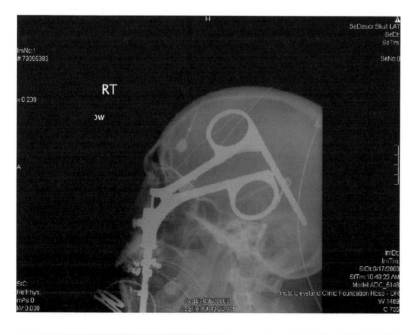

Figure 70.2. Lateral radiograph of the skull, without evidence of intraventricular air.

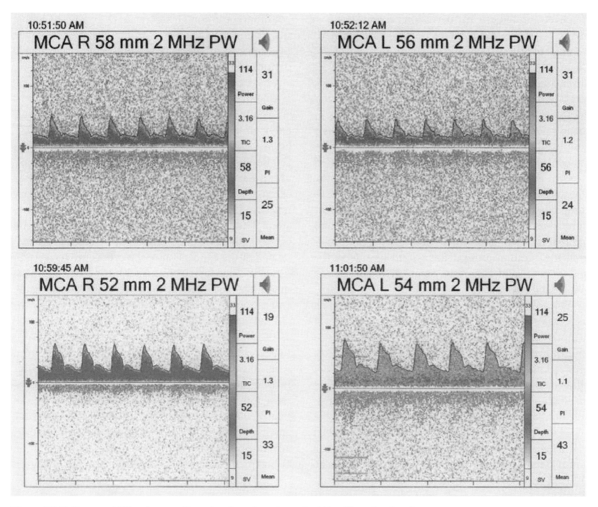

Figure 70.3. Transcranial Doppler recordings, showing adequate cerebral blood flow signal tracings.

Discussion

The presence of a VP shunt is not considered an absolute contraindication for laparoscopic surgery provided the shunt and its valvular mechanism are fully functional [1]. However, increases in intracranial pressure (ICP) are well known to occur during laparoscopy in VP shunt patients with less than normal cerebral compliance [2]. While there was no evidence preoperatively to suggest the presence of VP shunt malfunction or of decreased cerebral compliance, the rapid development of a reversible and reproducible blood pressure increase following the institution of the pneumoperitoneum suggested that the VP shunt valvular function was likely faulty, allowing the increase in intra-abdominal pressure during CO_2 insufflation to

be transmitted to the central nervous system. This, in turn, presumably caused a compensatory increase in mean arterial pressure in order to maintain sufficient cerebral perfusion pressure and blood flow. Absence of CO_2 gas pockets in the cerebral ventricles on the lateral skull X-ray did not rule out the possibility of valvular incontinence of the VP shunt since the patient was in a rather steep Trendelenburg position, presumably causing any pressurized gas within the shunt to be kept floating above a contiguous CSF fluid column that would have precluded any further tracking of gas while still effectively transmitting increased pressure to the cerebral ventricles. As soon as the rising ICP would have exceeded venous pressure it would have

235

effectively limited cerebral perfusion pressure (CPP = MAP – ICP), creating a (compensatory) need for MAP to increase proportionally in order to maintain CPP. Cushing in 1901 described the classical triad of physiologic responses to intracranial hypertension, consisting of apnea, increased blood pressure, and bradycardia. More recent observations during neuroendoscopic procedures under general anesthesia describe the rapid development of hypertension without concomitant bradycardia in response to increased ICP [3]. Based on the same physiologic rationale the anesthesia team considered it absolutely imperative to allow blood pressure to rise ("permissive hypertension") during periods of increased peritoneal pressure rather than trying to normalize blood pressure. However, the question arose if this would be safe in the present setting of abnormal coagulation due to von Willebrand's disease.

Von Willebrand's disease is known to carry an increased risk of bleeding, including that of cerebral hemorrhage [4, 5]. Is this risk increased in the presence of hypertension? It could be argued that the risk of bleeding was undoubtedly increased *in areas not affected by increased pressure* during abdominal gas insufflation. However, transmural pressure (the pressure gradient across the blood vessel wall between the vessel lumen and surrounding tissue) and the related risk of hemorrhage would not have been elevated to the same extent in all those tissues experiencing increased ambient tissue pressure from abdominal gas insufflation, including the surgical site itself and, indirectly, in this case, brain tissue, thus mitigating an otherwise increased risk of hemorrhage at these sites. On the other hand, the actual risk of hemorrhage at the surgical site was certainly higher in the presence of compensatory hypertension than it would have been otherwise, thus likely contributing to more severe surgical bleeding and, ultimately, the need for platelet transfusion. Yet, given the risk of cerebral ischemia (consequent to the rise in ICP) it was most likely preferable to accept an increased likelihood of abdominal hemorrhage at the surgical site rather than risking a (more likely ischemic rather than hemorrhagic) insult in the CNS. This anesthetic assessment and management plan was thoroughly discussed with the surgical team as part of the decision to proceed with surgery. The question arose as to whether the compensatory blood pressure increase occurring during abdominal insufflation would, in fact, *be sufficient* to maintain adequate cerebral perfusion. To address this critical question, continuous transcranial Doppler monitoring was instituted in an ad hoc fashion, demonstrating the maintenance of adequate cerebral blood flow during periods of abdominal inflation. Utility of this technology has been previously advocated in a similar clinical setting [6].

While unrecognized shunt malfunction was most likely already present preoperatively, it could possibly have developed *de novo* during the laparoscopy [7]. Because of these various possibilities of shunt failure, it has been suggested that VP shunts should be externalized prior to laparoscopy as a precautionary measure [8]. Another approach might have been to attempt to laparoscopically clamp off the distal end of the VP shunt tubing, followed by cutting the distal end at the conclusion of the procedure to reestablish CSF drainage. Problems with the latter approach might have included technical difficulties locating the end of the shunt tubing in the upper abdomen without having to completely disengage the robot, as well as the risk of gradual formation of a hydrocephalus that might conceivably have ensued over the prolonged surgical course typical for robot-assisted laparoscopic prostatectomy. Ultimately, it is most important to consider this entire range of possible complications and management options in VP shunt patients undergoing laparoscopic procedures, which require coordination, advanced planning, and continued close cooperation between the surgical and anesthesia teams if potentially serious adverse sequelae are to be averted.

References

1. S. V. Jackman, J. D. Weingart, S. G. Docimo. Laparoscopic surgery in patients with ventriculoperitoneal shunts: safety and monitoring. *J Urol* 2000; **164**: 1352–4.

2. R. G. Uzzo, M. Bilsky, D. T. Minimberg *et al.* Laparoscopic surgery in children with ventriculoperitoneal shunts: effect of pneumoperitoneum on intracranial pressure – preliminary experience. *Urology* 1997; **49**: 753–7.

3. A. F. Kalmar, J. Van Aken, J. Caemaert *et al.* Value of Cushing reflex as warning sign for brain ischaemia during neuroendoscopy. *Br J Anaesth* 2005; **94**: 791–9.

4. W. S. Almaani, A. S. Awidi. Spontaneous intracranial hemorrhage secondary to von Willebrand's disease. *Surg Neurol* 1986; **26**: 457–60.

5. R. Nakau, M. Nomura, S. Kida *et al.* Subarachnoid hemorrhage associated with von Willebrand's disease – case report. *N Neurol Med Chir* 2005; **45**: 631–4.

6. **J. Ravaoherisoa, P. Meyer, R. Afriat** *et al.*
Laparoscopic surgery in a patient with ventriculoperitoneal shunt: monitoring of shunt function with
transcranial Doppler. *Br J Anaesth* 2004; **92**: 434–7.

7. **J. J. Baskin, A. G. Vishteh, D. E. Wesche** *et al.*
Ventriculoperitoneal shunt failure as a complication

of laparoscopic surgery. *JSLS* 1998; **2**:
177–80.

8. **J. A. Brown, M. D. Medlock, D. M. Dahl**.
Ventriculoperitoneal shunt externalization during
laparoscopic prostatectomy. *Urology* 2004; **63**:
1183–5.

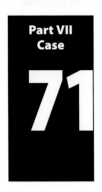

Neurologic sequelae in other patient populations. Miscellaneous

Perioperative acute ischemic stroke in general surgical procedures

Milad Sharifpour and George A. Mashour

Perioperative acute ischemic stroke (AIS) is a feared complication of surgery that is associated with increased in-hospital mortality, length of hospital stay, disability, and discharge to long-term care facilities [1]. The risk for AIS depends on a patient's preexisting co-morbidities, as well as the type and complexity of the planned surgical procedure. The incidence is reported to range from almost 1.0% in general surgical procedures to 4.5% in cardiovascular procedures [2, 3].

Case description

The patient was a 70-year-old female with a past medical history of hypertension, hypercholesterolemia, mitral stenosis, chronic atrial fibrillation (requiring anticoagulation therapy with coumadin), diabetes mellitus, myocardial infarction, and morbid obesity. She underwent an elective left total hip arthroplasty because of severe osteoarthritis. General anesthesia with endotracheal intubation was planned and the patient's coumadin was discontinued 5 days prior to surgery to allow the prothrombin time to return to normal. The intraoperative course was complicated by episodes of hypotension, which were treated with phenylephrine. The patient also had an episode of atrial fibrillation, which was treated with incremental boluses of esmolol. The remainder of the surgery was uneventful and the case was completed with approximately 500 mL of estimated blood loss. Emergence was smooth and the patient was neurologically intact. However, 3 hours after the procedure she had an acute onset of delirium with a new left-sided hemiparesis. A noncontrast computed tomography scan of the head demonstrated loss of gray and white matter differentiation in the insular region, as well as a hyperdensity in the right middle cerebral artery distribution, consistent with AIS. Since treatment with intravenous tissue plasminogen activator (tPA) is contraindicated

after major surgical procedures, the patient was taken to the interventional radiology suite and endovascular mechanical thrombolysis was performed.

Discussion

Perioperative AIS is a serious complication of surgery. The majority of perioperative strokes are embolic and associated with systemic atherosclerosis. Available data indicate that approximately 45% of strokes take place during the first day after surgery while the rest occur after recovery from anesthesia, from the second postoperative day onward [1]. A recent large-scale study found an incidence of 0.7% after hemicolectomy, 0.2% after hip arthroplasty, and 0.6% after lobectomy or segmental lung resection [2]. Even though the risk of stroke during the perioperative period is seemingly low, it is a significant source of increased morbidity and mortality. Therefore, it is important to identify modifiable risk factors for perioperative stroke and evaluate each patient's risk–benefit ratio prior to surgery in order to optimize care. The main risk factors for perioperative stroke include (1) female sex, (2) advanced age, (3) atrial fibrillation, (4) cardiac valvular disease, (5) congestive heart failure, (6) history of previous transient ischemic attack (TIA) or stroke, (7) renal disease, (8) diabetes mellitus, (9) hypertension, and (10) general anesthesia [1, 2, 4]. While female sex is protective against stroke in the general population, it is associated with a higher risk of stroke during the perioperative period [1, 2]. Advanced age is also associated with increased risk of perioperative stroke and Bateman et al. found that the incidence of perioperative AIS after hemicolectomy, total hip arthroplasty, and lobectomy was higher in patients >65 years old compared with that in patients <65 years old [2].

Atrial fibrillation is a significant and potentially modifiable risk factor and was identified as the most common co-morbidity associated with stroke after general surgery in a recent study of perioperative ischemic stroke [2]. It can lead to ischemic stroke by increasing the risk of cardioembolic events or by causing cerebral hypoperfusion in patients who develop rapid ventricular rate and hypotension. Therefore, patients should be closely monitored for perioperative arrhythmias. Electrolyte abnormalities and shifts in the intravascular volume should be corrected aggressively, and hyperadrenergic states and pulmonary complications should be treated promptly since they predispose patients to atrial fibrillation.

Prophylactic beta-adrenergic blocker therapy has been shown to decrease the incidence of atrial fibrillation after cardiovascular procedures. The POISE trial, however, examined patients undergoing noncardiac surgery and found a lower risk of atrial fibrillation but a higher risk of perioperative stroke and overall mortality associated with β-adrenergic blocker prophylaxis [5]. Currently the neuroprotective role of prophylactic beta-adrenergic blockade in noncardiac surgery remains unclear and more studies are required to better define this role.

Valvular heart diseases also increase the risk of perioperative stroke. Diseased or mechanical valves increase the risk of cardioembolic events, or can lead to decreased cardiac output and cerebral hypoperfusion. Furthermore, certain valvular diseases such as mitral stenosis increase the risk of atrial fibrillation and consequently the risk of perioperative stroke. Left ventricular dysfunction is another potentially modifiable risk factor of perioperative stroke. Preoperative evaluation with echocardiography may be required in order to assess left ventricular function and the presence of intracardiac emboli.

Proper anticoagulation is essential in order to decrease the risk of embolic stroke associated with atrial fibrillation and valvular heart disease. However, the potentially protective effect of anticoagulation should be weighed carefully against the risk of bleeding during the perioperative period. This is particularly important in patients with preexisting atrial fibrillation, in whom abrupt discontinuation of coumadin therapy leads to increased risk of perioperative stroke [1, 2, 4].

When oral anticoagulation must be withheld in anticipation of surgery, it is recommended that the time period during which anticoagulation is being withheld should be minimized and bridge therapy with heparin, as well as postoperative anticoagulation with coumadin, should be started as early as possible. This is of paramount importance in patients with increased risk of thromboembolism, namely those with chronic atrial fibrillation, valvular heart disease or mechanical valves, or those with left ventricular dysfunction.

Patients with a history of TIA or stroke are at a significantly higher risk of perioperative stroke. Thus, anesthesiologists must specifically inquire about history of such events and carefully assess neurologic status during the preoperative evaluation and document any deficits. Furthermore, they should investigate and possibly treat the causes of TIA and stroke prior to surgery.

Renal disease, diabetes mellitus, and hypertension are among the known risk factors of stroke in the general population and are also associated with increased risk of perioperative stroke. Renal disease predisposes patients to accelerated atherosclerosis and dialysis-dependent patients are at increased risk of hypotension and fluid shifts. Intraoperative and postoperative hyperglycemia is associated with increased risk of atrial fibrillation, stroke, and death. It is suggested to maintain blood glucose below 140 mg/dL to minimize the risk of these events. The optimal blood pressure during surgery is undetermined. However, it has been reported that deviations more than 20% or 20 mmHg from the preoperative baseline blood pressure for prolonged periods leads to increased perioperative complications.

Conclusion

Despite advances in surgical technique and perioperative monitoring, stroke remains a significant complication of general surgical procedures with considerable morbidity and mortality. Preoperative evaluation of patients should focus on identifying and correcting potentially modifiable risk factors to reduce the risk of this devastating complication.

References

1. **M. Selim**. Perioperative stroke. *N Engl J Med* 2007; **356**: 706–13.

2. **B. T. Bateman, H. C. Schumacher, S. Wang, S. Shaefi, M. F. Berman**. Perioperative acute ischemic stroke in noncardiac and nonvascular surgery. *Anesthesiology* 2009; **110**: 231–8.

3. **J. Bucerius, J. F. Gummert, M. A. Borger** *et al.* Stroke after cardiac surgery: a risk factor analysis of 16,184 consecutive adult patients. *Ann Thorac Surg* 2003; **75**: 472–8.

4. **V. Szeder, M. T. Torbey**. Prevention and treatment of perioperative stroke. *Neurologist* 2008; **14**: 30–6.

5. **P. J. Devereaux, H. Yang, S. Yusuf** *et al.* Effects of extended-release metoprolol succinate in patients undergoing noncardiac surgery (POISE trial): a randomized controlled trial. *Lancet* 2008; **371**: 1839–47.

Neurologic complications following cardiothoracic surgery

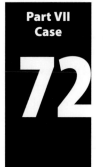

Donn Marciniak and Colleen G. Koch

Up to 79% of patients undergoing cardiac surgery utilizing cardiopulmonary bypass will demonstrate some degree of neuropsychiatric dysfunction and up to 5.4% will manifest perioperative stroke [1]. These statistics vary greatly in the literature and are influenced by procedure type and co-morbidities, but reflect a common problem in patients undergoing cardiac surgery. Perioperative neurologic disturbances are a major cause of morbidity and mortality in the cardiac surgery population and numerous methods and techniques have been developed to help minimize these occurrences.

Case description

The patient was a 34-year-old male seen in consultation for treatment of an ascending aortic aneurysm and fungal endocarditis. He had a mitral valve repair and an ascending aortic replacement with an aortic valve homograft 10 years prior to this admission. Approximately 6 months prior to the current admission, the patient underwent cardiac surgery for aortic homograft failure. On this most recent admission, the patient presented with fever, sternal wound drainage, and right leg pain. Computed tomography (CT) scan revealed a false aneurysm of the distal anastomosis of the prior aortic graft to the aorta. Distal pulses in the right foot were diminished and he was diagnosed with a fungal thromboembolus to the right tibial artery. The patient underwent a third reoperation with ascending aneurysm repair, with a distal ascending aortic graft and a cryopreserved homograft under deep hypothermic circulatory arrest. *Candida albicans* was cultured from the graft material and the patient was placed on appropriate antibiotic therapy.

On postoperative day 1 the patient developed seizures and no demonstrable movement of his upper extremities. A 24-hour electroencephalogram (EEG) recorded seizures arising from the left hemisphere and the occipital region. On discontinuation of propofol, the EEG demonstrated status epilepticus arising from

both hemispheres. A neurology consult attributed his status epilepticus to suspected anoxic brain injury secondary to intraoperative events. The seizure activity resolved with appropriate therapy. A CT of the brain revealed findings suggestive of diffuse cerebral edema related to a global anoxic event and a small acute anterior cerebral artery distribution cortical infarct without mass effect. Magnetic resonance imaging revealed diffuse signal changes worrisome for global hypoxic injury. A follow-up CT of the brain 3 days later reported a stable infarct, ischemia in the bifrontal lobes, and a punctate hyperdensity in the occipital lobes. The patient required tracheostomy for respiratory insufficiency, but was eventually weaned from ventilatory support. He demonstrated slow clinical improvement in neurologic activity, was eventually less confused, and able to reply to commands; with physical and occupational therapy, he slowly regained upper extremity motor strength. He was discharged to rehabilitation approximately 1 month after surgery.

Discussion

Our patient presented with both focal and global neurologic complications related to cardiac surgery. Fungal thromboemboli, air emboli, and circulatory arrest were thought to contribute to his motor deficit, diffuse hypoxic injury, altered sensorium, and seizure activity. Risk factors for neurologic complications following cardiac surgery in general include patient characteristics such as age, hypertension, and operative factors. Roach and colleagues reported the incidence of adverse cerebral outcomes to be 6.1% following cardiac surgery [1]. Neurologic injury was divided into type I, which constituted focal injury, stupor, or coma and type II, which constituted deterioration in intellectual function, memory deficit, or seizures. Predictors of type I outcomes were proximal aortic atherosclerosis, a history of neurologic disease, and advanced age. Predictors for type II outcomes were advanced age, hypertension, pulmonary disease and excessive alcohol use. Those who experienced adverse cerebral outcomes had higher in-hospital mortality and longer duration of hospitalization [1]. Because of variable definitions of what comprises a neurocognitive deficit and differences in measuring techniques, there is great variance of rates reported in the literature.

Focal ischemia during cardiopulmonary bypass is often a consequence of an embolic phenomenon from gaseous or atheromatous debris. In this case, the patient was also at risk for infectious fungal emboli. Various methods to identify and protect against regional neurologic injury are in use today but many are of questionable efficacy. Epiaortic ultrasound attempts to identify atheromatous regions of the aorta that can be avoided during the procedure, but data regarding its efficacy are mixed and embolic load may be unaffected [2]. This technique can evaluate transesophageal echocardiogram (TEE) 'blind spots' in zones three and four of the aorta and thus help guide the sites of cannulation and clamping. Surgical palpation of the ascending aorta is a poor indicator of the presence of atheroma. Changes in the site of cannulation may reduce the risk of atheromatous embolization initially, but the risk of a sand-blasting effect still exists. Improvements in the cardiopulmonary bypass machine, such as the incorporation of a 25 μm aortic inflow-line filter, the use of membrane oxygenators, and cardiotomy suction filters, are used in an attempt to reduce the embolic load delivered to the patient. Careful de-airing of the cardiac chambers with the help of TEE guidance is often employed to decrease the gaseous embolic load. Avoiding nitrous oxide will also likely reduce the size of gaseous emboli. Carotid artery compression during periods of expected embolic showering is not likely to be helpful.

Since our patient required surgery on the aortic arch, interruption of brain perfusion with circulatory arrest was necessary. Fleck and colleagues reported duration of circulatory arrest, in particular arrest times >30 minutes, as the most important determinant of postoperative temporary neurologic dysfunction (TND) defined as confusion, delirium, and agitation [3]. They reported an 18% incidence of TND and a 21% incidence of combined temporary and permanent neurologic deficit following surgery. Furthermore, TND led to impaired functional recovery due to impaired fine motor function and short-term memory loss [3]. Intraoperative factors utilized in our case

to mitigate risk of neurologic injury included use of retrograde cerebral perfusion, hypothermia, and TEE guided de-airing. Others have reported the prevalence of TND following circulatory arrest as between 16% and 43% and dependent on the type of cerebral protective strategies used [4, 5].

We used hypothermia as a technique for global cerebral protection during circulatory arrest. Our patient was cooled to 18 °C to decrease neuronal metabolic rate and therefore oxygen demand. Temperature was measured with a nasopharyngeal probe placed before heparinization with the thought that this site correlates reasonably well with jugular venous bulb temperature and is a good surrogate for more invasive locations. Regional temperature differences may occur during cooling and many centers pack the patient's head in ice to compensate for this, but there are scant data to support this maneuver and care must be taken to avoid injury to the skin and eyes. Rewarming must be carefully controlled. If this process is too rapid, an overshoot may occur and an increased risk of neuronal damage exists through mechanisms such as widening of ischemic penumbra, accelerated free radical formation, and increased acidosis [6]. Limiting arterial inflow temperature to 37 °C is one possible maneuver to avoid this complication. Sodium thiopental administration is often used during cooling to minimize neuronal damage by establishing an isoelectric state, along with a Bispectral Index value of zero, thereby further reducing metabolic demand. If thiopental is administered, it should be given 3–5 minutes before circulatory arrest.

We used retrograde cerebral perfusion as a brain-protective technique where the superior vena cava was cannulated and cooled; oxygenated blood flowed from the venous to arterial networks. The premise is that nutrient-rich blood will reach the brain, toxic metabolites will be washed out, and regional warming will be diminished. Additionally, air, atheroma, and in this case, fungal debris may have also been washed out. Antegrade cerebral perfusion may also be employed where blood flows in an anatomic manner, with the carotid or innominate arteries cannulated. There is ongoing debate as to whether one technique offers better outcomes than the other.

Hyperglycemia worsens both global and regional neurologic injuries in cardiac surgery. Maintenance of euglycemia is desirable in all cardiac surgical patients and more so in patients undergoing circulatory arrest considering their increased incidence of neurologic insult [7]. Whether one is to allow tight or permissive glucose control is unclear, as hypoglycemia may be more deleterious than hyperglycemia during circulatory arrest. Ultimately, blood glucose must be carefully regulated and it is likely a good practice to avoid introducing unnecessary exogenous sources of glucose.

Near infrared spectroscopy (NIRS) is often employed during circulatory arrest to allow assessment of regional oxygen saturation. Since this technology is highly regional in nature, it is speculative to use the data to assess global cerebral oxygenation. Regardless, its use is well-established in pediatric cardiac surgery and less so in adult circulatory arrest procedures [8]. Observing a drop in the NIRS may lead one to increase oxygen delivery by introducing antegrade or retrograde cerebral perfusion (presuming it is not in place), increasing cerebral flow pressures, or administering red blood cells. None of these approaches is benign in nature and great consideration must be used in allowing NIRS data to guide clinical management.

References

1. **G. W. Roach, M. Kanchuger, C. M. Mangano** *et al.* Adverse cerebral outcomes after coronary bypass surgery. Multicenter Study of Perioperative Ischemia Research Group and the Ischemia Research and Education Foundation Investigators. *N Engl J Med* 1996; **335**: 1857–63.

2. **G. Djaiani, M. Ali, M. A. Borger** *et al.* Epiaortic scanning modifies planned intraoperative surgical management but not cerebral embolic load during coronary artery bypass surgery. *Anesth Analg* 2008; **106**: 1611–18.

3. **T. M. Fleck, M. Czerny, D. Hutschala** *et al.* The incidence of transient neurologic dysfunction after ascending aortic replacement with circulatory arrest. *Ann Thorac Surg* 2003; **76**: 1198–202.

4. **E. Apostolakis, E. N. Koletsis, F. Dedeilias** *et al.* Antegrade versus retrograde cerebral perfusion in relation to postoperative complications following aortic arch surgery for acute aortic dissection type A. *J Card Surg* 2008; **23**: 480–7.

5. **A. Zierer, M. R. Moon, S. J. Melby** *et al.* Impact of perfusion strategy on neurologic recovery in acute type A aortic dissection. *Ann Thorac Surg* 2007; **83**: 2122–8.

6. **A. M. Grigore, C. F. Murray, F. Ramakrishna** *et al.* A core review of temperature regimens and neuroprotection during cardiopulmonary bypass: does rewarming rate matter? *Anesth Analg* 2009; **109**: 1741–51.

7. **A. K. Lipshutz, M. A. Gropper.** Perioperative glycemic control: an evidence-based review. *Anesthesiology* 2009; **110**: 408–21.

8. **M. C. Taillefer, A. Y. Denault.** Cerebral near-infrared spectroscopy in adult heart surgery: systematic review of its clinical efficacy. *Can J Anaesth* 2005; **52**: 79–87.

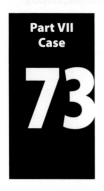

73

Anesthetic management for subdural hematoma evacuation in a patient with a left ventricular assist device

Marcos Gomes, Hesham Elsharkawy, Endrit Bala and Ehab Farag

Developments in ventricular assist devices (VADs) and the limited supply of donor hearts for transplantation have made the former an important method of treatment for patients with end-stage heart failure. As the use and life expectancy on a VAD increases, the probability increases that the anesthesiologist will provide anesthesia for noncardiac surgery in such patients. Here we present the case of a patient who underwent two surgical procedures for subdural hematoma evacuation while on left VAD (LVAD) support. Anesthetic management and potential problems such as coagulation status and hemodynamic stability in patients with an LVAD are presented and discussed.

Case description

The patient was a 72-year-old male who presented for an emergent subdural hematoma decompression after falling at home the night before and becoming unresponsive that morning. A computed tomography (CT) scan of the head done in the emergency department showed a large left subdural hematoma with approximately 1.7 cm midline shift, as well as evidence of herniation. He had a past medical history significant for nonischemic cardiomyopathy, congestive heart failure, with an ejection fraction of 5%, status post pacemaker-defibrillator implantation 10 months earlier, type 2 diabetes mellitus, chronic kidney disease (baseline creatinine 1.6), and an LVAD that had been implanted 4 months earlier, which improved his ejection fraction to 20%. The patient's LVAD was a model HeartMate® II, and required the patient to be continuously anticoagulated on coumadin. Upon arrival in the operating room and application of standard ASA monitors, an arterial line was placed and the patient had his defibrillator turned off for the procedure. The trachea had already been intubated in the emergency department for airway protection; therefore, induction was performed with sevoflurane inhalation as well

as intravenous rocuronium and fentanyl. A central line and two extra large-bore peripheral intravenous catheters were inserted afterwards. During the procedure, mean arterial pressures were maintained with norepinephrine infusion with a mean arterial pressure goal of ~80 mmHg. One unit of fresh frozen plasma and five units of platelets were given intraoperatively. Coagulopathy had also been treated in the emergency department with fresh frozen plasma and platelets, improving the International Normalized Ratio (INR) from 2.4 to 1.2. Two liters of crystalloids were also given throughout the procedure and the estimated blood loss was 200 mL. The patient was transferred to the intensive care unit, intubated, and sedated. The following day, a control CT scan of the head showed a new hemorrhagic contusion with surround edema in the posterotemporal lobe with a residual 2.6 cm epidural hematoma, and a second emergency evacuation was performed. For that procedure, a similar anesthetic technique was used, with the exception of using remifentanil infusion for analgesia instead of intravenous fentanyl. During the procedure the LVAD team was present to assist the management of LVAD. The surgery took place uneventfully and the patient returned to the cardiovascular intensive care unit. On postoperative day number 12, a tracheostomy and gastric tube placement were performed. Unfortunately, throughout the whole postoperative period, the patient never recovered from a neurologic point of view, and the family decided to change his status to comfort care without resuscitation. On postoperative day number 17, the LVAD was turned off and the patient passed away.

Discussion

According to the American Heart Association, approximately 500 000 new cases of congestive heart failure are diagnosed every year, affecting 4.6 million Americans [1]. It is estimated that 250 000–500 000 patients in the USA, and approximately 2.2 million worldwide, are currently in the terminal phase of heart failure and are refractory to maximized medical therapy. Each year approximately 30 000 patients are listed for cardiac transplantation, but only 3500 are performed, making it evident that there is a chronic shortage of donors [2]. Having said that, it is inevitable that we will watch an increasing number of patients with terminal congestive heart failure present to our hospitals in search of an alternative treatment.

The Randomized Evaluation of Mechanical Assistance for the Treatment of Congestive Heart failure (REMATCH) trial [3, 4], as well as other early clinical experiences [4], has shown that an implantable LVAD as a destination therapy prolongs and enhances the quality of life in heart failure patients [5]. This hemodynamic restoration therapy has increased the 1- and 2-year survival rates compared with pharmacologic interventions alone. There is also evidence that New York Heart Association Class IV patients improve to Class I or II post-LVAD treatment.

As the number of patients chronically supported with long-term implantable devices grows, general surgical problems that are commonly seen in other hospitalized patients are becoming more common and will eventually lead to an increase in the number of patients with LVADs coming in for noncardiac elective or emergency surgery. Anesthesiologists are required to have knowledge of the function of these devices and to understand its implications during anesthesia for noncardiac surgery. There are currently different models on the market. However, we are going to focus our discussion on the one used in our patient, the HeartMate® II. This device is smaller, more durable, and promotes continuous flow, which is why it has been used more often recently.

The HeartMate® II consists of an internal blood pump with a percutaneous lead that connects the pump to an external system driver and power source. The pump has an implant volume of 63 mL and generates up to 10 L/min of flow at a mean pressure of 100 mmHg. It drains blood from the left ventricle into a mechanical pump, which then ejects the blood via a conduit that links to the ascending aorta. The pump is driven by a small electric motor and the rotary action of the single moving part is responsible for its effect. The LVAD is normally powered electrically and can be connected to two rechargeable batteries worn in a waist pack, which could last for up to 3 hours. The blood flow generated by the LVAD is nonpulsatile and

for this reason these patients require anticoagulation. Low postoperative mortality rate, low incidence of adverse events, favorable low thrombogenicity and low thromboembolic risk make the HeartMate® II LVAD an ideal device to be used as a bridge to transplantation and destination therapy as well [6]. A third indication for LVADs is the patient with potentially reversible cardiac ischemia resulting in severe cardiogenic shock. In this scenario, the LVAD can serve to maintain systemic circulation while the myocardium is allowed time to recover [1].

Four aspects have to be considered in the management of patients with LVADs presenting for noncardiac surgery: (1) LVAD specialists, (2) power supply and electromagnetic interference, (3) hemodynamics, and (4) anticoagulation [5].

The first priority for the anesthesiologist caring for a patient with an LVAD is to identify the "LVAD team" in the institution. A specialized team of healthcare professionals that may include cardiothoracic surgeons, nurses, engineers, and cardiopulmonary perfusionists is usually responsible for the management of LVAD patients in the vast majority of medical centers. This team is an indispensable and valuable resource for information regarding the details of LVAD management.

Securing a reliable power supply to assure continuous operation of a mechanical assist device is the next consideration for the LVAD patient presenting for surgery, since the LVAD has a limited battery capacity (rechargeable batteries). An alternating current source in the operating room may be safe and more reliable [1]. The potential for electromagnetic interference with LVAD function by external defibrillation or electrocautery should be recognized. As a result, device settings and connections may require adjustment, but it must be emphasized that such maneuvers should only be done with consultation or supervision of the institution's LVAD team. The manufacturer recommends that the electric model be set to function in the fixed-rate mode as opposed to the "fill-to-empty" (auto) mode during surgical procedures in which the use of electrocautery is anticipated. Bipolar cautery should be used if possible, since current flows only between the tips of the bipolar instrument, but bipolar cautery is impractical for many surgical procedures because it is much less powerful than monopolar cautery [7].

The pumping mechanism of the LVAD depends on both *preload* and *afterload*. These devices do not obey Starling's law with respect to stroke volume or stroke work, and can only pump the delivered volume and therefore inadequate filling leads to inadequate flow. Optimal function is consequently achieved with increased intravascular volume and decreased vascular resistance. Maintenance of adequate preload is thus critically important. Direct decreases in pump flow occur when preload declines as a consequence of decreased venous return secondary to increased venous capacitance (including drug-induced venodilatation), alterations in body position that reduce venous return (e.g., lateral decubitus or reverse Trendelenburg position), inadequate administration of intravenous fluids, or uncontrolled surgical bleeding. Conventional inhalational and intravenous anesthetic techniques were well tolerated in these patients [8]. All commercially available assist devices exhibit sensitivity to changes in afterload. As a result, hypertension should be specifically avoided because emptying of the LVAD is reduced by increases in arterial pressure. Incomplete LVAD ejection not only decreases forward flow but also promotes blood stasis within the device and increases the risk of thrombus formation, even in the presence of systemic anticoagulation. Systemic responses to laryngoscopy and surgical stimulus should be attenuated and avoidance of hypertension should be the primary aim in the perioperative management of these patients. Hemodynamically significant arrhythmias should be treated appropriately with pharmacologic or electrical means. External chest compression should be avoided because of the risk of cannula dislodgement [9]. These objectives may be achieved by assurance of adequate anesthetic depth using volatile anesthetics in combination with an opioid or by the judicious administration of arterial vasodilators (e.g., sodium nitroprusside, fenoldopam) to treat increases in arterial pressure. The drugs should be added cautiously, paying careful attention to resultant increased venous capacitance and decreased venous return. In the absence of hypertension, most cases of low LVAD flow can be corrected by volume expansion. The fluid, inotropic, and vasopressor requirements do not appear to be significantly different than those required in other patients undergoing similar procedures [8]. Right ventricle dysfunction must also be considered and negative inotropic drugs (e.g., volatile anesthetics, adrenoceptor antagonists, calcium channel blockers), as well as factors that increase pulmonary vascular resistance (e.g., hypoxemia, hypercarbia, acidosis), should be

avoided [7]. In such cases, a positive inodilator (e.g., milrinone) or a selective pulmonary vasodilator (e.g., inhaled nitric oxide) may be required [7]. In our case, we managed hypotension throughout the case with norepinephrine, aiming at a target systolic blood pressure of 90 mmHg. Norepinephrine exerts its effects on alpha-1 and beta-1 adrenoreceptors, therefore it works as a vasopressor and an inotrope, usually with doses ranging from 0.05–1 mcg/kg/min. It is indicated for severe systemic hypotension, mostly related to profound vasodilatation, and it should be tapered off as the hemodynamics stabilize in order to prevent prolonged peripheral vasoconstriction resulting in limited perfusion to end organs [10].

Management of anticoagulant therapy is another major issue that requires attention in the perioperative care of the LVAD patient. Experience with surgery under anticoagulant conditions such as the ones found in patients with VADs is scarce. These patients require preoperative admission and conversion to heparin anticoagulation, which is stopped in the immediate preoperative period. Most procedures can be delayed until coagulation parameters are optimized; however, in emergency operations, in which oral anticoagulants (coumadin) have not been stopped, transfusion with fresh frozen plasma is required to acutely correct clotting parameters [1]. Transfusion of fresh frozen plasma and platelet concentrates can be started with liberal amounts at any time and will certainly relieve bleeding. Postponing resumption of full anticoagulation is advisable because it may reduce bleeding complications without increasing the risk for thromboembolism. On the other hand, in many institutions, treatment with heparin is indeed resumed to lower the risk of thromboembolism, when risk of bleeding is diminished [7].

Conclusion

The anesthetic management of patients with an LVAD who present for elective or emergent surgery represents a unique challenge for the anesthesiologist. A detailed understanding of the operation of the device, as well as the factors that affect its normal functioning are essential in order to promote successful surgical outcomes. A multidisciplinary approach, hemodynamic stability, and anticoagulation status are crucial issues for safe perioperative care in VAD patients.

References

1. **A. E. Eckhauser, W. V. Melvin, K. W. Sharp**. Management of general surgical problems in patients with left ventricular assist devices. *Am Surg* 2006; **72**: 158–61.

2. **A. Garatti, G. Bruschi, T. Colombo** *et al.* Noncardiac surgical procedures in patient supported with long-term implantable left ventricular assist device. *Am J Surg* 2009; **197**; 710–14.

3. **E. A Rose, A. C. Gelijns, A. J. Moskowitz** *et al.* Long-term mechanical left ventricular assistance for end-stage heart failure. *N Engl J Med* 2001; **345**: 1435–43.

4. **O. H. Frazier, C. Gemmato, T. J. Myers** *et al.* Initial clinical experience with the HeartMate II axial-flow left ventricular assist device. *Tex Heart Inst J* 2007; **34**: 275–81.

5. **V. Kartha, W. Gomez, B. Wu** *et al.* Laparoscopic cholecystectomy in a patient with an implantable left ventricular assist device. *Br J Anaesth* 2008; **100**: 652–5.

6. **R. John, F. Kamdar, K. Liao** *et al.* Improved survival and decreasing incidence of adverse events with the HeartMate II left ventricular assist device as bridge-to-transplant therapy. *Ann Thorac Surg* 2008; **86**: 1227–34.

7. **A. C. Nicolosi, P. S. Pagel**. Perioperative considerations in the patient with a left ventricular assist device. *Anesthesiology* 2003; **98**: 565–70.

8. **D. J. Goldstein, S. L. Mullis, E. S. Delphin** *et al.* Noncardiac surgery in long-term implantable left ventricular assist-device recipients. *Ann Surg* 1995; **222**: 203–7.

9. **S. T. Webb, V. Patil, A. Vuylsteke**. Anaesthesia for non-cardiac surgery in patient with Becker's muscular dystrophy supported with a left ventricular assist device. *Eur J Anaesthesiol* 2007; **24**: 640–2.

10. **N. C. Dang, Y. Naka**. Perioperative pharmacotherapy in patients with left ventricular assist devices. *Drugs Aging* 2004; **21**: 993–1012.

Neurocritical care

74

Hypotension

Edward Noguera

Hypotension is one of the most common findings in the intensive care unit (ICU) patient and requires prompt attention in order to avoid poor clinical outcomes.

Case description

A 42-year-old morbidly obese female (body mass index = 38) was transferred to the ICU after being diagnosed with a subarachnoid hemorrhage due to a ruptured aneurysm of the right middle cerebral artery. Her past medical history was relevant for hypertrophic cardiomyopathy with an ejection fraction of 30%, hypertension, and Crohn's disease. Her medications included digoxin, carvedilol, enalapril, and prednisone. Upon arrival to the ICU she was comatose and intubated. Her heart rate was 142 beats per minute and irregular, mean arterial blood pressure (MAP) was 40 mmHg, temperature was 39.6 °C, and pulse oximeter saturation was 93%. She had an 18-gauge peripheral line, 20-gauge radial artery line and a Foley catheter. A resident physician in the emergency room attempted central line placement before transport to the ICU, without success. After ICU admission a pulmonary artery catheter (PAC) was inserted via right internal jugular vein using ultrasound guidance. The first reading of her pulmonary capillary occlusion pressure (PCOP) was 10 mmHg and her cardiac output was 3 liter/min. Transthoracic echocardiogram (TTE) was ordered to assess her myocardial function due to her past medical history, the potential for ventricular dysfunction due to the subarachnoid hemorrhage and to rule out other causes for hypotension-like tamponade. The patient's hypotensive condition was corrected by fluid boluses to increase her filling pressure, guided by PCOP and by starting the patient on norepinephrine infusion to increase her cardiac output and maintain her perfusion pressure as well.

Discussion

Classically, blood pressure is determined by the product of cardiac output and systemic vascular resistance ($BP = CO \times SVR$). Cardiac output itself is determined by several interrelated factors: mainly preload, pump function, and afterload. Systemic vascular resistance is determined by a complex relationship of blood viscosity, vessel length, and vessel radius. In approaching the patient with hypotension, a focused history and physical examination should be performed, with attention to the "ABCs" of airway, breathing, and circulation. The goal is to identify an immediate cause of hypotension based on physiologic principles. However, many cases such as the one described above can have multiple causes based on clinical history. For example, our patient could have been hypotensive due to preexisting cardiomyopathy, ventricular dysfunction due to subarachnoid hemorrhage, hypovolemia, or sepsis. In these situations, a systematic approach is essential and tools such as the PAC or echocardiogram can be helpful. There is, of course, controversy regarding the value of the PAC in the ICU setting [1].

Preload

Disorders of preload relate primarily to hypovolemia, as can occur with inadequate oral intake, inadequate fluid administration, hemorrhage, excessive urine output, or insensible loss. In this situation physical examination might reveal poor skin turgor or dry mucous membranes; abnormal vital signs could include orthostatic hypotension. Pulmonary artery catheter data would demonstrate low PCOP and low cardiac output, with possibly increased SVR as compensation. Although a measured pressure, PCOP is used as a surrogate for left ventricular end-diastolic volume. In a patient with an arterial line and endotracheal tube, high systolic pressure variation might be seen due to the effects of positive pressure ventilation on venous return [2]. The treatment of choice in this situation is volume (crystalloid, colloid, blood), with temporizing measures including vasopressors such as phenylephrine (alpha-1 agonist) and norepinephrine (alpha-1 and beta-1 agonist).

Pump function

Ventricular failure syndromes present with hypotension due to inadequate ejection of blood. In this case patients may have a history of coronary artery disease or heart failure. Physical examination signs might include peripheral edema, jugular venous distension, or crackles upon auscultation. Either TTE or transesophageal echocardiogram are very good tools to assess myocardial contractility and valvular function. The presence of wall motion abnormality in an echocardiogram is considered the earliest sign of myocardial ischemia. Pulmonary artery catheter data would include a low cardiac output but, unlike hypovolemia, a high PCOP (since blood is not getting ejected). Vasopressors used for treatment in this situation include dobutamine and dopamine (for beta-1 adrenergic effects), as well as milrinone (a phosphodiesterase inhibitor).

Dysrhythmias are also a cause of hypotension. Electrical cardioversion, defibrillation or pacing capabilities are indicated according to the type. Cardiac dysrhythmias can be potentiated or induced by myocardial ischemia, hypoxia, acidosis, hypercarbia, electrolyte disturbances and mechanical irritation from intravascular devices in proximity to the myocardium.

Other causes of pump dysfunction that are external to the heart include pneumothorax and tamponade. Placement of a chest tube is indicated if a pneumothorax is suspected or documented; if this is not possible, needle decompression can be performed by the anesthesiologist. Our patient had an unsuccessful attempt of central line placement and therefore was at risk of pneumothorax. Cardiac tamponade can be another cause of hypotension, especially in trauma settings, and can be manifested by severe hypotension, distant heart sounds, tachycardia, jugular venous distension, and pulsus paradoxus. If one suspects cardiac tamponade, TTE should be ordered and a pericardiocentesis is indicated [3]. A PAC evaluation would show equalization of pressures.

Afterload

Afterload can be affected by processes such as sepsis, anaphylaxis, or (in part) neurogenic shock. In the septic patient, hypotension is thought to be caused by inflammatory mediators involved in the immune and humoral response to disseminated infection. The increased production of cytokines can cause severe peripheral vasodilation and severe hypotension. Pulmonary artery catheter numbers would reveal a potentially high cardiac output (unless there is myocardial stunning) and a very low SVR. Treatment involves eradication of the underlying infection and vasopressors of choice would be phenylephrine, norepinephrine, and vasopressin. Relative adrenal insufficiency is commonly seen in septic patients, which could be another cause of hypotension during sepsis. Steroids are indicated in septic shock once adequate fluid resuscitation is provided and the patient is vasopressor dependent [4]. A recent underpowered trial did not demonstrate that steroids are deleterious in septic shock patients [5].

Conclusion

There are multiple causes of hypotension in the ICU patient. Basic principles of physiology help with the differential diagnosis of hypotension. Prompt management of hypotension often requires invasive monitoring, fluid resuscitation, and the use of vasopressor or inotropic therapy.

References

1. **M. Hadian, M. R. Pinsky**. Evidence-based review of the use of the pulmonary artery catheter: impact data and complications. *Crit Care* 2006; **10** Suppl 3: S8.

2. **M. R. Minsky, D. Payen**. Functional hemodynamic monitoring. *Crit Care* 2005; **9**: 566–72.

3. **D. Spodick**. Acute cardiac tamponade. *N Engl J Med* 2003; **349**: 684–90.

4. **D. Annane, V. Sébille, C. Charpentier** et al. Effect of treatment with low doses of hydrocortisone and fludrocortisone in patients with septic shock. *J Am Med Assoc* 2002; **288**: 862–71.

5. **C. Sprung, D. Annane, D. Keh** et al. Hydrocortisone therapy for patients with septic shock. *N Engl J Med* 2008; **358**:111–24.

General topics in neurocritical care

Mechanical ventilation

Piyush Mathur and Vikram Dhawan

The need for mechanical ventilation in patients with acute or chronic neurologic disorders is not uncommon. Patients with neurologic disease are prone to hypoventilation, hypoxia, aspiration, atelectasis, and lung collapse. Decreased gag and cough reflex puts these patients at high risk for aspiration. Inability to clear orotracheal secretions is common with poor mental status.

Case description

A 55-year-old female presented to the emergency department with sudden onset of severe headache and deterioration in her level of consciousness. Her Glasgow Coma Scale on arrival to the emergency department was 5 and the trachea was therefore emergently intubated. After intubation, bilious fluid was suctioned out of the endotracheal tube. Mechanical ventilation was initiated with initial settings of synchronized intermittent mandatory ventilation, fraction of inspired oxygen (FiO_2) 50%, respiratory rate of 12/minute, positive end expiratory pressure (PEEP) 5 mmHg, pressure control 15 cmH_2O, and pressure support of 10 cmH_2O. Chest X-ray revealed a right middle lobe infiltrate. Arterial blood gas (ABG) was pH 7.39, $PaCO_2$ 40, PaO_2 156. A computed tomography scan of the brain showed diffuse subarachnoid blood in the right hemisphere. The patient was taken to the angiography suite and an aneurysm was coiled successfully with no intraoperative complications. On arrival to the neurointensive care unit, the patient had worsening oxygenation and ventilation. A repeat ABG revealed pH 7.22, $PaCO_2$ 61, PaO_2 65 on 100% FiO_2. A pulmonary artery catheter that was placed intraoperatively showed pulmonary artery wedge pressure of 8 mmHg. Repeat chest X-ray showed development of bilateral infiltrates consistent with acute respiratory distress syndrome. Mechanical ventilation mode was switched to pressure control ventilation and PEEP incrementally increased to 15 cmH_2O with improvement in both oxygenation and ventilation.

After enhancing the patient's urine output with diuretics, her oxygenation improved. She was subsequently weaned to pressure support ventilation with further improvement in both mental and respiratory status. The trachea was extubated by postoperative day 5. She developed worsening respiratory insufficiency 6 hours postextubation. She was found to have poor cough and gag reflexes and was unable to clear her secretions. A chest X-ray revealed a collapsed right lung. She was nasotracheally suctioned and placed on a noninvasive continuous positive airway pressure machine. Her mental status continued to decline and a decision was made to reintubate. Upon postintubation, both her mental status and respiratory status gradually improved. Failure to wean the patient from mechanical ventilation led to a tracheostomy by postoperative day 10. She was subsequently discharged to a long-term acute care facility for ventilator weaning and rehabilitation.

Discussion

Modes of mechanical ventilation

Multiple ventilation modes and nomenclature schemes are in existence. No one mode of ventilation has been proven to be superior. Mechanism of ventilation is characterized by the mode of ventilation delivery and type of breath sequencing. The *control* mode is the variable that is set on the ventilator as the mechanism of delivery of ventilation (i.e., pressure or volume). If the *pressure* mode is selected then the ventilator will generate breaths at that set pressure level and tidal volume can vary. If the *volume* mode is selected then the ventilator will deliver the set tidal volume and the pressure generated may vary [1].

Table 75.1. Classification of modes of ventilation based on mechanism of ventilation delivery and breath sequencing.

Mode	Control setting	Variable parameter	Breath sequencing
Pressure control	Pressure	Volume	Mandatory ventilator breaths
Volume control ventilation	Volume	Pressure	Mandatory ventilator breaths
Assist control	Pressure/volume	Pressure/volume	Mandatory ventilator breaths
Synchronized intermittent mandatory ventilation	Pressure/volume	Pressure/volume	Intermittent mandatory ventilator breaths+support spontaneous breaths
Pressure support ventilation/continuous positive airway pressure	Pressure	Volume	Support spontaneous breaths

Three types of breath sequences are possible (Table 75.1):

1. Continuous mandatory: all breaths are delivered by the ventilator, e.g., pressure control ventilation or controlled mechanical ventilation.
2. Intermittent mandatory: some mandatory breaths are delivered by the ventilator but the patient can also breathe spontaneously in between the mandatory breaths.
3. Continuous spontaneous: all breaths are spontaneously generated by the patient (e.g., pressure support ventilation).

In Assist Control mode, a preset tidal volume breath is delivered, which is either triggered by the patient or as a mandatory breath when not triggered in a specified time. Although this mode can decrease the work of breathing, it can also lead to high minute ventilation. Trigger refers to the mechanism that sets the ventilator to initiate inspiration. The trigger can be time, pressure, or flow. Ventilator cycling refers to the mechanism by which the ventilator switches from the inspiratory to the expiratory cycle. It can be flow, time, or volume cycled (Table 75.2).

Ventilator settings

The following parameters are required to be set by the operator of the ventilator on initiation of mechanical ventilation.

Mode: Determines the mechanism of delivery of ventilation.

Control: Sets the pressure or volume limits for mandatory ventilator breaths.

Support: As the name suggests, determines the pressure level of a spontaneously generated but supported breath.

Table 75.2. Alternative modes of mechanical ventilation.

Adaptive pressure control
Adaptive support ventilation
Proportional assist ventilation
Airway pressure-release ventilation and biphasic positive airway pressure
High-frequency oscillatory ventilation
Inverse ratio ventilation
Prone position ventilation

Tidal volume: Volume of inspiratory breath delivered. Usually set at 6–10 mL/kg of ideal body weight; 6–8 mL/kg tidal volume has been shown to have better outcomes in acute respiratory distress syndrome patients [2].

FiO_2: Allows delivery of oxygen at different fractions during inspiratory breaths.

PEEP: Positive end expiratory pressure is valuable in maintaining alveolar patency at end of expiration.

Respiratory rate: Rate of delivery of mandatory inspiratory breaths.

I:E ratio: The ratio of duration of inspiratory breath to expiratory breath. Normally set at 1:2, it can be changed to prolong the duration of either breath component depending on the disease process. The ratio can be reversed in the management of severe hypoxia.

Sensitivity: Level of negative pressure or flow required to trigger a ventilator breath. Usually, pressure is set at −1 to −2 cmH_2O and flow at 2–4 liters.

Ventilator weaning

Weaning from mechanical ventilation should be attempted as soon as possible. Patients who are on mechanical ventilation should meet the following criteria before ventilator weaning is undertaken [3].

- The underlying cause should have been reversed or under control.
- The patient should be able to initiate adequate respiratory breaths on his or her own. Respiratory rate <25, tidal volume >5 mL/kg, vital capacity >10 mL/kg, and negative inspiratory force <25 cm H_2O are useful guidelines.
- The patient should have adequate oxygenation and ventilation on minimal ventilator support. That includes PaO_2/FiO_2 ratio >150–200, PEEP of ≤5–8 cmH_2O, FiO_2 ≤0.4 and an acceptable pH, $PaCO_2$, and PaO_2.
- The patient should be hemodynamically stable. The patient should not have any acute illness which might lead to failure of extubation.
- Mental status should be good enough to be able to protect airway and participate in maintenance of bronchopulmonary hygiene.

Some patients may not meet all the criteria and may still be eligible for a weaning trial.

The Spontaneous Breathing Trial (SBT) has demonstrated efficacy in rapid discontinuation of mechanical ventilation. The trial consists of the patient on minimal ventilator support or a T-piece spontaneously breathing. The SBT is administered for 30–120 minutes. The patient is evaluated at the end of the SBT based upon the patient's stable respiratory, hemodynamic, and mental status. Multiple trials in one day have not shown any benefit.

The rapid shallow breathing index (RSBI) is the ratio of respiratory rate divided by tidal volume. An RSBI <105 is used as a weaning parameter which has been found to predict successful discontinuation of mechanical ventilation.

A cuff-leak test (air leak around the cuff) can be performed in patients who have been intubated for a prolonged period to determine if they have swollen upper airways.

Protocol-driven weaning ensures that weaning is attempted every day if possible. It has shown faster ventilator discontinuation rates when compared with the standard physician-driven weaning.

Patients who fail to wean off the ventilator despite best efforts will need a tracheostomy. The timing of tracheostomy is still controversial, but guidelines and meta-analysis suggest performing early tracheostomy in patients who are anticipated to be on mechanical ventilation for >21 days. Tracheostomy decreases the duration of mechanical ventilator use and shortens the length of stay in the intensive care unit. It is more comfortable for the patient and decreases the work of breathing and sedation requirements.

Noninvasive ventilation

Noninvasive mechanical ventilation is delivery of ventilation without endotracheal intubation. Either a face mask or a nasal device is used to deliver ventilation. It is suited for patients who have pulmonary insufficiency that is temporary, not very severe, and with the patient breathing spontaneously. The patient should be awake and able to protect his or her airway. It is not suited for patients with a high risk of aspiration or with ongoing hemodynamic instability.

In continuous positive airway pressure mode, a set constant airway pressure is maintained throughout inspiratory and expiratory cycles. With bi-level positive airway pressure, different levels of airway pressure settings can be set for inspiration and expiration.

Complications of mechanical ventilation

Mechanical ventilation has many complications such as barotrauma, volutrauma pneumothorax, ventilator associated pneumonia, acute lung injury, hypotension, and decreased cardiac output. Plateau pressure should be maintained at ≤30 cmH_2O. Auto-PEEP is the development of positive pressure at end expiration due to incomplete exhalation. This leads to subsequent build up of pressure which can lead to hemodynamic effects such as hypotension by decreasing cardiac output. Simply increasing the expiratory time might help eliminate auto-PEEP. Oxygen toxicity characterized mainly by either resorption atelectasis or acute lung injury is seen with use of high FiO_2 (>0.6) for prolonged periods of time.

Ventilator associated pneumonia is a common cause of morbidity and mortality in the intensive care unit. It can be decreased by keeping the head of the bed >30 degrees, administering gastrointestinal ulcer prophylaxis, maintaining oropharyngeal hygiene, and decreasing the number of days on the ventilator.

Mechanical ventilation in patients with neurologic disorders

Patients with neurologic illness often require intubation and mechanical ventilation secondary to decreased levels of consciousness, impaired airway protection, neuromuscular weakness, or pulmonary complications. Large ischemic strokes, intracranial hemorrhages, and subarachnoid hemorrhage are some examples in which consciousness is depressed, while conditions such as Guillain-Barré syndrome and myasthenia gravis lead to neuromuscular weakness. A Glasgow Coma Scale ≤8 is usually taken as a cut-off to secure the airway, although in some patients with a lower score successful extubation has been performed. The decision to intubate the trachea in patients with neuromuscular weakness should be based on both subjective and objective assessments. Poor inspiratory effort, dyspnea, diaphoresis, tachycardia, use of accessory muscles, vital capacity <15 mL/kg, maximal inspiratory pressure <−30 cmH$_2$O and nocturnal desaturation predict impending respiratory failure. Acute ischemic stroke patients with intact brain stem reflexes may do well in the long term and mechanical ventilation as a life-saving measure should be instituted. Hypercarbia increases intracranial pressure and can be deleterious in patients with brain injury. Mechanical ventilation can be very useful in decreasing PaCO$_2$ acutely for the short term and thus lowering the intracranial pressure. Patients with intracranial hypertension usually tolerate high levels of PEEP (even up to 20 mmHg), without any change in their intracranial pressure or cerebral perfusion pressure [4].

Conclusion

Mechanical ventilation is required frequently for patients with neurologic disorders for airway protection, pulmonary insufficiency, or management of intracranial pressure. No one mode of mechanical ventilation has proven to be superior in these patients. Mechanical ventilation strategies require optimizing oxygenation and ventilation with respect to the particular neurologic disorder.

References

1. **R. L. Chatburn**. Classification of ventilator modes: update and proposal for implementation. *Respir Care* 2007; **52**: 301–23.

2. Ventilation with lower tidal volumes as compared with traditional tidal volumes for acute lung injury and the acute respiratory distress syndrome. The Acute Respiratory Distress Syndrome Network. *N Engl J Med* 2000; **342**: 1301–8.

3. **N. R. MacIntyre, D. J. Cook, E. W. Ely, Jr** *et al.* Evidence-based guidelines for weaning and discontinuing ventilatory support: a collective task force facilitated by the American College of Chest Physicians; the American Association for Respiratory Care; and the American College of Critical Care Medicine. *Chest* 2001; **120**: 375S-95S.

4. **E. Muench, C. Bauhuf, H. Roth** *et al.* Effects of positive end-expiratory pressure on regional cerebral blood flow, intracranial pressure, and brain tissue oxygenation. *Crit Care Med* 2005; **33**: 2367–72.

General topics in neurocritical care

Mechanical ventilation for acute lung injury in the neurosurgical patient

James M. Blum

Acute lung injury/acute respiratory distress syndrome (ALI/ARDS) is a common problem faced by patients in the intensive care unit (ICU). The etiology of ALI is multifactorial and depends on the clinical situation; frequently ALI is the manifestation of bilateral pneumonia, transfusion reactions, or aspiration. The definition of ALI stems from the American–European consensus conference, which states that three criteria must be met to designate a patient as having ALI [1]. Although survival of ALI patients has improved greatly over the past 30 years, many of the modalities used to treat the syndrome have potential consequences in the neurosurgical population.

Case description

The patient was a 26-year-old female admitted for confusion, continuing headache, nausea, and vomiting at 10:00 pm. Noncontrast computed tomography of the head found mass effect consistent with possible tumor, minimal midline shift, left ventricular compression, and no intracranial blood. She was treated with antiemetics and admitted to a step-down unit for continuing observation while awaiting further neuroimaging; dexamethasone was administered and the patient's head was elevated in order to avoid further increases in intracranial pressure. Three hours after admission, the patient had a witnessed aspiration event and her trachea was rapidly intubated. During endotracheal intubation, the patient was noted to have copious amounts of particulate matter on the vocal cords. After intubation, the patient continued to have oxygen saturations in the range of 83–86% on 100% fraction of inspired oxygen (FiO$_2$). Aggressive endotracheal suctioning was performed and the patient's oxygen saturation increased to the range of 91–93%. The patient was transferred to the ICU, where therapeutic bronchoscopy was performed. Large particulate plugs were found and retrieved from tertiary bronchioles in both lungs. After bronchoscopy, the patient's oxygen satura-

tion further improved and she was taken for magnetic resonance imaging, which revealed a large mass in the temporal lobe consistent with a resectable tumor. The patient was scheduled for craniotomy and tumor resection as the first case in the morning.

Upon arrival for transport the anesthesia team noted that the oxygen saturation was 93% on 50% FiO$_2$. Arterial blood gas (ABG) analysis revealed a PaO$_2$ of 65 mmHg, PaCO$_2$ of 35 mmHg, and pH of 7.43. The patient was transported to the operating room uneventfully; however, after the cranial vault was opened, the patient was noted to have oxygen saturations in the low 90s despite having an FiO$_2$ of 80%. As the case continued, oxygenation continued to deteriorate with saturations into the mid 80s on 100% FiO$_2$, despite stable hemodynamics. Further ABG analysis revealed a PaO$_2$ of 55, PaCO$_2$ of 33, and pH of 7.34. The surgeon was informed of the ongoing hypoxia.

The primary concerns of the anesthesiology team were (1) management of potentially life-threatening hypoxia, (2) potential consequences of positive end expiratory pressure (PEEP) on cerebral hemodynamics and venous drainage, and (3) the potential effects of lung-protective ventilation on CO$_2$ and thus intracranial pressure. To address the hypoxia, the patient was started on propofol and remifentanil infusions and an ICU ventilator was employed. A recruitment maneuver of 40 cmH$_2$O for 40 seconds was performed, the ventilator parameters were changed to pressure control ventilation with a delta P of 15, and PEEP was increased to 15 cmH$_2$O with an I:E ratio of 3:1. These measures resulted in improvement of oxygen saturations into the high 90s on 100% FiO$_2$. Arterial blood gas revealed a PaO$_2$ of 130, PaCO$_2$ of 49, and pH of 7.31. The patient's respiratory rate was increased to 20 breaths/min and tidal volumes remained the same at about 350 mL. The surgeon placed a brain tissue oxygenation probe to assist with continuing management postoperatively. The case was completed and chest radiography revealed bilateral fluffy infiltrates.

The patient returned to the ICU where she was managed using similar ventilator settings. Slowly, her FiO_2 requirement began to wean, her PEEP was reduced, and the trachea was extubated on postoperative day 9.

Discussion

Acute lung injury is defined by the American–European consensus conference as acute hypoxia with a PaO_2/FiO_2 (P/F) ratio <300 (<200 for ARDS), bilateral infiltrates on chest radiograph, and absence of clinical signs of left atrial hypertension [1]. Mortality from ARDS overall is accepted to be around 30% currently; however, most patients that expire with ARDS do not die from hypoxia but rather sepsis or other causes [2, 3].

There are two different etiological categories of ALI: direct lung injury and indirect lung injury. Direct lung injury tends to include pneumonia and aspiration along with inhalational injury and pulmonary contusions. Indirect injury etiology includes sepsis, trauma, blood transfusions, and pancreatitis. Acute lung injury tends to occur with an initial phase that lasts 3–5 days, a subacute phase that lasts 5–7 days, and then a possible chronic phase that may result in long-term lung injury and pulmonary fibrosis.

Currently, the only well-supported treatment of ARDS is low tidal volume ventilation as prescribed by the ARMA trial conducted by ARDSNet [2]. In this trial, patients were randomized to receive either 12 mL/kg/predicted body weight (PBW) with maximal plateau pressures of 50 cmH_2O or 6 mL/kg/PBW. In the 6 mL/kg/PBW group if plateau pressures exceeded 30 cmH_2O, the volumes were reduced to 4 mL/kg/PBW. This trial used levels of PEEP not commonly seen in the operating room in order to enhance oxygenation. The ALVEOLI trial showed that even higher levels of PEEP and "open lung" ventilation was associated with fewer ventilator days although no mortality benefit [2].

The basic settings on a ventilator include the mode, respiratory rate, FiO_2, PEEP, and I:E ratio. From this basic point, one can then select either volume control or pressure control settings. In volume control, one selects a set tidal volume to be delivered to the patient. For example, one could select a 400 mL tidal volume. In pressure control, one generally selects PEEP and a drive pressure to generate the peak inspiratory pressure (PIP). For example, one may set PEEP at

Table 76.1. Predicted body weight (PBW) calculations (www.ardsnet.org).

Males	PBW (kg) = 50 + 2.3 (height (in) − 60)
Females	PBW (kg) = 45.5 + 2.3 (height (in) − 60)

5 cmH_2O and a drive pressure of 20 cmH_2O which will result in peak pressures of 25 cmH_2O. Ventilator settings that directly affect oxygenation are the FiO_2 and the combination of PEEP, PIP, and I:E ratio, all of which contribute to the mean airway pressure. By increasing PEEP to 10 and PIP to 30, the mean airway pressure, with an I:E ratio of 1:2 (common on most OR ventilators) is 30/3 + (10 × 2)/3 or 17. By using extended inverse ratio ventilation, with an I:E ratio of 3:1, the mean airway pressure increases to 25 ((30 × 3/4) + (10/4)). The advantage of these settings is that the patient is exposed to higher mean airway pressures without profoundly increased PIP, which would present increased risk of barotrauma. However, one must be careful in this situation that the patient has sufficiently compliant lungs and a sufficient amount of time to exhale in order to prevent profound auto-PEEP.

In general, the use of 10 mL/kg tidal volumes is still espoused in the anesthesia community as appropriate ventilation. Typically, anesthesiologists attempt to target an end-tidal CO_2 of around 35 mmHg to attempt to prevent spontaneous respiration during anesthesia and maintain normal pH. To address hypoxia, it is reasonable to provide increased amounts of PEEP. In the ARDSNet trials, PEEP levels >20 cmH_2O were not uncommon. Another key component of the ARDSNet ventilation strategy is the use of low tidal volume ventilation based on 6 mL/kg/PBW. The PBW calculation is shown in Table 76.1. One should note that the calculation varies based on the individual's sex.

The use of PEEP and low tidal volume ventilation in the neurosurgical population is problematic, as a key component of ventilator management in this population is appropriate CO_2 removal. Low tidal volume ventilation is frequently associated with increased $PaCO_2$, which results in increased blood flow to the brain and potential increases in intracranial pressure and consequent ischemia to the brain parenchyma. Furthermore, an increase in intrathoracic pressure by PEEP and/or increased mean airway pressure reduces venous return and potentially increases intracranial pressure to an even greater extent. These concerns led to the exclusion of neurosurgical and intracranial pathology patients from the initial ARDSNet studies.

Despite these concerns, it is possible to safely improve oxygenation and potentially reduce mortality using ARDSNet settings and open lung ventilation in the critically ill neurosurgical patient. Wolf *et al.* demonstrated the safety of the open lung approach in 2002 using mean PEEP levels of 15 cmH$_2$O [4]. Despite using this relatively high level of PEEP, ICP declined over 24 hours despite a moderate increase in PaCO$_2$. In 2005, Wolf *et al.* used brain tissue oxygenation probes to determine the oxygen delivery to brain tissue at risk in 13 neurosurgical patients [5]. In this study, patients received recruitment maneuvers at a level of 30–40 cmH$_2$O for 40 seconds and increased PEEP. Cerebral oxygenation improved using this technique, demonstrating overall improved oxygen delivery to the brain tissue in question.

Conclusion

The management of the hypoxic neurosurgical patient is challenging and requires the balancing of multiple organ systems needs. No one technique is appropriate in every patient, as some patients may develop increased intracranial pressure with even minimal changes in their ventilation. Despite these challenges, good outcomes are possible with attentive management.

References

1. **G. R. Bernard, A. Artigas, K. L. Brigham** *et al.* Report of the American-European Consensus conference on acute respiratory distress syndrome: definitions, mechanisms, relevant outcomes, and clinical trial coordination. Consensus Committee. *J Crit Care* 1994; **9**: 72–81.

2. Ventilation with lower tidal volumes as compared with traditional tidal volumes for acute lung injury and the acute respiratory distress syndrome. The Acute Respiratory Distress Syndrome Network. *N Engl J Med* 2000; **342**: 1301–8.

3. **R. Brower, P. Lanken, N. MacIntyre** *et al.* Higher versus lower positive end-expiratory pressures in patients with the acute respiratory distress syndrome. *N Engl J Med* 2004; **351**: 327–36.

4. **S. Wolf, L. Schurer, H. A. Trost** *et al.* The safety of the open lung approach in neurosurgical patients. *Acta Neurochir Suppl* 2002; **81**: 99–101.

5. **S. Wolf, D. V. Plev, H. A. Trost** *et al.* Open lung ventilation in neurosurgery: an update on brain tissue oxygenation. *Acta Neurochir Suppl* 2005; **95**: 103–5.

Encephalopathies are commonly encountered in the intensive care unit (ICU) and portend worse outcomes. The etiology of these encephalopathies is incompletely understood and treatment is oftentimes based on the presumed underlying mechanisms.

Case description

A 54-year-old man with a history of alcohol abuse and cirrhosis was admitted to the neurologic ICU after drainage of a large right-sided subdural hematoma. On arrival the patient was awake and alert without a focal neurologic deficit. His postoperative course was uneventful until postoperative day 3 when he became progressively obtunded and stuporous, with a low-grade fever. A repeat head computed tomography (CT) revealed no recurrence of his hematoma. An electroencephalogram (EEG) was diffusely slow without epileptiform activity. His liver function tests and serum ammonia levels were quite elevated. The patient was therefore given a flumazenil challenge under EEG monitoring and he became immediately responsive. His mental status returned to baseline after treatment with lactulose and neomycin.

Discussion

Consciousness is a product of an individual's degree of arousal (or wakefulness) and awareness. Arousal is regulated through a series of interconnecting neuronal circuits in the reticular activating system (RAS). The RAS consists of three groups of neuronal cell bodies (norepinephrine, serotonin, dopamine) that originate throughout the brainstem and project to various regions in the diencephalon and telencephalon [1]. Awareness or subjective experience is thought to be maintained diffusely through the cerebral cortex and its interconnections with the thalamus and basal ganglia structures. A change in consciousness requires a process that affects the RAS or bilateral cerebral hemispheres or both [1].

The above patient has many possible etiologies that could underlie his change in mental status. The most obvious would be a recurrence of his space-occupying lesion that could lead to distortion of the brainstem thus directly affecting the RAS. Subclinical seizures secondary to alcohol withdrawal is a possibility. Both of these appear unlikely given the CT evidence of lack of a structural cause and for lack of EEG evidence for seizure activity (although a previous seizure could have been missed). A low-grade fever raises the possibility of an underlying infection and a possible early septic encephalopathy. However, his elevated liver function tests and response to treatment argue strongly that the source of his mental status decline was secondary to hepatic failure. Alteration in consciousness is one of the most common issues found in all ICUs. Due to the many potential causes, a systematic approach to the evaluation of the patient is mandated.

The initial evaluation should include a thorough history and physical. Does the patient have any underlying medical issue that could lead to deterioration in mental status? Is there a history of trauma, substance abuse, depression with previous overdose attempts? Is there a previous history of seizures? What were the circumstances under which the patient was admitted? The history may need to be obtained (or verified) from a witness, emergency medical services, friends, or family.

A general physical examination should search for evidence of trauma or intoxication. Meningismus should be evaluated. A fundoscopic examination may reveal papilledema. The breath may suggest intoxication or ketoacidosis. Subtle findings such as nystagmus, eyelid, finger or lip twitching may indicate subclinical seizure activity. Vital signs can also provide diagnostic clues as to the etiology of changes in mental status. Elevated temperatures can suggest an underlying infection and hypothermia is commonly seen after cold exposure, Addison's disease, hypoglycemia, and/or pituitary disease. Hypotension and hypertension can also impact a patient's mental status. Mean arterial blood pressures below and above the level of a patient's cerebral autoregulation can lead to cerebral hypoperfusion or the development of cerebral edema, respectively.

A complete laboratory evaluation is mandatory and should include serum electrolytes, liver and thyroid function tests, arterial blood gases, complete blood count with differential, toxicology evaluations, and a sedimentation rate. Infectious sources as well as vasculitic processes should also be evaluated. Drug levels should be evaluated and sedation limited as much as possible. A very common cause of decreased mental status is poor hepatic clearance of sedative drugs. A routine chest X-ray should be obtained to evaluate for pneumonia or other acute processes. Additional body imaging may also be required.

The neurologic examination often will provide clues as to whether the alteration of consciousness is due to a structural or metabolic source. Obviously, neuroimaging is crucial in this evaluation [2]. The clinical situation should suggest whether lumbar puncture or neurophysiologic monitoring is needed. Common encephalopathies encountered in the ICUs include septic and hepatic encephalopathies. The exact mechanism by which sepsis impairs consciousness is not known. It is speculated that the release of cytokines and interleukins during the early inflammatory response can cause direct blood–brain barrier damage. This can subsequently alter the internal milieu of the brain, affecting neuronal transmission [3].

The etiology of hepatic encephalopathies has been discussed extensively, with ammonia levels and the development of false neurotransmitters claimed to be the source of the encephalopathy. More recent evidence has suggested that the development of endogenous benzodiazepines may contribute to the encephalopathy. However, this is not the complete answer since only about 40% of patients will respond to intravenously administered flumazenil. Electroencephalographic monitoring during administration of flumazenil can be used to determine if an occasional subclinical seizure can be detected. Inflammatory mediators have also been implicated in the etiology of hepatic encephalopathy [4].

Conclusion

Change in mental status and encephalopathy are common occurrences in the ICU. Ruling out physiologic, pharmacologic, and neurologic etiologies requires a thorough history, careful physical examination, and the appropriate use of laboratory and imaging tests. Treatment should be tailored to the underlying etiology of the encephalopathy.

References

1.	F. Plum, J. B. Posner. The pathologic physiology of signs and symptoms of coma. In Plum F., Posner J. B., eds. The Diagnosis of Stupor and Coma, 3rd edition. Philadelphia, PA: F.A. Davis Company, 1982; 1–86.

2.	G. B. Young. Initial assessment and management of the patient with impaired alertness. In Young G. B., Ropper A. H., Bolton C. F., eds. Coma and Impaired Consciousness. A Clinical Perspective. New York, NY: McGraw-Hill, 1998; 79–118.

3.	J. Mahler, G. B. Young. Septic encephalopathy. Intensive Care Med 1993; 38: 177–87.

4.	V. Sundaram, O. S. Shaikh. Hepatic encephalopathy. Pathophysiology and emerging therapies. Med Clin North Am 2009; 93: 819–36.

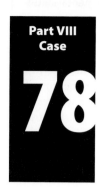

Therapeutic hypothermia using an endovascular approach in the neurocritical care patient

Anupa Deogaonkar and Andrea Kurz

Therapeutic hypothermia for cerebral protection was first used in the 1950s [1] and its use has waxed and waned since then. Previous trials in brain trauma [2], ischemic stroke [3], and stroke due to subarachnoid hemorrhage [4] have examined the neuroprotective effect of mild to moderate hypothermia. The Intra-operative Hypothermia for Aneurysm Surgery Trial (IHAST) was a well-matched, prospective, international, multicenter, randomized study of 1001 patients with good-grade subarachnoid hemorrhage (SAH). This trial showed that there was no difference in outcome between the mild intraoperative hypothermic and normothermic groups [5]. However, in the following case we decided to use hypothermia as a neuroprotective method due to a high-grade SAH and persistent unconsciousness after cardiac arrest.

Case description

A 56-year-old female patient was admitted to the neurocritical care unit after being resuscitated by the Emergency Medical Services team that was called by the family when the patient arrested at home. On arrival, the patient's blood pressure was 210/120 mmHg, heart rate was 86/min, body temperature was 35.9 °C, Glasgow Coma Scale score was 3. The patient's pupils were miotic and unreactive to light. The patient arrived intubated and mechanically ventilated. An electrocardiogram showed diffuse elevation of the ST segment, and serum cardiac markers were mildly elevated, including creatine-kinase and troponin T. A computed tomography scan of the brain showed diffuse SAH. The Hunt–Hess Scale score was IV with Fisher's score of 3. A ventriculostomy was performed that showed an elevated opening pressure. Approximately 20 mL of cerebrospinal fluid (CSF) were removed to reduce the intracranial pressure (ICP). The CSF was xanthrochromic on inspection with numerous red blood cells. ICP was measured using an intraparenchymal sensor (Camino, USA) that showed an ICP of

>40 mmHg. After obtaining informed consent from the patient's family, mild hypothermia therapy was initiated using the Reprieve Endovascular Temperature Management Systems (Radiant Medical, CA). This consists of a triple-lobed, helically wound, heat-exchange balloon catheter that was placed in the inferior vena cava through the femoral vein via a 10 French femoral introducer sheath and a microprocessor-driven controller. The distal tip of the catheter was at the level of the diaphragm and was connected to a pump that circulated cold saline. The target core temperature of 33 °C was achieved in 1 hour. Midazolam and vecuronium were continuously used for sedation and muscle relaxation, respectively. A Foley temperature catheter was used to monitor body core temperature. Cerebral angiography 1 day after the admission revealed an intracranial aneurysm. The patient was then taken for endovascular coiling on the same day. Hypothermia was maintained during the procedure and for up to 2 days after the procedure. The patient was gradually decooled to 37.5 °C at a rate of 0.2 °C/hour. Shivering was suppressed using a forced-air warming blanket, oral buspirone, and intravenous meperidine. The patient slowly regained consciousness over the next 2 days and, after being treated in a rehabilitation program for another 3 months, the patient was discharged home. Modified Rankin Score at the time of discharge from the rehabilitation center was 4.

Discussion

Cooling a patient to mild or moderate hypothermia is usually performed by conductive (liquid-circulating water mattress), convective (forced air cooling via full body blankets or air beds) surface cooling, cold infusions, gastric lavage, passive cooling by leaving the anesthetized patient uncovered in a cool environment (e.g., operating room, intensive care unit), or through a combination of these methods. Studies using convective and/or conductive techniques to cool subjects presenting with traumatic brain injury, stroke, and cardiac arrest found that the time required to cool subjects to the desired temperature was often 6–8 hours and that the cooling process was not very precise. A more recent approach to controlling temperature in critically ill patients uses intravascular cooling devices. The intravascular cooling device connects to an external cooling system. The system circulates temperature-controlled sterile saline through heat exchangers mounted on the distal end of the catheter. The patient's blood is gently cooled as it passes over the balloons. Similar to cooling blanket equipment, the system responds to probes measuring the patient's rising temperature and adjusts the temperature of the sterile saline flowing within the catheter. Endovascular cooling techniques seem to be superior for rapid induction of hypothermia and for maintenance of stable temperature as compared with surface cooling techniques. Furthermore, during slow rewarming, body core temperature is comparatively easier to control with endovascular cooling/warming.

The majority of therapeutic hypothermia trials for brain protection have involved surface-cooling techniques that require mechanical ventilation in intubated and paralyzed patients. Therapeutic hypothermia using the endovascular technique has distinct advantages, such as rapid cooling in an awake patient with intact shivering response and without using neuromuscular blockade, stability of temperature during treatment, and controlled decooling [6]. Currently, two endovascular heat-exchange catheters are available for use: Celsius Control System (Innercool, Inc, San Diego, CA) and Cool Line System (Alsius Inc, Irvine, CA). The RapidBlue™ system by Innercool Inc. automatically cools or warms the patient as necessary to maintain the desired body temperature. It includes a programmable console with an enhanced user interface and can be used with InnerCool's Standard and Accutrol™ catheters to quickly modulate patient temperature in association with surgery or other medical procedures. Similarly, the new Thermogard XP™ temperature management system and new Quattro™ catheter by Alsius Inc. together team up to deliver more power and control for both cooling and warming applications. Heat exchange occurs between cooled saline that passes through the heat exchange portion of the catheter in a coil with large surface area for heat exchange and the blood that flows over the outer surface of the catheter. This closed-circuit circulation of a chilled solution through a flexible metallic heat-exchange element is connected to a programmable external heat exchange bath and recirculates the saline returning from the catheter. Venous blood is thus cooled on its way back to the heart as it passes the cooled element. An intravascular thermometer built in the catheter provides feedback to precisely cool core blood to a target temperature.

These devices are generally placed in the femoral vein and are associated with a low rate of complications. Endovascular cooling allows rapid cooling with tight control of target temperature, minimal shivering, and the possibility of avoiding paralysis of the patient. There are other techniques involving internal cooling methods using infusion of cold fluids for the induction of mild-to-moderate hypothermia. The rates of induction are variable but are otherwise considered to be rapid. Cold fluid infusion with concomitant use of cooling blankets has also been shown to be efficacious. Typically, the infusion volume is 30 mL/kg of normal saline or lactated Ringer solution.

All anesthetics so far tested markedly decrease the shivering threshold as well as the maximum intensity of shivering. Reduction in the cold responses is especially important if hypothermia is induced for therapeutic reasons. Thus, induction of therapeutic hypothermia in awake patients is complicated by the need to overcome arteriovenous shunt vasoconstriction and shivering, and to do so without provoking extreme thermal discomfort. The search continues for a drug or drug combination that sufficiently impairs thermoregulatory defenses without simultaneously producing unacceptable toxicity. Drugs such as meperidine, dexmedetomidine, clonidine, nefopam, and buspirone alone, as well as in various combinations, reduce the shivering threshold and thus complement external and internal cooling.

Conclusion

Therapeutic hypothermia has been shown to improve outcome in patients after cardiopulmonary resuscitation and might prove helpful for other circumstances in which a compromise of neurologic function is expected. External (convective or conductive) as well as internal cooling can be used for induction of therapeutic hypothermia. However, internal (endovascular) cooling induction of hypothermia is more rapid with a more precisely controlled maintenance and decooling phase. If certain aspects of its use such as timing, rate of rewarming, and selective perfusion strategies are optimized, the neuroprotective effects can likely be enhanced.

References

1. **W. G. Bigelow, J. C. Callaghan, J. A. Hopps**. General hypothermia for experimental intracardiac surgery; the use of electrophrenic respirations, an artificial pacemaker for cardiac standstill, and radio-frequency rewarming in general hypothermia. *Trans Meet Am Surg Assoc Am Surg Assoc* 1950; **68**: 211–219.

2. **D. W. Marion, L. E. Penrod, S. F. Kelsey** *et al.* Treatment of traumatic brain injury with moderate hypothermia. *N Engl J Med* 1997; **336**: 540–546.

3. **M. A. De Georgia, D. W. Krieger, A. Abou-Chebl** *et al.* Cooling for Acute Ischemic Brain Damage (COOL AID): a feasibility trial of endovascular cooling. *Neurology* 2004; **63**: 312–317.

4. **B. J. Hindman, M. M. Todd, A. W. Gelb** *et al.* Mild hypothermia as a protective therapy during intracranial aneurysm surgery: a randomized prospective pilot trial. *Neurosurgery* 1999; **44**: 23–32.

5. **M. M. Todd, B. J. Hindman, W. R. Clarke** *et al.* Mild intraoperative hypothermia during surgery for intracranial aneurysm. *N Engl J Med* 2005; **325**: 135–145.

6. **E. Keller, H. G. Imhof, S. Gasser** *et al.* Endovascular cooling with heat exchange catheters: a new method to induce and maintain hypothermia. *Intens Care Med* 2003; **29**: 939–943.

Therapeutic hypothermia after cardiac arrest

James W. Jones and Piyush Mathur

Each year in the USA, approximately 450 000 men and women suffer cardiac arrest due to various causes, most commonly myocardial injury secondary to coronary artery disease. The vast majority of the victims do not survive to hospital admission, and more than two-thirds of all survivors suffer major neurologic dysfunction ranging from disabling cognitive deficits to permanent coma. The major factors in predicting neurologic dysfunction secondary to cardiac arrest involve the extent of brain insult as a function of time to return of circulation. Even with early resuscitation, neurologic outcomes have remained poor. Cerebral ischemia and reperfusion trigger multiple metabolic cascades that ultimately result in permanent neuronal loss. The use of induced hypothermia has been studied as a way to combat neurologic injury for nearly five decades.

Case description

A 37-year-old female with a history of chronic back pain and depression arrived at the emergency department following a witnessed cardiac arrest 1 week after beginning risperidone therapy. Bystanders at the scene performed cardiopulmonary resuscitation for 12 minutes until paramedics arrived, at which time the trachea was promptly intubated and 1 mg epinephrine was administered intravenously. Her cardiac rhythm on the defibrillator monitor was ventricular fibrillation. Following two biphasic shocks at 200 Joules, she was noted to have a spontaneous return of circulation by carotid artery palpation. Subsequent blood pressure cuff readings consistently demonstrated mean arterial pressures between 70 and 95 mmHg. However, her neurologic exam upon arrival at the emergency department was remarkable for a Glasgow Coma Scale score of 6, including bilateral withdrawal from pain and twitching of the right eye and mouth. Urgent head computed tomography scan demonstrated early signs of global ischemia consistent with anoxic brain injury. Propofol and atracurium infusions were started and

an automated intravascular cooling device was placed into the femoral vein and a target temperature of 33 °C was obtained within 6 hours of arrest. Hypokalemia and hyperglycemia were corrected. After 24 hours, the patient was decooled slowly to 36.0 °C over the subsequent 12 hours. Propofol and atracurium infusions were interrupted and the patient was noted to be moving all extremities and following simple commands. She was extubated on day 3 and discharged on day 7. A 6-month follow-up visit with her neurologist demonstrated minimal cognitive deficits, mostly with word recall.

Discussion

Following Dr. Peter Safar's 1965 publication, *Management of the Comatose Patient*, in which he proposed the benefits of therapeutic hypothermia in comatose patients following restoration of blood flow, multiple subsequent studies have confirmed these findings and demonstrated a clear improvement in those patients who are resuscitated quickly and cooled early. The mechanism by which cooling improves neurologic function is not clear, and the benefits of cooling demonstrated with anoxic type injuries have not been replicated for other types of brain injury including traumatic, or ischemic and hemorrhagic stroke [1]. Suggested mechanisms include a reduction in cerebral oxygen consumption especially in low flow areas, slowing of damaging enzymatic reactions, maintenance of the lipoprotein fluidity of the neurons and blood–brain barrier, suppression of free radicals, reduced intracellular acidosis, and inhibition of the synthesis, release, and uptake of neurotransmitters such as glutamate and dopamine [2, 3].

Today, the use of therapeutic hypothermia is widely accepted as the standard of care for preserving neurologic function following cardiac arrest. Goals for therapy include attaining a core temperature of 32–34 °C within 8 hours of the return of spontaneous

Table 79.1. Phases of therapeutic hypothermia.

Precooling
 Restore circulation
 Neurologic assessment
 Intubation, sedation, and paralysis as needed
 Placement of cooling device

Initiation of cooling
 Target 32–34 °C within 8 hours
 Management of metabolic abnormalities

Maintenance
 Stabilize core temperature at 32–34 °C
 Keep mean arterial pressure >65 mmHg
 Monitor for tissue injury
 Management of metabolic abnormalities

Decooling
 Gradual (0.2–0.3 °C /hour) restoration of normothermia
 Management of hemodynamics (fluids and vasopressors)
 Management of metabolic abnormalities
 Discontinuation of sedation and paralysis
 Reassess neurologic status and consider extubation

circulation (Table 79.1). This should be maintained for 12–24 hours [1, 3]. Multiple small studies have examined the efficacy of various cooling modalities but none has proven superior. Also, data suggest a potential benefit in attaining target core temperatures earlier via infusion of cold intravenous fluids (2 liters normal saline at 4 °C) both during and after return of circulation, however this remains controversial as fluids may increase the risk of pulmonary edema in those with cardiac dysfunction. Current research focuses on the use of intranasal catheters, which deliver a cooling mixture of gas to localize cooling to the brain as well as decrease time to achieve target brain temperatures.

Evidence for cooling

Two landmark randomized clinical trials published in 2002 demonstrate a clear benefit in the therapeutic use of mild hypothermia following cardiac arrest [1, 3]. Both studies randomized patients to receive either hypothermia or maintenance of normothermia. The Hypothermia after Cardiac Arrest Study Group (HACA) found that 55% of the hypothermic group had a favorable neurologic outcome (e.g., ability to live independently) compared with 39% in the normothermic control group [1]. This was echoed by Bernard *et al.*, which found a 49% vs 29% favorable neurologic outcome [3]. Furthermore, the HACA Group showed decreased 6-month mortality for the hypothermic group (41%) vs the normothermic group (55%) [1]. In light of this evidence, the American Heart Association, as well as the International Liaison

Committee on Resuscitation, currently recommend therapeutic hypothermia in their published resuscitation guidelines [4]. A 2009 Cochrane review focusing on neurologic outcomes, survival, and adverse events further supports these guidelines as the "best medical practice" [5].

Choice of cooling device

Therapeutic hypothermia is simple to perform. Numerous cooling devices are available on the market today, which utilize the principles of conduction, convection, and evaporation [6]. Devices such as cool water or air-circulating blankets, gel-coated adhesive pads, blood-cooling central venous catheters, and ice-packs effectively cool via conduction. Less commonly, misting in combination with a fan effectively uses convection and evaporation to cool the patient. No single device has been proven superior in terms of patient outcomes, but devices with feedback temperature controls meet target temperatures sooner and more effectively maintain this temperature throughout the cooling and decooling phase.

Initiation of cooling

Cooling should be performed in all postcardiac arrest patients regardless of documented dysrhythmia, but supportive data are strongest for patients who are post ventricular fibrillation [7]. Initiation of cooling should ideally begin within 8 hours following return of spontaneous circulation in all patients who do not follow verbal commands, are free from life-threatening bleeding or infection, and are not at risk for imminent cardiopulmonary collapse. Sedation, paralysis, and mechanical ventilation are generally required to protect the airway and prevent shivering. The optimal time to achieve target hypothermic temperatures is unknown – most major studies target a core temperature of 32–34 °C for 12–24 hours [1, 3]. Electrolytes should be checked frequently during the initiation and maintenance of cooling to monitor for hypokalemia and hyperglycemia; potassium and insulin should be supplemented.

The negative physiologic effects of cooling include decreased cardiac output and coagulopathy as well as complications from the cooling device, specifically hypothermic tissue injury from surface cooling and infection from intravascular catheters. Such complications are more common with cooling below 32 °C. Positive physiologic effects of mild cooling, in addition to long-term neurologic benefits, include antiseizure activity and improved response to electrical defibrillation in the setting of re-arrest.

Decooling

Decooling is the most hemodynamically unstable phase (Table 79.1) and is defined by the decreased removal of patient-generated heat until normothermia is reached. This is better tolerated in contrast to "rewarming," in which heat from an external energy source is added to the patient. Cooling devices with feedback temperature control allow the patient to achieve normothermia gradually, preventing the patient's intrinsic thermoregulatory mechanisms from generating a deleterious rebound hyperthermia, which can occur for up to 72 hours. Gradual decooling at 0.2 to 0.33 °C per hour until normothermia is reached helps diminish hemodynamic instability as well as the occurrence of "post-resuscitation syndrome," characterized by systemic inflammation, vasodilation, and hypotension [6]. Patients may require fluid administration and vasopressor support during the decooling phase, as well as continued sedation and paralysis to prevent shivering. Hypokalemia and hyperglycemia may persist during this phase and should be corrected.

Conclusion

Victims of cardiac arrest are at risk for neurologic injury. Institution of therapeutic hypothermia within 8 hours of return of circulation, targeting a goal of 32–34 °C for 12–24 hours, has been shown to improve neurologic outcomes and mortality [1, 3]. Therapeutic hypothermia has been shown to be relatively safe and effective, and should be considered in the treatment of comatose patients following cardiac arrest. Multiple devices are available to assist with active cooling, none of which has been proven over others to improve patient outcomes. However, automated devices with feedback temperature controls have improved attainment of target temperatures and reduced the hemodynamic instability associated with uncontrolled decooling. Electrolyte abnormalities are common and should be corrected.

Acknowledgments

Appreciation to Jessica E. Bollinger, Critical Care Pharmacist, Cleveland Clinic.

References

1. **Hypothermia After Cardiac Arrest Study Group.** Mild therapeutic hypothermia to improve the neurologic outcome after cardiac arrest. *N Engl J Med* 2002; **346**: 549–53.

2. **L. A. McIntyre, D. A. Fergusson, P. C. Hébert** *et al.* Prolonged therapeutic hypothermia after traumatic brain injury in adults: a systematic review. *J Am Med Assoc* 2003; **289**: 2992–9.

3. **S. A. Bernard, T. W. Gray, M. D. Buist** *et al.* Treatment of comatose survivors of out-of-hospital cardiac arrest with induced hypothermia. *N Engl J Med* 2002; **346**: 557–63.

4. **J. P. Nolan, P. T. Morely, T. L. Hock** *et al.* Therapeutic hypothermia after cardiac arrest. An advisory statement by the Advancement Life support Task Force of the International Liaison committee on Resuscitation. *Resuscitation* 2003; **57**: 231–5.

5. **J. Arrich, M. Holzer, H. Herkner** *et al.* Hypothermia for neuroprotection in adults after cardiopulmonary resuscitation. *Cochrane Database Syst Rev* 2009; **4**: CD004128.

6. **D. B. Sedar, T. E. Van Der Kloor.** Methods of cooling: practical aspects of therapeutic temperature management. *Crit Care Med* 2009; **37**: S211–22.

7. **M. Oddo, V. Ribordy, F. Feihl** *et al.* Early predictors of outcome in comatose survivors of ventricular fibrillation and non-ventricular fibrillation cardiac arrest treated with hypothermia: a prospective study. *Crit Care Med* 2008; **36**: 2296–301.

80

Subarachnoid hemorrhage

Cerebral vasospasm

Edward Manno

Subarachnoid hemorrhage (SAH) represents bleeding into the subarachnoid space, most commonly from a ruptured cerebral aneurysm. There are approximately 30 000 patients with SAH per year in the USA making it a commonly encountered disease in the neurologic intensive care unit (ICU).

Case description

A 52-year-old right-handed female with a medical history of smoking and hypertension developed the abrupt onset of a severe bifrontal headache. She was taken to a local emergency department where a head computed tomography (CT) revealed a Fisher 3 SAH with moderate hydrocephalus. Her initial exam was stuporous but arousable with intact cranial nerve responses. She was able to follow commands with stimulation. An external ventricular drain was placed with improvement in her mental status. Cerebral angiography revealed an 8 mm anterior communicating artery aneurysm that was treated with coil embolization. The patient was then transferred to the neurologic ICU. Intravenous magnesium and oral nimodipine were started for cerebral vasospasm prophylaxis.

Five days posthemorrhage she developed a worsening of her headache. Her serum sodium decreased from 143 mOsm/L to 132 mOsm/L. The following day she developed progressive right-sided weakness and word-finding difficulties. Repeat cerebral angiography revealed severe vessel narrowing of the left middle and anterior cerebral arteries (Figure 80.1). She was given aggressive volume replacement with normal saline and her mean arterial blood pressure was increased to 110 mmHg with intravenous phenylephrine. She had improvement but not complete resolution of her signs and symptoms. The decision was made to proceed with angioplasty of the narrowed cerebral vessels. Her symptoms resolved and she was returned to the neurologic ICU. She made a good recovery and she was discharged home 2 weeks later.

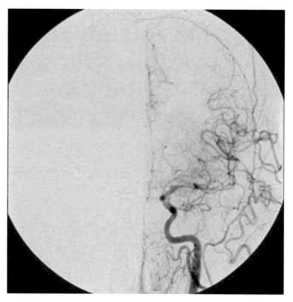

Figure 80.1. Cerebral angiography 5 days after a patient had a subarachnoid hemorrhage. The image reveals severe vessel narrowing of both the middle and anterior cerebral arteries.

Discussion

Aneurysmal SAH is a disease with a devastating natural history. Epidemiologically, it is a disease of middle-aged women with a 3:2 female to male predominance in the 40–60 year age group. Major risk factors for the development and rupture of cerebral aneurysms include hypertension and cigarette smoking.

Two major interventions over the past 20 years have had a significant impact on the treatment of SAH. The development of the operative microscope and interventional procedures has allowed for the early treatment of cerebral aneurysms to prevent rebleeding. Rebleeding occurs within the first few weeks of the initial hemorrhage in one-third of patients with SAH and acutely worsens outcomes. The other intervention is the development of critical care strategies based on an improved understanding of the cerebrovascular and hemodynamic changes that occur after SAH.

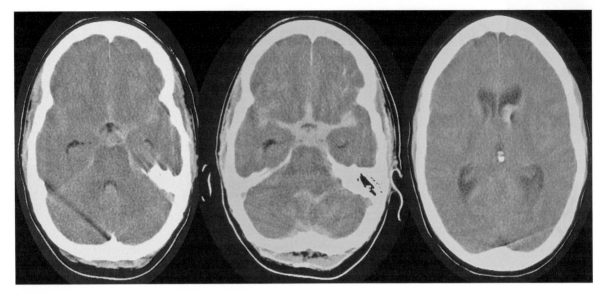

Figure 80.2. Serial computed tomographic images of subarachnoid hemorrhages (SAH). The left image is a Fisher 2 SAH with thin layered blood in the basal cisterns. The center image is a Fisher 3 SAH with thick clots in the cisterns. The image on the right is categorized as a Fisher 4 SAH with no or little blood in the cisterns but some intraventricular blood.

Patients are categorized into clinical and radiological groups. The Hunt–Hess scale is a subjective clinical grouping of patients ranging from 1 (asymptomatic) to 5 (moribund) [1]. The World Federation of Neurological Surgeons scale incorporates the Glasgow Coma Scale into a similar 1–5 scale in an attempt to increase the objectivity and reliability of the score. Long-term patient outcome correlates best with the initial presentation of the patient [2].

The risk of the development of cerebral vasospasm is estimated by the amount of subarachnoid blood in the basal cisterns determined on a 24–48 hour CT scan. Fisher described the original grouping of patients with group 1 having no subarachnoid blood on the initial scan, group 2 having thin layered blood in the basal cisterns, group 3 having thick clots in the cisterns, and group 4 having no blood or thin layered blood in the cisterns with either additional intracerebral or intraventricular blood (Figure 80.2) [3]. Patients with thick clots were found to be at very high risk for developing cerebral vasospasm with subsequent neurologic deficits.

Cerebral vasospasm is a self-limited vasculopathy that develops 4–14 days after SAH. Pathologically, the basal cerebral arteries exhibit a T-cell infiltrate, collagen remodeling and smooth muscle proliferation. The process is initiated by an unidentified metabolic product of oxyhemoglobin and leads to the vessels becoming stiff and narrowed. Complications can be significant as severe vessel narrowing can lead to stroke and death. Specific neurologic signs and symptoms are dependent upon the involved vessels [4].

Treatment of patients with SAH, once an aneurysm is secured, includes generous use of intravenous isotonic fluids. A cerebrally induced salt wasting nephropathy can develop in some patients, which may be related to the release of the B-type of natriuretic peptide. In some instances hypertonic intravenous fluids may be necessary to avoid hyponatremia and volume depletion [4].

Cerebral autoregulation is lost as cerebral vasospasm develops. Decreases in cerebral blood flow secondary to vessel narrowing can be attenuated and reversed with the application of induced hypertension. Clinical studies have suggested that a majority of neurologic deficits can be reversed with the application of the above hemodynamic techniques [5]. Cerebral angioplasty and direct vasodilator application is reserved for patients that do not respond to hemodynamic augmentation.

Conclusion

The application of interventions for vasospasm may be guided by noninvasive measures of vessel narrowing and cerebral blood flow. Transcranial Doppler ultrasound is a noninvasive device used to measure blood flow velocities in the basal cerebral arteries. Rising flow velocities may portend vessel narrowing. Subsequent measures of cerebral blood flow may be needed to verify decreases in blood flow requiring treatment [4]. Further work is required for a better understanding of cerebral vasospasm, the leading cause of delayed cerebral ischemia after SAH.

References

1. **W. E. Hunt**, **R. M. Hess**. Surgical risk as related to time of intervention in the repair of intracranial aneurysms. *J Neurosurg* 1968; **1**: 14–20.

2. **Anonymous**. Report of World Federation of Neurological Surgeons Committee on a universal subarachnoid hemorrhage grading scale. *J Neurosurg* 1988; **68**: 985–6.

3. **J. P. Kistler**, **R. M. Crowell**, **K. R. Davis**. The relation of cerebral vasospasm to the extent and location of subarachnoid blood visualized by CT scan: a prospective study. *Neurology* 1983; **33**: 424–36.

4. **E. M. Manno**. Subarachnoid hemorrhage. *Neurol Clin* 2004; **22**: 347–66.

5. **N. F. Kassell**, **S. J. Peerless**, **Q. J. Durwaed** *et al.* Treatment of ischemic deficits from vasospasm with intravascular volume expansion and induced arterial hypertension. *Neurosurgery* 1982; **11**: 337–43.

Subarachnoid hemorrhage

Ventriculoperitoneal shunt dependence

Vivek Sabharwal and Asma Zakaria

Chronic hydrocephalus as a sequela of subarachnoid hemorrhage is a complication that neurosurgeons battle with every day. These patients often have a difficult recovery period, requiring shunt revisions due to malfunction and infections.

Case description

A 49-year-old female presented to the hospital with fever and altered mental status. The patient had a past medical history significant for traumatic subarachnoid hemorrhage and subdural hematoma after a motor vehicle collision 2 months prior. The patient developed hydrocephalus after the incident, which required placement of an external ventricular drain (EVD). The patient continued to have high drain output several days after her injury, which mandated placement of a ventriculoperitoneal shunt (VPS). The patient was transferred to an inpatient rehabilitation facility where she was noted to be more somnolent and intermittently febrile over the last several days. Physical examination revealed a fluctuant area under the craniotomy scar. Computed tomography (CT) scan of the head revealed scalp tissue edema and a fluid collection under the bone flap (Figure 81.1). The patient was taken to the operating room and the infected bone flap and VPS removed. The patient was extubated postoperatively and returned to the neurosurgical intensive care unit for observation. Six hours later, the patient became progressively more obtunded and had difficulty protecting her airway; her cranial skin flap was noted to be tight and bulging. A CT scan of the head revealed acute hydrocephalus, with ventriculomegaly and hypodensity in the surrounding white matter representing transependymal translocation of cerebrospinal fluid (CSF) (Figure 81.2). An EVD was inserted emergently and 20 mL of CSF were drained. The drain was then left open at 10 cmH$_2$O. The patient's examination returned to baseline a few hours later.

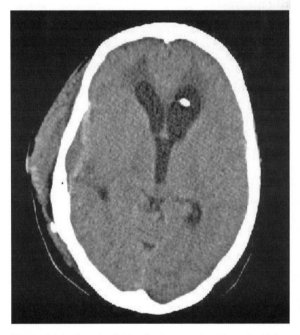

Figure 81.1. There is a fluid collection over the right parietal lobe. The bright spot in the left lateral ventricle is the tip of the ventriculoperitoneal shunt.

Discussion

The incidence of hydrocephalus after aneurysmal subarachnoid hemorrhage (SAH) has been reported to range from 6–67% in the literature [1]. This may occur acutely (day 0–3), subacutely (day 4–13) or chronically (>14 days) after the bleed and can be obstructive or nonobstructive in nature. Several pathophysiologic mechanisms for this impediment to CSF flow have been postulated, but no clear etiology has been identified. Most theories seem to suggest a role in the alteration of CSF flow dynamics within the ventricular system.

Cerebrospinal fluid is produced by active secretion from the cerebral arterial blood. It is generated at a constant rate, largely from the choroid plexus, and circulates through the ventricular system, exiting into

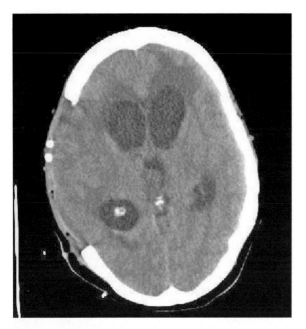

Figure 81.2. The ventricles are grossly enlarged upon removal of the ventriculoperitoneal shunt with hypodensities around the frontal poles suggesting transependymal flow of cerebrospinal fluid from elevated pressures.

the subarachnoid space via the foramina of Luschka and Magendie. It is then propelled upwards towards the superior sagittal sinus where most of it is reabsorbed. Some CSF flows down towards the lumbar subarachnoid space and is reabsorbed through the spinal venous plexus. The rate of absorption is dependent on the pressure gradient between the subarachnoid space and venous system. Absorption ceases if venous pressure exceeds the intracranial pressure. The presence of blood or adhesions within the ventricular system or subarachnoid space can result in acute obstructive hydrocephalus. Alternatively, a nonobstructive pattern can be seen when the arachnoid granulations draining CSF into the sagittal sinus are plugged with posthemorrhagic or postinflammatory debris. The resistance to CSF outflow through the arachnoid granulations may be increased 3-fold after SAH and may not return to physiologic parameters until 40–50 days post-SAH [1]. In some cases scarring may occur resulting in chronic hydrocephalus.

The diagnosis of acute hydrocephalus is made based on CT scan evidence of SAH or intraventricular blood, with or without the presence of enlarged ventricles, as well as a declining mental status. An EVD is emergently placed to relieve the elevated intracranial pressure and is subsequently rapidly or gradually weaned off based on the patient's progress. Chronic hydrocephalus, defined as shunt-dependent hydrocephalus, affects between 6–37% of patients with SAH [2]. Acute hydrocephalus at presentation is the biggest predictor of the development of shunt-dependent hydrocephalus followed by the need for ventilator support on admission [3]. Other predictors of shunt dependency include: higher Hunt–Hess grade, higher Fisher grade, advanced age, female sex, larger third ventricular and bicaudate diameter, posterior circulation location of the ruptured aneurysm, endovascular treatment, high CSF protein levels, and prolonged duration of EVD [2, 4].

Patients who require an EVD for a longer duration, or have multiple EVD revisions are more likely to develop chronic hydrocephalus [3]. This may be a reflection of the persistent failure of return to normal CSF dynamics in these patients. Multiple EVD revisions can be predictive of high CSF protein from inflammation or infection, or a high clot burden, both of which clog the draining tubes and are independent predictors of chronic hydrocephalus. Alternatively, numerous passes with the EVD can increase the risk of infection or intracerebral hemorrhage resulting in a prolonged need for ventricular drainage.

As the popularity of endovascular treatment of ruptured cerebral aneurysms has grown, there has been speculation that this treatment modality results in a higher incidence of shunt-dependent hydrocephalus. However, most studies comparing the two treatment modalities are retrospective and have not matched the patient groups for grade of SAH [2, 5]. Aggressive irrigation and early clot evacuation in patients undergoing microsurgery may be responsible for this trend. In addition, some surgeons routinely perform fenestration of the lamina terminalis during aneurysm clipping to facilitate CSF flow. While this is helpful in patients with ventricular obstruction, it has not been found to be beneficial in nonobstructive forms of hydrocephalus and has not been shown to reduce the incidence of chronic hydrocephalus.

Age is a strong predictor for shunt-dependent hydrocephalus with a 2% per year of age increase in risk [3]. This may be due to an expanded subarachnoid space and an ability to accommodate more blood, causing greater CSF flow disturbances, increased meningeal fibrosis in the elderly resulting in impaired absorption and decreased ventricular compliance causing early symptomatic hydrocephalus.

Although necessary for the treatment of chronic hydrocephalus, VPS are fraught with complications. Patients with shunt-dependent hydrocephalus have longer length of stays in the ICU. Approximately 4% of insertions are associated with intracerebral hemorrhage and 8–10% become infected – requiring removal, placement of a temporary EVD and intravenous antibiotics before the shunt can be replaced. The 1- and 5-year rates of shunt longevity are 57% and 37%, respectively, requiring a shunt revision. In one series, almost one-third of the patients undergoing shunt placement required a revision procedure and 43% of these required a second revision [3]. Almost half of the shunt failures occurred within 14 days postoperatively and 90% failed within the first 60 days. Shunt failure after 6 months of insertion was exceedingly rare. This may be because normal CSF dynamics are restored by this time making shunt failure less noticeable clinically.

Conclusion

Shunt-dependent hydrocephalus is a multifactorial disease and many researchers have tried to formulate a mathematical model to predict its occurrence [2, 4]. This would allow for early shunt placement in patients at risk and reduce hospital lengths of stay. Unfortunately, no such scale exists at this time and patients must undergo a prolonged EVD wean before they can be deemed shunt-dependent. The fact that shunt failure rates are minimal after 6 months of insertion suggests that this is a transient phenomenon and some surgeons propose a more conservative wean or serial lumbar drainage to avoid the placement of and morbidity associated with ventriculoperitoneal shunts. What is known is that untreated hydrocephalus can result in significant disability and cognitive decline, which may become irreversible if not relieved in a timely manner.

References

1. **A. R. Dehdashti, B. Rilliet, D. A. Rufenacht** et al. Shunt dependent hydrocephalus after rupture of intracranial aneurysms: a prospective study of the influence of treatment modality. *J Neurosurg* 2004; **101**: 402–7.

2. **Z. Dorai, L. S. Hynan, T. A. Kopitnik** et al. Factors related to hydrocephalus after aneurysmal subarachnoid hemorrhage. *Neurosurgery* 2003; **52**: 763–71.

3. **C. J. O'Kelly, A. V. Kulkarni, P. C. Austin** et al. Shunt-dependent hydrocephalus after aneurysmal subarachnoid hemorrhage: incidence, predictors, and revision rates. *J Neurosurg* 2009; **111**: 1029–35.

4. **M. Chan, A. Alaraj, M. Calderon** et al. Prediction of ventriculo-peritoneal shunt dependency in patients with aneurysmal subarachnoid hemorrhage. *J Neurosurg* 2009; **110**: 44–9.

5. **P. Varelas, A. Helms, G. Sinson** et al. Clipping or coiling of ruptured cerebral aneurysms and shunt-dependent hydrocephalus. *Neurocrit Care* 2006; **4**: 223–8.

Subarachnoid hemorrhage

Ventriculostomy infection

Samuel A. Irefin

Ventriculostomies and external ventricular drainage devices are common in neurosurgical and neurocritical care practice. The potential for infection of this low-flow system is significant and the consequences can be severe.

Case description

A 45-year-old male was admitted to the neurosurgical intensive care unit after an endovascular treatment with complete coil occlusion of basilar artery aneurysm. Twenty-four hours after admission, a computed tomography scan revealed acute obstructive hydrocephalus and an external ventriculostomy catheter was placed. On postoperative day 5 the patient developed a fever and an increase in inflammatory biomarkers. Analysis of cerebrospinal fluid (CSF) demonstrated a 10-fold increase in cell index; white blood cells 1526, protein 70, glucose 77. Multiresistant coagulase-negative *Staphylococci* were isolated from CSF culture. Vancomycin therapy was initiated intravenously.

Discussion

Ventriculostomy catheters are vital in caring for neurosurgical patients. They provide continuous intracranial pressure monitoring and external CSF drainage. First introduced in 1875, they did not gain wide acceptance until the 1960s, when Lundberg *et al.* refined the technique and demonstrated its usefulness for bedside analysis [1]. Ventriculostomy catheters are commonly used to allow invasive monitoring of elevated intracranial pressure (ICP) secondary to acute hydrocephalus in various neurosurgical disorders such as severe head trauma, subarachnoid hemorrhage, intracranial hypertension, or intraventricular hemorrhage. The primary aim of these catheters is to detect elevated ICP and thereby guide medical or surgical therapies to maintain an adequate cerebral perfusion pressure. Since they are foreign bodies, ventriculitis

related to intraventricular drainage systems is a common complication. It is often difficult to make a diagnosis of ventriculitis with a ventriculostomy catheter in place. There are often signs of cerebral infection because of underlying illness. Some patients may be asymptomatic or show only minor signs of infection such as fever, anemia, or leucocytosis [2]. Diagnosis of catheter-related infection can be made according to criteria advocated by Mayhall *et al.* [3]. These include positive CSF culture obtained from the ventricular catheter or from CSF drawn via lumbar puncture. In addition, CSF pleocytosis, low glucose level, or high protein level may indicate CSF infections [4].

The reported incidence of ventriculostomy-related catheter infection varies between 0% and 45% of patients depending on technique of insertion and management of the catheter [5]. As common with the use of percutaneous catheters, Gram-positive infections traditionally have been predominant in patients who present with ventriculitis. However, Gram-negative infections have been reported in ventriculostomy catheter use and have resulted in higher mortality rates [6]. The risk factors for catheter-related ventriculitis can be categorized into three groups: (1) patient characteristics and the underlying mechanism of injury, (2) events that break the integrity of a closed system, and (3) environmental influences [7]. As far as patient characteristics are concerned, neither age, sex, nor race increase the risk of developing catheter infections [6].

As a result of potential pitfalls in diagnosis and subsequent delayed initiation of appropriate antimicrobial therapy contributing to morbidity or mortality, prevention of catheter-related ventriculitis is of paramount importance. Special emphasis should be placed on avoiding modifiable risk factors [8]. Review of the literature does not support prophylactic exchange of catheters in reducing the incidence of catheter-related ventriculitis [2]. However, the duration of the ventriculostomy catheter is a significant risk factor in developing catheter-related infection. Therefore, efforts must be made to identify clinically relevant CSF infections and suspected or confirmed infections must be differentiated from contamination and catheter colonization. The administration of prophylactic antibiotics decreases the incidence of CSF infections at the expense of predisposing the patient to infection by more resistant organisms when infections do occur [4]. It is prudent to administer prophylactic antibiotics before the catheter insertion to protect against the skin flora contamination of the wound site. Consideration may be given to Gram-negative coverage in selected patients who may require prolonged hospitalizations. These agents may be provided for the entire duration of catheter use. The selected antibiotics must penetrate the blood–brain barrier and knowledge of local resistance patterns is of paramount importance.

Conclusion

Ventriculostomy-related infections remain a serious complication of intraventricular catheter use. Causes of these infections are multifactorial in nature. Close monitoring and rigorous catheter maintenance remain the mainstay of catheter care. Assessment of risk factors is crucial to determine changes in microbial infection and to identify ways to prevent future complications.

References

1. **N. Lundberg, H. Troupp, H. Lorin**. Continuous recording of ventricular-fluid pressure in patients with severe traumatic brain injury: a preliminary report. *J Neurosurg* 1965; **22**: 581–90.

2. **Y. Arabi, Z. A. Memish, H. H. Balkhy** *et al.* Ventriculostomy-associated infections: incidence and risk factors. *Am J Infect Control* 2005; **33**: 137–43.

3. **C. G. Mayhall, N. H. Archer, V. A. Lamb** *et al.* Ventriculostomy-related infections. A prospective epidemiologic study. *N Engl J Med* 1984; **310**: 553–9.

4. **K. E. Lyke, O. O. Obasanjo, M. A. Williams** *et al.* Ventriculitis complicating use of intraventricular catheters in adult neurosurgical patients. *Clin Infect Dis* 2001; **33**: 2028–33.

5. **K. L. Holloway, T. Barnes, S. Choi** *et al.* Ventriculostomy infections: the effect of monitoring duration and catheter exchange in 584 patients. *J Neurosurg* 1996; **85**: 419–24.

6. **F. J. Buckwold, R. Hand, R. R. Hansebout**. Hospital-acquired bacterial meningitis in neurosurgical patients. *J Neurosurg* 1977; **46**: 494–500.

7. **J. K. Ohrström, J. K. Skou, T. Ejlertsen** *et al.* Infected ventriculostomy: bacteriology and treatment. *Acta Neurochir (Wien)* 1989; **100**: 67–9.

8. **A. M. Korinek, M. Reina, A. L. Boch** *et al.* Prevention of external ventricular drain-related ventriculitis. *Acta Neurochir (Wien)* 2005; **147**: 39–45.

Subarachnoid hemorrhage

Sodium abnormalities in neurocritical care

William R. Stetler and George A. Mashour

Disorders of sodium and water balance are frequent complications encountered in the care of critically ill neurologic patients. Common dysnatremias include hyponatremia caused by syndrome of inappropriate antidiuretic hormone (SIADH) and cerebral salt wasting syndrome (CSWS), as well as hypernatremia caused by central diabetes insipidus (CDI). Proper diagnosis of the cause of each sodium abnormality is critical, as treatment varies widely among etiologies.

Case description

The patient was a 45-year-old female with a 30 pack-year history of tobacco use who had the "worst headache of [her] life" while at dinner and then immediately slumped over in her chair. Family alerted emergency medical services; the patient was unresponsive so the trachea was intubated and she was taken to the emergency department. A computed tomography (CT) scan of the head revealed a large amount of subarachnoid hemorrhage (SAH) with ventricular extension. Neurosurgery was consulted and a ventriculostomy catheter was placed with opening pressure of 36 cmH$_2$O above the tragus. The following morning the patient was taken to the angiography suite where a basilar apex aneurysm was found and embolized using endovascular coils. The patient was then transported to the neurosurgical intensive care unit and stabilized. On neurologic examination she was noted to briskly localize with all four extremities.

On admission the patient's serum sodium was 144 mmol/L. By postoperative day 1 her sodium dropped to 135, and by postoperative day 2 to 129. A urine osmolality was found to be 405 mOsm/kg and the urine sodium was 45 mmol/L. Urine output was noted to be 12 liters over 48 hours and total intake had been only 6 liters and central venous pressure dropped from 10 mmHg on admission to 4 mmHg. The neurocritical care team pursued fluid rehydration with normal saline, however the sodium continued to drop to 123 mmol/L. Therefore, on postoperative day 4, 3% NaCl was begun at 50 mL/hour. By postoperative day 5 the patient's serum sodium rose to 131 mmol/L, but she was now noted to be extensor posturing with her left upper and lower extremities. A noncontrast CT scan of the head did not reveal appreciable change, but CT angiography revealed diffuse right anterior circulation vasospasm. Fluids were increased and the patient was taken emergently to angiography where intra-arterial administration of nicardipine and selective angioplasty of the right anterior circulation was employed to achieve angiographic resolution of vasospasm.

Over the following 3 weeks the patient's serum sodium stabilized to approximately 135 mmol/L on an oral regimen of NaCl tablets, and she was discharged from the hospital to a rehabilitation facility following commands on her right side and localizing to noxious stimuli on her left. At her 2-year follow-up the patient walked into the clinic with the use of a cane.

Discussion

As the major extracellular cation, sodium is one of the most important osmotic agents in the body. Disorders of sodium and water balance are common among the critical care patient and are especially common among neurocritical care patients. Hyponatremia is one of the most common electrolyte disorders in the neurologic patient and is frequently encountered in patients following SAH, traumatic brain injury, and many neurosurgical procedures. Patients with hyponatremia are often thought to suffer from cerebral edema [1], however, other complications such as mental status changes, seizures, vasospasm, and even death occur more frequently following hyponatremia. Hyponatremia has also been shown to be an independent risk factor for all-cause morbidity and mortality, even when controlling for the original pathology. Furthermore, correction of serum sodium may help improve mortality [2].

Table 83.1. Comparison of common dysnatremias in neurocritical care.

	SIADH	CSW	CDI
Hyponatremia vs hypernatremia	Hyponatremia	Hyponatremia	Hypernatremia
Euvolemia vs hypovolemia	Euvolemia	Hypovolemia	Hypovolemia
Serum osmolarity	<285 mOsm/L	<285 mOsm/L	>300 mOsm/L
Urine osmolarity	>200 mOsm/L	>200 mOsm/L	<350 mOsm/L
Urine sodium	↑	↑	↓

SIADH, syndrome of inappropriate antidiuretic hormone secretion; CSWS, cerebral salt wasting syndrome; CDI, central diabetes insipidus.

Despite its well-accepted complications, the etiology of hyponatremia in SAH is still debated with the most common causes cited as SIADH and CSWS. In SIADH, there is an inappropriate or excessive release of antidiuretic hormone, which acts on the distal renal tubule to increase water permeability and therefore create a concentrated urine and dilutional, euvolemic hyponatremia. Thus, SIADH is a problem of *water balance*. In CSWS, there is a renal loss of sodium (and consequently a loss of water), leading to a hypovolemic hyponatremia [1, 3]. Cerebral salt wasting syndrome is therefore a problem of *sodium balance*. The exact pathophysiology of CSWS is not known. However, it is hypothesized that the increase in sympathetic tone following SAH may increase blood pressure, increase systemic vascular resistance/venous capacitance vasculature tone, and possibly cause direct natriuretic effects on the kidney, all contributing to increased naturesis [4]. There is some evidence that release of natriuretic peptides following SAH (most notably atrial (A-type) natriuretic peptide and brain (B-type) natriuretic peptide) could cause either a direct or indirect renal sodium loss [5]. Nevertheless, the circulating levels of these peptides have not been shown to correlate with natriuresis [2, 5].

The distinction between the two pathologies is important as the treatment is typically opposite (Table 83.1). In SIADH, hyponatremia is controlled with fluid restriction, while CSWS is treated with fluid replacement. In fact, the key distinguishing feature between the two is volume status of the patient. The hyponatremia in SIADH is euvolemic or hypervolemic hyponatremia, whereas in CSWS it is a hypovolemic hyponatremia. Many laboratory investigations show similar trends in CSWS and SIADH, including serum osmolarity <285 mOsm/L, urine osmolarity >200 mOsm/L, urine sodium >25 mmol/L. However, there is often an associated fall in central venous pressure and pulmonary capillary wedge pressure in CSWS. Physical exam should focus on skin turgor, jugular venous distention, and mucous membranes to help determine volume status. Additionally, an elevation in hematocrit may be observed from the concentrating effects of CSWS. Secondary to the need for hypervolemic therapy in SAH, it is imperative that the two etiologies be distinguished [1, 2]. Hyponatremia alone has been shown to increase vasospasm risk and cerebral infarction in SAH patients [2]. Therefore, aggressive fluid resuscitation even before serum sodium drops appreciably may not only treat, but offset the drop of serum sodium associated with CSWS [4]. Because of the risk of vasospasm in SAH patients, SIADH is often not treated with fluid restriction in the neurocritical care setting.

In this case, the patient most likely developed CSWS as her urine output increased while her central venous pressure dropped precipitously. Unfortunately the patient went on to develop vasospasm in her right anterior circulation, an event more common in hyponatremic patients with SAH (especially in patients with hyponatremia caused by CSWS) [2].

Treatment of hyponatremia depends upon patient symptomatology. Mild cases of SIADH traditionally respond to fluid restriction; use of diuretics and demeclocycline, which has been shown to block ADH receptors, may augment fluid restriction. For more severe symptoms, hypertonic (3% NaCl) saline should be considered, especially in patients who may not tolerate diuresis or fluid restriction because of the risk for vasospasm. Rapid correction of hyponatremia (>12 mmol/L/day) should be avoided to help prevent pontine myelinolysis, especially in cases of chronic hyponatremia. The foundation for treatment of CSW is fluid resuscitation. Isotonic saline is often sufficient to correct both the volume deficit as well as the hyponatremia in CSW. Hypertonic saline may be used in more refractory cases. Additionally, mineralocorticoid therapy such as fludrocortisone may help treat the sodium loss [2]. In this case, 3% NaCl was used to treat the hyponatremia because conventional aggressive fluid resuscitation failed. Furthermore, aggressive correction of the patient's serum sodium was warranted because the patient developed cerebral vasospasm [2].

Hypernatremia is often defined as a serum sodium >145 mmol/L, and usually represents a loss of total body water. Common causes of hypernatremia include reduced intake of water, extrarenal water loss, intrarenal water loss, mineralocorticoid excess, and iatrogenic. Central diabetes insipidus represents intrarenal loss of water and is the most common cause of hypernatremia in the neurologic patient. As opposed to its counterpart nephrogenic diabetes insipidus, in which the kidneys are insensitive to antidiuretic hormone (ADH), in CDI there is a failure of release of ADH from the hypothalamopituitary axis. This is most commonly seen in patients after pituitary surgery, following traumatic brain injury (which can shear the pituitary stalk) or SAH, and in patients that are brain dead [3]. Antidiuretic hormone acts on the distal tubule and medullary collecting ducts to increase the permeability of water and therefore help reabsorb water through protein channels [1]. In the absence of ADH water is not reabsorbed but rather lost in a dilute urine resulting in hypovolemic hypernatremia. Serum osmolarity is often >305 mOsm/L while urine osmolarity is <350 mOsm/L (and urine specific gravity is often <1.005) in CDI (Table 83.1).

Treatment of CDI depends upon both severity of symptoms and level of consciousness of the patient. If the patient is conscious then increasing oral intake to balance urine output is ideal. If the patient is unable to drink orally, free water may be administered via a nasogastric tube. However, if the patient is unable to maintain a balanced intake and output or serum sodium continues to increase despite all efforts to increase free water intake, medical therapy may be considered. Intravenous or intranasal administration of vasopressin (1-deamino-8-D-arginine or DDAVP) may be administered and titrated to decrease urine output to <200 mL/hour in the short term [2].

Conclusion

In conclusion, dysnatremia is a common occurrence among critically ill neurologic patients. In particular, hyponatremia from either CSW or SIADH may increase the rate of complications and, in the case of SAH, predispose patients to cerebral vasospasm. Therefore, prompt recognition of hyponatremia and institution of appropriate, aggressive therapy is warranted to avoid complications [2].

References

1. **M. R. Harrigan**. Cerebral salt wasting syndrome. *Crit Care Clin* 2001; **17**: 125–38.

2. **M. Rahman, W. A. Friedman**. Hyponatremia in neurosurgical patients: clinical guidelines development. *Neurosurgery* 2009; **65**: 925–36.

3. **M. Tisdall, M. Crocker, J. Watkiss** et al. Disturbances of sodium in critically ill adult neurologic patients: a clinical review. *J Neurosurg Anesthesiol* 2006; **18**: 57–63.

4. **S. Singh, D. Bohn, A. P. Carlotti** et al. Cerebral salt wasting: truths, fallacies, theories, and challenges. *Crit Care Med* 2002; **30**: 2575–9.

5. **G. Audibert, G. Steinmann, N. de Talance** et al. Endocrine response after severe subarachnoid hemorrhage related to sodium and blood volume regulation. *Anesth Analg* 2009; **108**: 1922–8.

Initial management

Lauryn R. Rochlen

Stroke is classified into two major types [1]. Ischemic strokes represent 80% of cerebral vascular events and occur as a result of thrombosis, embolism, or hypoperfusion. The remainder are hemorrhagic in nature, due to either intracerebral or subarachnoid hemorrhage. This chapter will focus on the initial management of patients with ischemic stroke.

Case description

The patient was a 54-year-old female with a past medical history significant for hypertension and bilateral carotid stenosis. She presented to the hospital complaining of fatigue and pallor, and was found to have a hemoglobin of 4 g/dL due to a lower gastrointestinal bleed. She was receiving a packed red blood cell transfusion when she had acute onset of dysarthria, left hemiparesis, right gaze deviation, and left-sided neglect. Immediate evaluation revealed an intact airway, appropriate ventilatory pattern and oxygenation, and a blood pressure of 144/69. Neurologic exam was consistent with a National Institutes of Health (NIH) Stroke Scale (NIHSS) of 22. Labs were collected. A head computed tomography (CT) scan was significant for evidence of a large right middle cerebral artery (MCA) infarct. Given the recent history of lower gastrointestinal bleed, this patient was not a candidate to receive recombinant tissue plasminogen activator (rtPA). The patient was transferred to an institution capable of performing intra-arterial thrombolysis.

Upon arrival at the tertiary center, exam was unchanged except for an NIHSS of 16. She was transferred to the interventional radiology suite for intra-arterial thrombolysis. Following successful dissolution of a thrombus in the right MCA, she was brought to the neurosurgical intensive care unit for further monitoring.

Discussion

The main goals of the immediate evaluation of a patient with an acute neurologic change are to determine whether the patient's symptoms are due to a stroke and to establish potential contraindications for thrombolysis. Emergency evaluation of a patient with possible ischemic stroke should initially focus on rapid assessment and stabilization of the airway, breathing, and circulation. This is quickly followed by the secondary assessment of neurologic deficits and comorbidities. Pertinent history is essential in order to determine time of symptom onset and potential causes in order to provide for early secondary prevention and options for intervention [2]. The NIHSS (Table 84.1) is particularly useful for quantifying the degree of deficit, facilitating communication between practitioners, identifying possible location of vessel occlusion, providing early prognosis, and identifying patient eligibility for certain interventions. Diagnostic tests, including electrolytes, glucose, complete blood count, and coagulation profiles should be performed to rule out conditions that imitate acute stroke. However, as time is critical in these situations, thrombolytic therapy should not be delayed unless there is high suspicion for a hypocoagulable state.

Early diagnosis of acute ischemic stroke is facilitated with the widespread use of neuroimaging. A noncontrast enhanced CT scan of the head identifies most cases of intracranial hemorrhage and aides in diagnosing nonvascular causes of symptoms, but is insensitive in detecting small, acute infarctions. Signs of severe ischemic stroke seen on CT, such as loss of gray–white matter differentiation and sulcal effacement, are associated with poorer outcomes and may correlate with a higher risk of hemorrhagic transformation following thrombolysis. Magnetic resonance imaging (MRI) is more accurate for identifying ischemic lesions, as well as distinguishing between acute and chronic infarcts. Due to cost limitations, limited availability, and patient

Table 84.1. The National Institutes of Health Stroke Scale [2].

Tested item	Title	Responses and scores
1A	Level of consciousness	0 – alert 1 – drowsy 2 – obtunded 3 – coma/unresponsive
1B	Orientation questions (2)	0 – answers both correctly 1 – answers one correctly 2 – answers neither correctly
1C	Response to commands (2)	0 – performs both tasks correctly 1 – performs one task correctly 2 – performs neither
2	Gaze	0 – normal horizontal movements 1 – partial gaze palsy 2 – complete gaze palsy
3	Visual fields	0 – no visual field defect 1 – partial hemianopia 2 – complete hemianopia 3 – bilateral hemianopia
4	Facial movement	0 – normal 1 – minor facial weakness 2 – partial facial weakness 3 – complete unilateral palsy
5	Motor function (arm) a. left b. Right	0 – no drift 1 – drift before 5 seconds 2 – falls before 5 seconds 3 – no effort against gravity 4 – no movement
6	Motor function (leg) a. left b. Right	0 – no drift 1 – drift before 5 seconds 2 – falls before 5 seconds 3 – no effort against gravity 4 – no movement
7	Limb ataxia	0 – no ataxia 1 – ataxia in 1 limb 2 – ataxia in 2 limbs
8	Sensory	0 – no sensory loss 1 – mild sensory loss 2 – severe sensory loss
9	Language	0 – normal 1 – mild aphasia 2 – severe aphasia 3 – mute or global aphasia
10	Articulation	0 – normal 1 – mild dysarthria 2 – severe dysarthria
11	Extinction or inattention	0 – absent 1 – mild (loss 1 sensory modality) 2 – severe (loss 2 modalities)

contraindications with MRI, CT scan remains the standard mode of imaging and will provide sufficient information needed to proceed with decisions regarding treatment.

Once the diagnosis of acute ischemic stroke is established, focus should shift on management strategies to prevent secondary neurologic injury and determine treatment options. The main tenets of secondary injury prevention are to maintain adequate oxygenation, cellular homeostasis, and appropriate cerebral perfusion. Patients with a considerable extent of neuronal damage are at risk for airway obstruction, hypoventilation, aspiration pneumonia, and atelectasis, which can all result in desaturation and decreased oxygen delivery to already compromised neurons. Need for tracheal intubation should be evaluated in every patient. Avoiding hyperthermia, hypo- and hyperglycemia are also important for maintaining optimal neuronal function.

In the immediate poststroke period, blood pressure is often elevated, which may represent a protective response attributed to the Cushing reflex [3]. Higher blood pressure is beneficial for maintaining perfusion to the pressure-dependent peri-infarct penumbra. However, hypertension will increase the risk of hemorrhagic transformation of the infarcted area. Arguments for lowering blood pressure include prevention of hemorrhagic conversion, minimizing cerebral edema and preventing secondary ischemic events due to hypoperfusion of the at-risk penumbra. Data regarding blood pressure management are currently inconclusive, but recommendations are available. Patients who are not candidates for rtPA should not receive medications to lower blood pressure until systolic pressure is >220 mmHg or diastolic pressure is >120 mmHg. Treatment goal is to lower blood pressure by 15% during the first 24 hours of stroke onset. For those patients who are eligible to receive rtPA, blood pressure should be lowered to a systolic pressure <185 mmHg and a diastolic pressure <110 mmHg before thrombolysis is initiated.

Intravenous thrombolytic therapy with rtPA has been shown to improve outcomes following ischemic stroke [4]. Risk of adverse events following rtPA administration, such as intracranial or systemic hemorrhage, correlate directly with time since onset of neurologic symptoms. Current guidelines limit its use to within 3 hours of symptom onset. Other contraindications include evidence of intracranial or systemic hemorrhage, stroke or myocardial infarction in the previous 3 months, major surgery in the previous 14 days, elevated blood pressure, current anticoagulation or hypocoagulable state and patient/family refusal of treatment. No other IV thrombolytic agent is approved for use in the USA.

Intra-arterial thrombolysis may be an alternative for patients unable to receive IV rtPA. With IA thrombolysis, a high concentration of thrombolytic agent is deposited directly into the thrombus. Intra-arterial thrombolysis is presently limited to patients who have presented <6 hours from symptom onset due to MCA occlusion, are otherwise not candidates to receive rtPA, and are at a treatment center with qualified interventionalists and immediate access to cerebral angiography.

Conclusion

Treatment of patients with acute ischemic stroke can be challenging. Initial goals are to prevent secondary neurologic injury and determine eligibility for thrombolysis. As new data on management of ischemic stroke continue to emerge, guidelines will be updated with the latest evidence-based recommendations.

References

1. **P. Amarenco, J. Bogousslavsky, L. R. Caplan** *et al.* Classification of stroke subtypes. *Cerebrovasc Dis* 2009; **27**: 493–501.

2. **H. P. Adams Jr, G. del Zoppo, M. J. Alberts** *et al.* Guidelines for the early management of adults with ischemic stroke: a guideline from the American Heart Association/American Stroke Association Stroke Council, Clinical Cardiology Council, Cardiovascular Radiology and Intervention Council, and the Atherosclerotic Peripheral Vascular Disease and Quality of Care Outcomes in Research Interdisciplinary Working Groups: The American Academy of Neurology affirms the value of this guideline as an educational tool for neurologists. *Circulation* 2007; **115**: e478–534.

3. **E. Cumbler, J. Glasheen**. Management of blood pressure after acute ischemic stroke: an evidence-based guide for the hospitalist. *J Hosp Med* 2007; **2**: 261–7.

4. Tissue plasminogen activator for acute ischemic stroke. The National Institute of Neurological Disorders and Stroke rt-PA Stroke Study Group. *N Engl J Med* 1995; **333**: 1581–7.

85

Increased intracranial pressure at 48 hours poststroke

Lauryn R. Rochlen

Intracranial pressure (ICP) reflects the cumulative pressures of the intracranial contents – brain tissue, cerebral blood volume (CBV), and cerebrospinal fluid (CSF). Normal values for ICP are <20 mmHg [1]. The primary concern when ICP is elevated is that cerebral perfusion pressure (CPP) will be reduced, resulting in ischemia and irreversible cellular damage. Patients with intracranial pathology have decreased intracranial elastance and are at risk for exaggerated increases in ICP with small changes in intracranial volume.

Case description

Please refer to Case 84 for the patient's original presentation.

A 54-year-old female with a past medical history significant for hypertension and bilateral carotid artery stenosis presented with an acute right middle cerebral artery (MCA) ischemic infarct. She was not eligible to receive intravenous recombinant tissue plasminogen activator (rtPA), but did undergo intra-arterial rtPA administration under fluoroscopic guidance by an interventional radiologist.

During the first postoperative day, the patient remained hemodynamically stable with an intact airway. Neurologically she was alert and oriented, with hemiparesis in the left upper and lower extremity. A follow-up noncontrast head computed tomography (CT) scan revealed minor cerebral edema with a 9-mm midline shift, no evidence of hydrocephalus, and small areas of hemorrhagic conversion.

Over the course of the second postoperative day, the patient's neurologic examination deteriorated and she became increasingly somnolent and aphasic. Mannitol 0.5 g/kg was administered intravenously, and a head CT was obtained. Results from the head CT showed worsened mass effect on the right side with increased midline shift. The trachea was intubated for airway protection and hyperventilated to a PaCO$_2$ of

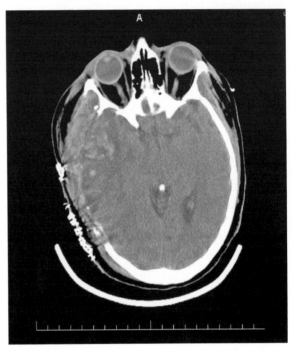

Figure 85.1. Head computed tomography scan following right hemicraniectomy.

30 mmHg. The decision was made to proceed to the operating room for emergent decompressive hemicraniectomy (Figure 85.1).

Discussion

When ICP becomes elevated following intracranial trauma of any cause, global cerebral blood flow (CBF) becomes compromised to levels that cannot support brain metabolism, ultimately resulting in neurologic changes and irreversible damage. The mechanism of increased ICP can be attributed to cytotoxic and vasogenic edema [2]. Cytotoxic edema refers to the shift of water from extracellular to intracellular compartments. Cellular swelling and electrolyte imbalances eventually result in cellular death. Vasogenic edema refers to the phenomenon of water shifting from intravascular to extravascular compartments due to a breakdown of the blood–brain barrier. Cerebral edema typically occurs during the first 24–48 hours following injury, and peaks approximately 3–5 days after an ischemic insult [3]. Patients with large hemispheric infarctions are at increased risk for malignant cerebral swelling [4]. In addition to reduction of CPP, increased ICP leads to tissue shifts that can eventually result in herniation and further irreversible damage.

An integrated approach is suggested for management of elevated ICP, beginning with conservative maneuvers prior to proceeding to more aggressive interventions. As with any acute change in patient status, it is necessary to re-evaluate airway, breathing, and circulation (the "ABCs"). Avoidance of hypoxemia and hypotension are essential to prevent further neuronal destruction. Intubation may be required both for airway protection and maintenance of adequate oxygenation. In the setting of increased ICP, it will be necessary to increase the mean arterial pressure in order to maintain CPP.

A few simple maneuvers can be attempted initially. Elevating the head and neck >30 degrees and avoiding jugular venous compression enhance intracranial venous outflow and allow gravity to assist in reduction of CBV. If the trachea is intubated, manual hyperventilation will quickly lower CO_2 levels resulting in cerebral vasoconstriction and decreased cerebral blood volume and ICP. The CSF is able to regulate pH and will therefore return to normal pH within 12–36 hours, limiting the beneficial effects of hyperventilation [5].

The next step in treatment of increased ICP is to institute hyperosmolar therapy. The two most common agents used are mannitol, an osmotic diuretic, and 3% sodium chloride. Increasing the serum osmolality creates an osmotic gradient across the blood–brain barrier and therefore efficacy depends on an intact blood–brain barrier. Free water will follow its concentration gradient, moving from the edematous intracellular environment to the more concentrated intravascular compartment, thereby improving intracranial elastance. Another potential advantage seen with mannitol is that it reduces blood viscosity, which improves CBF and leads to vasoconstriction. The initial dose for mannitol is 0.25–1 g/kg. Treatment should be targeted to a goal serum osmolality of ≤320 mOsm/kg. Systemic complications of hyperosmolar therapy include congestive heart failure due to initial intravascular volume expansion, electrolyte disturbances, rebound cerebral edema, and acute tubular necrosis [3].

High-dose intravenous steroids reduce the permeability of the blood–brain barrier and have been effective in reducing edema surrounding intracranial tumors. However, the use of steroids in patients with edema due to ischemic stroke has not been shown to result in any improvement in outcome.

If the above measures are ineffective, more aggressive options should be considered. Decompressive surgery involves removal of part of the cranium to allow space for the swollen brain tissue to expand. Goals of decompression are to prevent herniation, increase CPP to areas that are still viable, and preserve CBF. Hemicraniectomy has been shown to be especially effective in patients with malignant MCA infarcts who have failed conventional therapies [2]. Exact timing of when to proceed with decompression has not been established.

Induction of moderate hypothermia (32–34 °C) will reduce cerebral metabolic rate and ICP. Experimentally, hypothermia has been shown to decrease the volume of infarcted area. Prospective studies are needed to determine the overall effect of hypothermia on patient outcomes. The more important concept may be to avoid hyperthermia, which causes an increase in cerebral metabolic rate.

Pharmacologic coma is reserved for the patient in whom all other interventions have been unsuccessful. By reducing cerebral metabolic rate, pharmacologic coma reduces cellular oxygen requirements and therefore decreases CBF, CBV, and ICP. Maximum reductions are thought to occur when a burst-suppression pattern is evident on continuous electroencephalographic monitoring. Agents used include pentobarbital, thiopental, propofol, and benzodiazepines. While pharmacologic coma has been shown to reduce ICP, there are currently no proven benefits on overall morbidity and mortality.

Pharmacologic coma and hypothermia are potentially associated with more extensive care and sequelae. Both usually require mechanical ventilation, muscle paralysis, and use of vasopressors. High levels of sedation and paralysis make it difficult to follow clinical examinations. Patients are also at higher risk for adverse events such as pneumonia and coagulopathy, as well as cardiovascular and electrolyte disturbances.

The interventions discussed above are not without adverse effects. The risk of intervention must be balanced against the risk of prolonged, untreated increases in ICP. Unfortunately, current guidelines do not have specific recommendations regarding when to initiate treatment – decisions must be specific for the individual patient's clinical status.

References

1. **M. Czosnyka, J. D. Pickard**. Monitoring and interpretation of intracranial pressure. *J Neurol Neurosurg Psychiatry* 2004; **75**: 813–21.

2. **C. Ayata, A. H. Ropper**. Ischaemic brain oedema. *J Clin Neurosci* 2002; **9**: 113–24.

3. **V. Singh**. Critical care assessment and management of acute ischemic stroke. *J Vasc Interv Radiol* 2004; **15**: S21–7.

4. **M. Kohrmann, S. Schwab**. Hemicraniectomy for malignant middle cerebral artery infarction. *Curr Opin Crit Care* 2009; **15**: 125–30.

5. **N. Stocchetti, A. I. Maas, A. Chieregato** *et al.* Hyperventilation in head injury: a review. *Chest* 2005; **127**: 1812–27.

Intraparenchymal hemorrhage

Hypertensive intracerebral hemorrhage

James F. Burke and Teresa L. Jacobs

Intracerebral hemorrhage (ICH) accounts for 10–15% of all strokes and is associated with significant mortality [1]. Hypertension is, by far, the most important risk factor.

Case description

The patient was a 45-year-old male with a history of severe hypertension on a multidrug regimen for blood pressure control who alerted his spouse shortly after acutely developing an acute onset headache associated with severe nausea. The patient's spouse noted that the patient's gait was grossly unsteady and immediately activated emergency medical services. On arrival in the emergency room, the patient had a blood pressure of 210/105. The patient was awake, but minimally somnolent, requiring that questions and commands be repeated in order to respond appropriately. On examination, the patient was oriented to person, place, and time and able to participate with a neurologic examination, albeit with some difficulty. His speech was moderately dysarthric. On cranial nerve evaluation, he was noted to have spontaneous left-beating nystagmus with saccadic pursuit movements. No facial asymmetry was detected and no significant motor or sensory deficits were noted. The patient had difficulty maintaining seated balance with a tendency to sway back and forth unless supported. The patient had mild dysmetria on finger-nose-finger testing bilaterally. Reflexes were symmetric throughout with an upgoing plantar response bilaterally.

Noncontrast head computed tomography (CT) scan (Figure 86.1) revealed a midline cerebellar hemorrhage with maximal diameter of 4 cm, perpendicular diameter of 3 cm and was visualized on 6 slices with a 5.0 mm slice thickness (hemorrhage volume estimated at $4 \times 3 \times (6 \times 0.5)/3 = 12$ mL) In the emergency room, the patient's blood pressure spontaneously decreased to 180/105 and he subsequently received two small boluses of labetalol (10 mg and then

20 mg) which transiently lowered his blood pressure to 150/90. However, his blood pressure subsequently increased and he was started on a nicardipine infusion (starting dose 5 mg/hour) which was titrated to a goal mean arterial pressure (MAP) of 110.

The patient was admitted to the neurologic intensive care unit (ICU) where the nicardipine infusion was continued and the patient's neurologic status was closely monitored. The patient failed a bedside swallow evaluation and a Dobhoff tube was inserted. He was clinically stable for almost 24 hours before his level of alertness declined further. At this time, concern emerged that the patient was not protecting his airway, and he underwent endotracheal intubation with initiation of mechanical ventilation. Head CT was emergently repeated and demonstrated a stable hemorrhage with the interval development of significant edema, fourth ventricular compression, and hydrocephalus. A ventriculostomy was performed at bedside and an external ventricular drain (EVD) was inserted. Over the next several hours, the patient's level of alertness improved to his admission baseline.

The patient remained hospitalized in the neurologic ICU for the next 3 days as oral antihypertensives were initiated and he was progressively weaned from the ventilator, nicardipine drip, and EVD. The patient was transferred to the general care ward where he was evaluated by physical, occupational, and speech therapists. His swallowing function progressively improved and he was progressively transitioned to an oral diet. After demonstrating the ability to maintain his caloric intake orally he was transferred to the inpatient rehabilitation service where therapy was focused on gait training. He was ultimately discharged home.

Discussion

Hypertensive ICH results from rupture of small penetrating arteries leading to intraparenchymal hematoma formation. Ongoing brain injury is

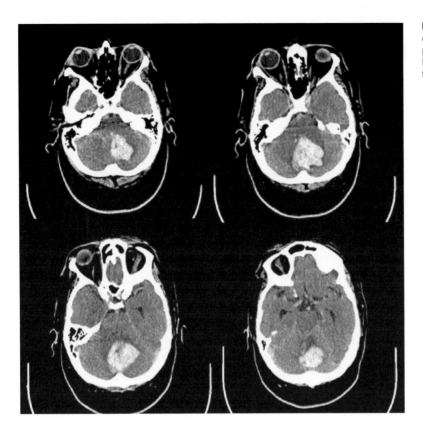

Figure 86.1. A noncontrast head computed tomography scan in the axial plane showing a large cerebellar hemorrhage with mass effect upon the fourth ventricle.

mediated by a host of pathologic processes including mass effect, edema, inflammation, and direct toxicity of blood products [2]. Intracerebral hemorrhage most commonly occurs in subcortical regions predominantly perfused by small penetrating arteries – basal ganglia, pons, thalamus, cerebellum. For ICH outside these regions (i.e., lobar hemorrhage), a broader differential diagnosis should be considered, including vascular malformation, primary brain tumor, metastasis, venous infarction, or amyloid angiopathy.

Hematoma location largely determines the presenting symptoms. Similar to ischemic stroke, ICH typically presents with acute onset focal neurologic symptoms. Deterioration in the level of consciousness and headache are more common in ICH than in ischemic stroke with alteration in level of consciousness being particularly common with ICH in the posterior fossa. Despite these differences, it is often difficult to distinguish ICH from ischemic stroke on clinical grounds alone and consequently emergent neuroimaging with CT or magnetic resonance imaging is essential. While hypertension is the most significant risk factor for ICH, male sex, age, smoking,

and excessive alcohol consumption also constitute risk factors.

For most patients, deficits are maximal at onset. However, early neurologic deterioration occurs in approximately one-quarter of patients [3]. Hematoma expansion is a common mechanism associated with early deterioration. Elevated blood pressures have been associated with hematoma expansion and a recent pilot trial demonstrated a decrease in hematoma size with early, intensive blood pressure lowering [4]. However, aggressive blood pressure lowering may potentially cause clinical deterioration either through failure to perfuse the ischemic perihematomal region or through decreasing cerebral perfusion pressure (CPP) in the context of elevated intracranial pressure (ICP). Consequently, current guidelines do not strongly recommend for or against aggressive blood pressure management, instead urging selection of blood pressure targets on the basis of the totality of clinical circumstances including the potential presence of elevated ICP and the patient's baseline blood pressure [5]. Factor VIIa has been shown to decrease rate of hematoma growth, but has

Table 86.1. Most common potential agents for blood pressure control along with typical initial dosages.

Initial agents	
Labetalol	5–10 mg intravenous (IV), may repeat
Hydralazine	5–10 mg IV, may repeat
Continuous infusions	
Nicardipine	5 mg/hour IV drip, titrate to effect
Clevidipine	1–2 mg/hour IV drip, titrate to effect
Nitroprusside	0.5–1 mcg/kg/min, titrate to effect
Esmolol	as per local routine

not shown benefit on survival or functional outcomes [6].

Medical management

Supportive care, close neurologic monitoring and attention to potential complications form the basis of ICH management. In contrast, early surgical management in the form of hematoma evacuation is not superior to conservative management in unselected patients, but may be beneficial in certain subsets of patients – for example, those with superficial lobar hemorrhages [7]. For subtentorial hemorrhages, posterior fossa decompression and clot evacuation are reasonable measures in the patient undergoing neurologic decline. Standard conservative measures in ICH consist of blood pressure (see Table 86.1) and ICP management in combination with control of hyperglycemia and hyperpyrexia, attention to common medical complications such as deep venous thrombosis and consideration of antiepileptic therapy. Seizures are not uncommon after ICH – occurring in 8.1% of patients by 30 days and most commonly in patients with lobar hemorrhages [8]. There is general consensus that patients with seizures should be treated with antiepileptics and uncertainty about the role of prophylactic antiepileptics [5].

Close monitoring of neurologic status in an ICU is essential in ICH and for patients with elevated ICP invasive monitoring may be beneficial. Elevated ICP is common after ICH as a consequence of variable combinations of mass effect, edema, hydrocephalus, and intraventricular hemorrhage. No specific ICP management strategies have been shown to be preferentially beneficial in this context. Most commonly a graded increase in invasiveness is utilized starting with less invasive measures (elevating the head of the bed, adequately managing pain) and progressively escalating the degree of invasiveness and risk (hyperventilation, osmolar therapy, cerebrospinal fluid drainage, barbiturate coma) [5].

Prognosis

Intracerebral hemorrhage is associated with significant mortality – between 35–50% of patients die within 1 month of presentation [1]. A number of variables predict mortality – Glasgow Coma Scale at presentation, age, infratentorial ICH, presence of intraventricular hemorrhage, and ICH volume – these variables can be combined into a single prognostic index, the ICH score, which strongly predicts 30-day mortality [9]. Of patients who survive their acute presentation, only about half are functionally independent 6 months after presentation.

Conclusion

In summary, hypertensive ICH is a relatively common reason for neurologic ICU admission and is associated with significant morbidity and mortality. Conservative management is the core principle with close attention to preventing and managing neurologic and medical complications. There are a number of significant unanswered questions in the care of these patients, including blood pressure management.

References

1. **V. L. Feigin, C. M. Lawes, D. A. Bennett** *et al.* Stroke epidemiology: a review of population-based studies of incidence, prevalence, and case-fatality in the late 20th century. *Lancet Neurol* 2003; **2**: 43–53.

2. **G. Xi, R. F. Keep, J. T. Hoff.** Mechanisms of brain injury after intracerebral haemorrhage. *Lancet Neurol* 2006; **5**: 53–63.

3. **R. Leira, A. Dávalos, Y. Silva** *et al.* Early neurologic deterioration in intracerebral hemorrhage: predictors and associated factors. *Neurology* 2004; **63**: 461–7.

4. **C. S. Anderson, Y. Huang, J. G. Wang** *et al.* Intensive blood pressure reduction in acute cerebral haemorrhage trial (INTERACT): a randomised pilot trial. *Lancet Neurol* 2008; **7**: 391–9.

5. **J. Broderick, S. Connolly, E. Feldmann** *et al.* Guidelines for the management of spontaneous intracerebral hemorrhage in adults: 2007 update: a guideline from the American Heart Association/ American Stroke Association Stroke Council, High Blood Pressure Research Council, and the Quality of Care and Outcomes in Research Interdisciplinary Working Group. *Stroke* 2007; **38**: 2001–23.

6. **S. A. Mayer, N. C. Brun, K. Begtrup** *et al.* Efficacy and safety of recombinant activated factor VII for acute intracerebral hemorrhage. *N Engl J Med* 2008; **358**: 2127–37.

7. **A. D. Mendelow, B. A. Gregson, H. M. Fernandes** *et al.* Early surgery versus initial conservative treatment in patients with spontaneous supratentorial intracerebral haematomas in the International Surgical Trial in Intracerebral Haemorrhage (STICH): a randomised trial. *Lancet* 2005; **365**: 387–97.

8. **S. Passero, R. Rocchi, S. Rossi** *et al.* Seizures after spontaneous supratentorial intracerebral hemorrhage. *Epilepsia* 2002; **43**: 1175–80.

9. **J. C. Hemphill, D. C. Bonovich, L. Besmertis** *et al.* The ICH score: a simple, reliable grading scale for intracerebral hemorrhage. *Stroke* 2001; **32**: 891–7.

Intracerebral hemorrhage and anticoagulation

Eric E. Adelman and Teresa L. Jacobs

Anticoagulation is used to prevent and treat thromboembolic disease. While anticoagulation is effective, adverse events from the treatment can be devastating. One of the most serious complications of anticoagulation is intracerebral hemorrhage (ICH).

Case description

The patient was a 66-year-old male with a history of prior ischemic stroke, atrial fibrillation (for which he took coumadin), hypertension, and type 2 diabetes, who developed the acute onset of right arm and leg weakness. He also had difficulty speaking and his wife noted a right facial droop. He presented to the emergency room with a systolic blood pressure of 225 and right hemiparesis. A noncontrast head computed tomography (CT) scan was performed that showed a hemorrhage in the posterior limb of the left internal capsule (Figure 87.1A). His blood counts were normal and his International Normalized Ratio (INR) was 2.7. He was treated with vitamin K 10 mg intravenously (IV), fresh frozen plasma (FFP) 1000 mL IV, and was admitted to the neurologic intensive care unit. His clinical condition deteriorated during the FFP infusion and a repeat noncontrast head CT, 53 minutes after the initial scan, showed growth of the hemorrhage with extension into the left lateral ventricle (Figure 87.1B). His blood pressure was controlled and his ICH remained stable on serial imaging. Ten days after his ICH, coumadin was restarted, and he was discharged to a subacute rehabilitation facility.

Discussion

Anticoagulants

In the USA, vitamin K antagonists, such as coumadin, are the most commonly used oral anticoagulants. Vitamin K antagonists, which inhibit vitamin K dependent cofactors (II, VII, IX, and X), can be difficult to use because they have a narrow therapeutic window, mul-

tiple drug and food interactions, and genetic factors impact dosing [1].

Coumadin's anticoagulation intensity is measured with the INR. This measure standardizes values across different laboratories, though there is still some variability [1]. The goal INR varies depending on the indication for anticoagulation and the individual patient. Typically, for nonvalvular atrial fibrillation the goal is 2–3. When the INR is supratherapeutic without bleeding, it can be managed with vitamin K administration. However, in the setting of bleeding, more intensive reversal is required and FFP, prothrombin complex concentrate (PCC), or recombinant factor VIIa (rFVIIa) are used.

Unfractionated heparin and low molecular weight heparins (LMWHs) are the most commonly used parenteral anticoagulants, though fondaparinux and direct thrombin inhibitors (hirudin and argatroban) are also used [2]. All of the parenteral anticoagulants, except the direct thrombin inhibitors, bind to antithrombin and exert downstream anticoagulant effects.

Unfractionated heparin's anticoagulant activity is monitored using the activated partial thromboplastin time (aPTT or PTT). The activated clotting time (ACT), is used primarily during procedures and surgeries. There is no uniform PTT goal, but 1.5–2.5 times the upper limit of normal is often used. There are multiple nomograms available to help guide dosing. The anticoagulant effects of unfractionated heparin are reversed by protamine.

Low molecular weight heparins bind to antithrombin but also act directly against factor Xa. They have a more predictable anticoagulant effect than heparin. Monitoring of anticoagulation intensity for LMWHs can be done by measuring anti-Xa levels, but this is of uncertain clinical benefit and only done in special circumstances [2]. There are no agents that completely reverse the anticoagulant effects of LMWHs, though protamine has limited efficacy. Fondaparinux is a

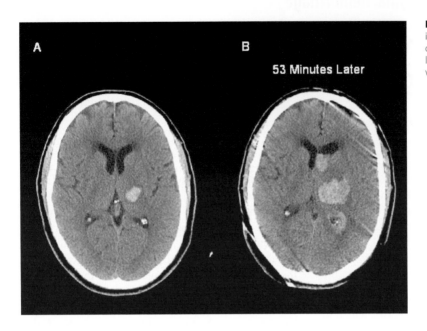

Figure 87.1. A. Intracranial hemorrhage in the posterior limb of the left internal capsule. B. Repeat imaging, 53 minutes later shows growth of the hematoma with extension in the left lateral ventricle.

synthetic pentasaccharide that binds to the heparin binding site on antithrombin. There is no specific reversal agent.

The direct thrombin inhibitors, often used in the setting of heparin-induced thrombocytopenia, bind to thrombin leading to downstream anticoagulant effects. These agents increase the PTT, but the response is nonlinear so it is not useful for monitoring [2]. Direct thrombin inhibitors also increase the INR, which can cause difficulties when transitioning from a direct thrombin inhibitor to coumadin. Some authors recommend using factor X levels instead of INR for monitoring [2]. Although there are no agents that specifically reverse the direct thrombin inhibitors, some have used rFVIIa.

Intracerebral hemorrhages and anticoagulation

While ICH are not common in anticoagulated patients, the mortality is high at about 60% [3]. As the indications for anticoagulation have expanded and as the population has aged, there are more patients taking anticoagulants.

The pathophysiology of anticoagulant-associated ICH is not entirely clear, but it is thought that microbleeds, which would be asymptomatic in a patient without a coagulopathy, become clinically significant in anticoagulated patients [3]. Risk factors for ICH

in anticoagulated patients are similar to patients not receiving anticoagulation, but increasing anticoagulation intensity also contributes.

Most hemorrhages occur when patients' anticoagulation is in the therapeutic range [4]. An INR of 3.5–3.9 increases the odds of hemorrhage by 3.6; conversely, an INR of <2 does not offer protection against intracerebral hemorrhage and is less effective in preventing thromboembolism [4]. The combination of coumadin and aspirin likely increases the risk of ICH [5], but there are also data arguing against an association [6].

Hematoma size and growth of the hematoma are predictors of poor outcome [7]. In comparison to unanticoagulated patients, the anticoagulated patient typically has a larger initial hematoma with an increased chance of expansion over a longer period of time [7, 8].

Reversal of anticoagulation

The mainstay of treatment for anticoagulant-associated ICH is correction of the coagulopathy to reduce the potential for hematoma expansion (Table 87.1). There are multiple agents that reverse coumadin and their uses are guided by expert opinion, rather than comparative data. Agents that are used to reverse coumadin include: vitamin K, FFP, PCC, and rFVIIa. As mentioned previously, heparin and LMWH are reversed with protamine. There are no

Table 87.1. Reversal of anticoagulation.

Coumadin	1. Vitamin K 10 mg intravenously 2. Fresh frozen plasma 15–20 mL/kg Consider: 3. Prothrombin complex concentrate 4. Recombinant activated factor VII 15–90 mcg/kg
Intravenous heparin	1. Protamine 1 mg per 100 U of heparin
LMWH	1. Protamine 1 mg per 100 anti-Xa units of LMWH (1 mg of enoxaparin is ~100 anti-Xa units), if the LMWH was given within 8 hours

LMWH, low molecular weight heparins.
Adapted from references [2, 9].

agents that directly correct the coagulopathy induced by direct thrombin inhibitors or fondaparinux.

Vitamin K reverses the coagulopathy caused by coumadin. Vitamin K can be given by a variety of routes, though the IV formulation is recommended for life-threatening bleeding, such as an ICH [9]. Others feel that the IV preparation may cause severe anaphylaxis, and thus recommend a subcutaneous route. The recommended dose is 10 mg and it can be hours, up to 24 hours, before it effectively corrects the coagulopathy [10].

While waiting for vitamin K to take effect, many patients are treated with FFP. Fresh frozen plasma is a collection of donor plasma that contains all clotting factors. The cost is low and it is readily available – though it must be unfrozen and may need to be blood type matched [10]. Fresh frozen plasma is given in a dose of 15–20 mL/kg [9]. The precise concentration of clotting factors varies between batches of FFP leading to unpredictable responses [9]. A large volume of fluid may need to be infused and, thus, there is a potential to precipitate congestive heart failure [9, 10]. Additionally, there are concerns about transmission of infection and transfusion-related lung injury with FFP [10].

Though not commonly used in the USA, PCC is used internationally to correct coagulopathy due to coumadin. Prothrombin complex concentrates are a heterogenous group of products that contain factor IX and variable amounts of factors II, VII, and X [10]. They correct the INR within minutes – with a minimal amount of volume infused. There are concerns because of thrombotic complications and different PCC products contain differing amount of coagulation factors [10].

While there has not been a randomized control trial for patients with coumadin-associated ICH,

rFVIIa is used in this setting [10], often with the combination of vitamin K and FFP. Recombinant factor VIIa acts by binding to tissue factor and activating thrombin. Concerns regarding rFVIIa include: correcting the INR without reversing the coagulopathy (i.e., the lab value is normal, but patient remains coagulopathic), thrombotic complications, and high costs [10].

Finally, the anticoagulation effects of heparin are reversed by protamine. Heparin has a half life of 60–90 minutes and the dose of protamine needs to be adjusted to account for heparin's metabolism. If heparin was immediately given, 1 mg of protamine reverses 100 U of heparin [9]. The dose of protamine is proportionally decreased as time has elapsed since the last heparin dose [9]. Protamine dose not fully reverse LMWH, but it can still be given as a one-time dose of 1 mg per 100 anti-Xa units (1 mg of enoxaparin equals 100 anti-Xa units) [2]. Protamine is given intravenously by slow injection (5 mg/min) as faster administration rates can cause hypotension [9].

Anticoagulation in patients with an intracerebral hemorrhage

After an ICH, the initial indication for anticoagulation remains and the balance between prevention of thromboembolism and further ICH can be difficult. Patients with ICH also suffer complications such as deep vein thrombosis and pulmonary embolus that necessitate anticoagulation.

There are no high-quality prospective data to guide restarting anticoagulation in these patients. Much of the decision making depends on the underlying reason for anticoagulation. For instance, the risk of thromboembolism is greater for patients with mechanical heart valves than in patients with atrial fibrillation without a prior stroke or vascular risk factors. The presence of microbleeds on T2* imaging may increase the risk of future hemorrhages [9]. Ultimately, the decision to restart anticoagulation is one that should be made in collaboration with the patient. If anticoagulation is to be restarted it is typically done 1–2 weeks after the initial ICH after serial neuroimaging has shown stability of the hematoma.

Conclusions

In conclusion, anticoagulation is effective in treating and preventing thromboembolic disease, but there is

293

a risk of ICH. Most anticoagulation agents can be reversed. Correction of the coagulopathy should occur quickly to prevent hematoma growth, a predictor of poor outcome.

References

1. **J. Ansell, J. Hirsh, E. Hylek** *et al.* Pharmacology and management of the vitamin K antagonists: American College of Chest Physicians Evidence-Based Clinical Practice Guidelines. *Chest* 2008; **133**: 160S–98S.

2. **J. Hirsh, K. A. Bauer, M. B. Donati** *et al.* Parenteral anticoagulants: American College of Chest Physicians Evidence-Based Clinical Practice Guidelines. *Chest* 2008; **133**: 141S–59S.

3. **R. G. Hart, B. S. Boop, D. C. Anderson**. Oral anticoagulants and intracranial hemorrhage: facts and hypotheses. *Stroke* 1995; **26**: 1471–7.

4. **M. C. Fang, Y. Chang, E. M. Hyleck** *et al.* Advanced age, anticoagulation intensity, and risk for intracranial hemorrhage among patients taking warfarin for atrial fibrillation. *Ann Intern Med* 2004; **141**: 745–52.

5. **R. G. Hart, S. B. Tonarelli, L. A. Pearce**. Avoiding central nervous system bleeding during antithrombotic therapy: recent data and ideas. *Stroke* 2005; **36**: 1588–93.

6. **J. Rosand, M. H. Eckman, K. A. Knudsen** *et al.* The effect of warfarin and intensity of anticoagulation on outcome of intracerebral hemorrhage. *Arch Intern Med* 2004; **164**: 800–4.

7. **J. J. Filbotte, N. Hagan, J. O'Donnell** *et al.* Warfarin, hematoma expansion, and outcome of intracerebral hemorrhage. *Neurology* 2004; **63**: 1059–64.

8. **M. L. Flaherty, H Tao, M. Heverbusch** *et al.* Warfarin use leads to larger intracerebral hematomas. *Neurology* 2008; **71**: 1084–9.

9. **J. Broderick, S. Connolly, E. Feldmann** *et al.* Guidelines for the management of spontaneous intracerebral hemorrhage in adults: 2007 update: a guideline from the American Heart Association/American Stroke Association Stroke Council, High Blood Pressure Research Council, and the Quality of Care and Outcomes in Research Interdisciplinary Working Group. *Stroke* 2007; **38**: 2001–23.

10. **J. N. Goldstein, J. Rosand, L. H. Schwamm**. Warfarin reversal in anticoagulant-associated intracerebral hemorrhage. *Neurocrit Care* 2008; **9**: 277–83.

Intraparenchymal hemorrhage

88

Cerebral amyloid angiopathy-related intracranial hemorrhage

Lesli E. Skolarus and Teresa L. Jacobs

Intracerebral hemorrhage (ICH) accounts for approximately 10% of the almost 800 000 strokes that occur in the USA annually. The most common risk factors associated with ICH are hypertension and cerebral amyloid angiopathy (CAA). While hemorrhages located in the thalamus, putamen, globus pallidus, pons and cerebellum are often attributed to hypertension, lobar hemorrhages are thought to be caused by CAA.

Case description

An 80-year-old male presented to the emergency department after being found fallen by his wife. His blood pressure was slightly elevated at 150/90 mmHg and his pulse was 70 beats/minute. On examination, his level of consciousness was diminished and he required constant noxious stimulation to remain alert. He had a decreased right nasolabial fold, a weak cough and gag reflex as well as a notable right hemiparesis. His trachea was intubated for airway protection. A noncontrast head computed tomography (CT) scan revealed a 3.4 × 3.0 cm area of hyperdensity in his left parietal lobe with no evidence of intraventricular extension of the hematoma. His coagulation panel and platelets were within normal limits. He was admitted to the neurologic intensive care unit (ICU) for close neurologic monitoring and ventilatory support. Management of presumed increased intracranial pressure (ICP) was initiated with head of the bed placed at 30 degrees to facilitate venous drainage.

On hospital day 2, the patient appeared more somnolent and a repeat head CT revealed increased mass effect on the right lateral ventricle. Mannitol 20% was given at 0.25 g/kg and serum osmolarity was checked for the next 48 hours.

On hospital day 4, the patient's level of awareness had improved and repeat head CT revealed decreasing edema; the trachea was extubated. Magnetic resonance imaging (MRI) was performed, showing multiple areas of microhemorrhage and macrohemorrhage

on gradient echo as well as the acute left parietal hemorrhage (Figure 88.1). The following day, he was stable and transferred to a general medical ward to continue vigorous rehabilitation.

Discussion

Cerebral amyloid angiopathy is the most common cause of spontaneous lobar ICH. It is characterized by the deposition of beta-amyloid peptide into the media and adventitia of small arteries and capillaries. The beta-amyloid peptide is toxic to the vascular smooth muscle cells leading to damage to the blood vessel wall and consequent hemorrhage. Not surprisingly, advancing age is the strongest risk factor for CAA. In addition, the presence of *APOE2* and *APOE4* alleles, which result in increased beta-amyloid peptide deposition and degeneration of vessel walls, are also risk factors for CAA [1].

Presentation and diagnosis

The presentation of CAA-related ICH is comparable to all lobar hemorrhages. Patients present with acute onset of headache, decreased level of consciousness, focal neurologic signs, especially cortical signs such as aphasia, neglect, or seizures. Currently, diagnosis is based on the Boston Criteria utilizing clinical data, autopsy, surgical pathology, or MRI (Table 88.1) [2]. The criteria rely on detecting the late manifestations of CAA-related vascular damage such as hemorrhage and microbleeding rather than the vascular amyloid itself. Recently, two potential biomarkers have been identified that detect the presence of the disease without having to rely on the presence of microhemorrhages, a late consequence of the disease. Pittsburgh Compound B, a beta-amyloid-binding compound used with positron emission tomography imaging, distinguished patients with CAA from healthy volunteers and patients with Alzheimer's disease via localization of the compound's

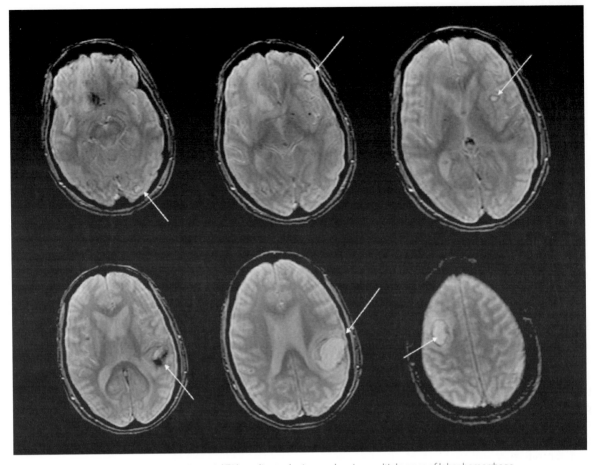

Figure 88.1. A magnetic resonance imaging, axial T2* gradient echo image showing multiple areas of lobar hemorrhage.

retention [3]. In addition, cerebral spinal fluid analysis of amyloid beta 40 and amyloid beta 42 also distinguished CAA from healthy controls and Alzheimer's disease patients [4].

Medical management

As with all critically ill patients, assessment and stabilization of the airway, breathing, and circulation are the essential first steps. This is followed by rapid diagnosis. Because it is difficult to clinically distinguish ICH from ischemic stroke, emergent diagnostic imaging with either a head CT or MRI is recommended [5]. If available, admission to a neurologic or neurosurgical ICU is preferred as it has been associated with decreased mortality [5].

Medical treatment of CAA-related ICH is based on control of the hemorrhage, management of blood pressure, management of elevated ICP, and treatment of seizures, fevers, and hyperglycemia. The Factor Seven for Acute Hemorrhagic Stroke (FAST) trial compared two doses of recombinant factor VII (rFVIIa) to placebo within 4 hours of onset of spontaneous ICH. While both doses of rFVIIa resulted in the reduction of hematoma volume, the small hematoma volume reductions did not result in improved outcome following ICH [6]. Unfortunately, at this time there are no effective treatments to reduce hematoma expansion.

The data on blood pressure management in acute ICH are inconclusive. Currently underway are the Antihypertensive Treatment in Acute Cerebral Hemorrhage (ATACH) and Intensive Blood Pressure Reduction in Acute Cerebral Hemorrhage (INTER-ACT) trials evaluating blood pressure management in the setting of acute ICH. Until the results of these

Table 88.1. Boston Criteria for diagnosis of cerebral amyloid angiopathy-related hemorrhage.

Definite CAA	Postmortem examination shows lobar cortical, or corticosubcortical hemorrhage ICH, severe CAA and no other diagnostic lesion
Probable CAA with supporting pathology	Clinical data and pathologic tissue (evacuated hematoma or cortical biopsy) showing some lobar, cortical, or corticosubcortical hemorrhage, some degree of CAA and absence of other diagnostic lesion
Probable CAA	Clinical data and MRI or CT with multiple hemorrhages restricted to lobar, cortical, or corticosubcortical regions (cerebellar hemorrhage allowed), age ≥55 years and no other cause of hemorrhage
Possible CAA	Clinical data and MRI or CT with single lobar, cortical, or corticosubcortical hemorrhage, age ≥55 years and no other cause of hemorrhage

CAA, cerebral amyloid angiopathy; MRI, magnetic resonance imaging; CT, computed tomography.

trials are published, we recommend mean arterial pressures of 70–110 mmHg based on our clinical experience. In our neurologic ICU, this is achieved via intravenous labetalol as needed or an intravenous infusion of nicardipine.

With regards to ICP management in the setting of ICH, no randomized clinical trial has demonstrated the efficacy of monitoring intracerebral pressure or cerebral perfusion pressure [5]. We recommend a stepwise approach starting with the patient's head midline and elevated to 30° in order to improve venous outflow, followed by osmotic therapy with either mannitol or hypertonic saline. As a temporizing measure for the acute patient in danger of herniation, hyperventilation with target CO_2 of 30–35 mmHg is an effective method for rapid reduction of ICP. Finally, for patients with refractory intracranial hypertension, barbiturate coma is initiated with electroencephalography monitoring in order to titrate the barbiturate dosing to burst suppression.

Clinical or electrographic seizures should be treated with intravenous antiepileptic. Euglycemia should be targeted for all patients and may require insulin. Finally, fevers should be aggressively controlled with acetaminophen and other measures such as a cooling blanket if needed.

Surgical management

The International Surgical Trial in Intracerebral Hemorrhage (STICH), published in 2005, was a multicenter randomized clinical trial comparing surgery within 96 hours of ICH onset to best medical treatment for patients with spontaneous supratentorial ICH. Patients were enrolled if their treating neurosurgeon felt clinical equipoise between surgery and medical management. Overall, no difference in functional outcome or mortality were found [7]. Subgroup analysis revealed that surgery may be beneficial in treating patients with lobar hematomas within 1 cm of the surface of the brain [7]. Presently a randomized trial, Surgical Trial in Intracerebral Hemorrhage II (STICH II), is underway evaluating this limited population. At the present time, surgery is reserved for a highly select group of patients at the discretion of the treating neurosurgeon and neurointensivist.

Prognosis

Unfortunately, the prognosis is poor for many ICH patients. Limitations in life-sustaining care may confound our current prognostication system for ICH patients [5]. In our opinion, prognosis after ICH may be clouded by the self-fulfilling prophecy of withdrawal of care. We encourage aggressive full support at least for the first 24 hours after acute ICH.

Risk of recurrent hemorrhage

Following the initial CAA-related ICH, the presence of additional areas of microhemorrhage on the baseline MRI Gradient Echo sequence, new areas of microhemorrhage on subsequent scans and presence of the *APOE2* or *APOE4* alleles result in increased rates of recurrent hemorrhage [8, 9]. The risk of recurrent hemorrhage is important to take into account because decision models for initiation of anticoagulation after ICH are based on estimates of this risk. For example, when clinicians contemplate restarting anticoagulation in a patient with CAA-related ICH and atrial fibrillation, an accurate assessment of the risk of recurrent hemorrhage is required to weigh the risks and benefits of anticoagulation.

Conclusion

The management of CAA-related ICH is complex and close neurologic monitoring is essential. With the development of new potential biomarkers for the disease, we may begin to explore therapeutic options before patients develop ICH.

References

1. **S. M. Greenberg, J. P. Vonsattel, A. Z. Segal** *et al.* Association of apolipoprotein E epsilon2 and vasculopathy in cerebral amyloid angiopathy. *Neurology* 1998; **50**: 961–5.

2. **K. A. Knudsen, J. Rosand, D. Karluk** *et al.* Clinical diagnosis of cerebral amyloid angiopathy: validation of the Boston criteria. *Neurology* 2001; **56**: 537–9.

3. **K. A. Johnson, M. Gregas, J. A. Becker** *et al.* Imaging of amyloid burden and distribution in cerebral amyloid angiopathy. *Ann Neurol* 2007; **62**: 229–34.

4. **M. M. Verbeek, B. P. Kremer, M. O. Rikkert** *et al.* Cerebrospinal fluid amyloid beta(40) is decreased in cerebral amyloid angiopathy. *Ann Neurol* 2009; **66**: 245–9.

5. **J. Broderick, S. Connolly, E. Feldmann** *et al.* Guidelines for the management of spontaneous intracerebral hemorrhage in adults: 2007 update: a guideline from the American Heart Association/American Stroke Association Stroke Council, High Blood Pressure Research Council, and the Quality of Care and Outcomes in Research Interdisciplinary Working Group. *Stroke* 2007; **38**: 2001–23.

6. **S. A. Mayer, N. C. Brun, K. Begtrup** *et al.* Efficacy and safety of recombinant activated factor VII for acute intracerebral hemorrhage. *N Engl J Med* 2008; **358**: 2127–37.

7. **A. D. Mendelow, B. A. Gregson, H. M. Fernandes** *et al.* Early surgery versus initial conservative treatment in patients with spontaneous supratentorial intracerebral haematomas in the International Surgical Trial in Intracerebral Haemorrhage (STICH): a randomised trial. *Lancet* 2005; **365**: 387–97.

8. **S. M. Greenberg, J. A. Eng, M. Ning** *et al.* Hemorrhage burden predicts recurrent intracerebral hemorrhage after lobar hemorrhage. *Stroke* 2004; **35**: 1415–20.

9. **H. C. O'Donnell, J. Rosand, K. A. Knudsen** *et al.* Apolipoprotein E genotype and the risk of recurrent lobar intracerebral hemorrhage. *N Engl J Med* 2000; **342**: 240–5.

Traumatic brain injury

Venkatakrishna Rajajee

Traumatic brain injury (TBI) is the leading cause of death and disability in children and adults from ages 1 to 44 [1]. The primary goal of management of the patient with severe TBI (Glasgow Coma Scale (GCS) 3–8) in the intensive care unit (ICU) is to prevent secondary brain injury.

Case description

A 26-year-old female was brought to the emergency room after a motor vehicle collision. In the emergency room, her GCS was 6 (E1M3V2). Her pupils were 3 mm on the left, unreactive, and 6 mm on the right, reactive. Following endotracheal intubation the patient was given mannitol 1 g/kg and a noncontrast computed tomography (CT) scan of the brain was urgently obtained. This revealed a right temporoparietal epidural hematoma 3.5 cm in greatest diameter with a 1.6 cm shift of the midline (Figure 89.1).

The patient was taken to the operating room (OR) immediately. Under general anesthesia, a craniotomy was performed and the epidural clot evacuated. The craniotomy bone flap was replaced. A right-sided external ventricular drain (EVD) was placed. A postoperative CT revealed an effective decompression and a CT of the cervical spine revealed no bony abnormality. The patient was admitted to the ICU.

In the ICU, her GCS was 6T, with an intracranial pressure (ICP) of 6 mmHg. She was mechanically ventilated with the Assist Control mode. She was given a phenytoin loading dose followed by a maintenance dose for seizure prophylaxis. By the next morning, she was seen to withdraw with the right side and frequently "buck" the ventilator. At this time her GCS was 6T (E1M4V1T), with an ICP of 28 mmHg. Propofol and fentanyl infusions were started. Following initiation of the sedative infusion the mean arterial pressure dropped to 60 mmHg and the ICP was 18 mmHg, resulting in a cerebral perfusion pressure (CPP) of $60 - 18 = 42$ mmHg. A norepinephrine infusion was

started to maintain the CPP >60 mmHg. A nasogastric feeding tube was placed and feeding was advanced to goal daily caloric requirement over the next 48 hours. Heparin 5000 U subcutaneously three times daily was started 24 hours postoperatively. Through the next 48 hours her ICP increased to 24 mmHg despite the sedation and analgesia. The ventricular catheter was opened to drain on several occasions for an ICP >20 cm; 3–5 mL of cerebrospinal fluid (CSF) was drained each time, followed by cessation of drainage. Eventually, on postoperative day 3, the ICP was 30 mmHg despite intermittent CSF drainage and sedation. She was given a 0.25 g/kg intravenous push of mannitol and her ICP decreased to 12 mmHg within 30 minutes. Repeat CT scans revealed no new hematoma. The set ventilator rate was adjusted to maintain the $PaCO_2$ 30–35 mmHg. Over the next 24 hours, bolus doses of mannitol were required every 4 hours for ICP >20 mmHg, while maintaining a serum osmolality 300–320 mOsm/kg. On postoperative day 4 the ICP was 30 mmHg despite the use of osmotherapy. The patient was taken back to the OR and the craniotomy flap removed, the dura opened and a duroplasty performed (Figure 89.2). Postoperatively, the ICP was 6 mmHg and remained <20 mmHg for the duration of the patient's ICU stay. No further use of mannitol was required. On postoperative day 7, the patient was following commands. She had 5/5 strength on the right side and 2/5 strength on the left. The trachea was extubated successfully and the ventricular catheter removed. She was transferred out of the ICU 24 hours later.

Discussion

The guidelines for the management of the patient with severe TBI published by the Brain Trauma Foundation (BTF) [2] form the basis for the following discussion. Management of TBI often begins with a decision to perform endotracheal intubation in the

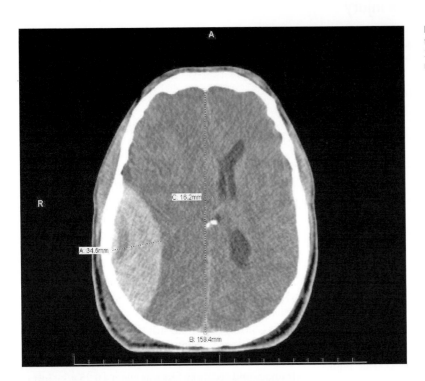

Figure 89.1. Right-sided temporoparietal epidural hematoma, 3.5 cm maximum thickness, 1.6 cm midline shift.

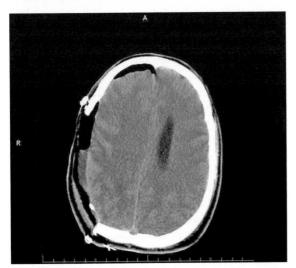

Figure 89.2. Right craniotomy bone flap removed with effective decompression.

emergency room. A widely used rule of thumb is "eight-intubate," with intubation performed when the GCS is 8 or less. Other factors such as intoxication and the risk of aspiration may need to be considered even if the GCS is greater than 8. Hypotension (a systolic blood pressure less than 90 mmHg) has most consistently been associated with poor neurologic outcome

following severe TBI. Hypoxia (SpO$_2$ <90%) is also associated with poor outcome. Early aggressive resuscitation of low blood pressure and poor oxygenation is therefore of critical importance. Clinical signs of transtentorial herniation (dilated pupil) warrant the immediate use of a bolus of mannitol IV. The next step in management is the removal of specific mass lesions, most commonly subdural, extradural, and intracerebral hematomas (contusions) guided by urgent noncontrast head CT. Guidelines for the surgical management of TBI and removal of mass lesions have also been published by the BTF (Table 89.1) [3]. The epidural hematoma in the case discussed was >2 cm in greatest thickness and resulted in >0.5 cm of midline shift in an individual with GCS ≤8; surgical evacuation is therefore urgently indicated. A decision was then made to place an ICP monitor, as monitoring of intracranial pressure is necessary in patients with TBI likely to have or develop intracranial hypertension (ICP >20 mmHg). This consists of patients with GCS ≤8 with an abnormal head CT as well as patients with GCS ≤8 and a normal head CT who are older than 40, hypotensive (SBP <90 mmHg) or have posturing on neurologic examination (Table 89.2). This patient with GCS 6 prior to transport to the operating room therefore had an EVD placed. The advantage of using an EVD, or ventriculostomy catheter, is

Table 89.1. Indications for surgical evacuation of traumatic mass lesions [3].

Epidural hematoma

An epidural hematoma (EDH) greater than 30 cm^3 should be surgically evacuated regardless of the patient's GCS score

An EDH less than 30 cm^3 and with less than a 15-mm thickness and with less than a 5-mm midline shift in patients with a GCS score greater than 8 without focal deficit can be managed nonoperatively with serial CT scanning and close neurologic observation in a neurosurgical center

Subdural hematoma

An acute subdural hematoma (SDH) with a thickness greater than 10 mm or a midline shift greater than 5 mm on CT scan should be surgically evacuated, regardless of the patient's GCS score

All patients with acute SDH in coma (GCS score less than 9) should undergo ICP monitoring

A comatose patient (GCS score less than 9) with an SDH less than 10-mm thick and a midline shift less than 5 mm should undergo surgical evacuation of the lesion if the GCS score decreased between the time of injury and hospital admission by 2 or more points on the GCS and/or the patient presents with asymmetric or fixed and dilated pupils and/or the ICP exceeds 20 mmHg

Traumatic parenchymal lesion (contusion)

Patients with parenchymal mass lesions and signs of progressive neurologic deterioration referable to the lesion, medically refractory intracranial hypertension, or signs of mass effect on CT scan should be treated operatively

Patients with GCS scores of 6 to 8 with frontal or temporal contusions greater than 20 cm^3 in volume with midline shift of at least 5 mm and/or cisternal compression on CT scan, and patients with any lesion greater than 50 cm^3 in volume should be treated operatively.

Patients with parenchymal mass lesions who do not show evidence for neurologic compromise, have controlled ICP, and no significant signs of mass effect on CT scan may be managed nonoperatively with intensive monitoring and serial imaging

Decompressive procedures, including subtemporal decompression, temporal lobectomy, and hemispheric decompressive craniectomy, are treatment options for patients with refractory intracranial hypertension and diffuse parenchymal injury with clinical and radiographic evidence for impending transtentorial herniation

Table 89.2. Indications for intracranial pressure monitoring in severe TBI [2].

GCS 3–8 plus abnormal CT

or

GCS 3–8 plus

Normal CT and any two of the following

Age > 40

Systolic blood pressure <90

Unilateral or bilateral posturing

that the catheter can also be used as a first-line therapeutic tool to reduce ICP (via drainage of CSF). The major alternative is an intraparenchymal ICP monitor (such as the Codman and Camino monitors). While these catheters cannot drain CSF, they are technically easier to place and carry a significantly lower risk of hemorrhage and infection. Anticonvulsant use is indicated for prophylaxis against early (<7 days) posttraumatic seizures, however, there is no value in primary prophylaxis beyond that period. Early seizures do not seem to correlate with poor long-term neurologic outcome. Once in the ICU, a decision often needs to be made about continued use of a semi-rigid collar for immobilization of the cervical spine. In the patient with severe TBI in whom a valid clinical examination to clear the cervical spine cannot be performed, a noncontrast CT of the cervical spine is generally adequate to clear the cervical spine and remove the collar [4]. Some physicians prefer to continue use of the semi-rigid collar until an adequate clinical examination, a flexion-extension X-ray or magnetic resonance image of the cervical spine can be obtained to exclude ligamentous and other soft tissue injury.

Sedation and analgesia is of critical importance in the TBI patient, not only to permit safe and effective mechanical ventilation and avoid unintended tracheal extubation or line removal but also to adequately control ICP. In the case discussed, a combination of propofol and fentanyl was used. Propofol has the advantage of having a short half life to permit neurologic examination as required and is a very effective sedative. Caution should be employed with long-term use, as propofol infusion syndrome may occur. Analgesia is important, particularly in the postoperative TBI patient. The goal is to maintain the ICP <20 mmHg and the CPP >60 mmHg, since the risk of secondary neurologic injury is considered to be significant outside these values. A vasopressor infusion was therefore warranted to maintain a CPP >60 mmHg. Maintaining the CPP >70 mmHg is no longer recommended, since the risk of acute respiratory distress syndrome appears to be greater when measures are taken to attain this goal, without a corresponding benefit in mortality or neurologic outcome. In the case discussed, when the patient's ICP remained consistently >20 mmHg, the first step taken was to drain some CSF through the EVD. In general, CSF drainage is performed on an intermittent, as-needed basis for 5–10 minutes for ICP >20 mmHg, with the catheter monitoring pressures at baseline. Early initiation of nutritional support is recommended, with enteral feeding the preferred route and the total daily calorific requirement goal attained within 7 days, usually sooner (within 72 hours for the patient discussed). Deep venous thrombosis prophylaxis is necessary in all patients with severe TBI in the ICU. A combination of immediate use of a sequential compression device and subcutaneous heparin (either unfractionated or low molecular weight) after 24–48 hours is safe and effective even in patients admitted with intracranial hematomas.

If the ICP cannot be controlled with the use of appropriate sedation/analgesia and intermittent CSF drainage, then as-needed osmotherapy is used. Mannitol and hypertonic saline are both reasonable options for this purpose. Mannitol often begins to act within 10–30 minutes with a clinical effect that lasts for 2–6 hours. The use of mannitol carries the risk of dehydration, renal injury, and hypotension. This should be judiciously avoided with the use of fluid resuscitation, usually crystalloid. While using mannitol the serum osmolality is typically not pushed beyond 310–320 mOsm/kg, to avoid the risk of renal injury. Prolonged or continuous use of mannitol may also result in rebound cerebral edema and intracranial hypertension. Hypertonic saline does not cause dehydration or hypotension but may result in fluid overload. Osmotherapy in general should be used only for episodes of elevated ICP or, prior to the placement of an ICP monitor, for clinical signs of herniation.

Hyperventilation to $PaCO_2$ <30–35 mmHg is rapidly effective in reducing ICP but may result in cerebral ischemia and worsened neurologic outcomes. The fall in ICP with hyperventilation is transient and rebound intracranial hypertension may result from a too-rapid increase in the $PaCO_2$ following initial hyperventilation. Hyperventilation to <30–35 mmHg should generally be avoided in TBI and, if used,

should be done so in conjunction with ancillary brain oxygenation monitoring to detect ischemia. There is no role for high-dose corticosteroid therapy in the management of severe TBI. Mild hypothermia (to 32–34 °C) lowers ICP and, on the basis of pooled data, may result in improved Glasgow Outcome Scales with an improvement in mortality when used for >48 hours. In the absence of conclusive evidence of benefit from large randomized controlled trials, however, the routine use of hypothermia in all patients with severe TBI is not recommended by the BTF. Similarly, although the use of jugular bulb oximetry and brain tissue oxygenation monitors to detect brain hypoperfusion/ischemia shows significant promise, in the absence of conclusive outcome data, the routine use of these techniques in severe TBI is not specifically recommended by the BTF.

For the patient who develops intracranial hypertension refractory to the above measures, the available options include mild hypothermia, barbiturate (pentobarbital or thiopental) infusion titrated to electroencephalogram burst suppression, and decompressive craniectomy. Increasingly, decompressive craniectomy is being used in patients with severe TBI and intracranial hypertension. In the case discussed, the original craniotomy flap was removed with subsequent excellent control of ICP followed by neurologic improvement. Frequently, the bone flap is not replaced at the time of initial hematoma evacuation when significant edema and intracranial hypertension is anticipated. The durotomy (with duroplasty) plays an important role in reduction of ICP. While this technique is very effective in controlling ICP, outcome data from large randomized controlled trials are not yet available [5]. Performing a decompressive craniectomy commits the patient to a subsequent cranioplasty to replace the bone flap and carries with it the risks of acute hemorrhage, extra-axial fluid accumulation and infection, among others. Once the patient's neurologic condition improves, tracheal extubation must not be delayed, with consideration given primarily to the patient's ability to cough and clear secretions spontaneously rather than a specific GCS number. Performing tracheostomy in TBI patients prior to 7 days will decrease the number of days on mechanical ventilation but may not reduce the risk of ventilator-associated pneumonia or alter mortality. The management of patients with TBI is often challenging but rewarding, with a significant number of patients achieving a good long-term neurologic outcome.

References

1. **J. A. Langlois, W. Rutland-Brown, M. M. Wald**. The epidemiology and impact of traumatic brain injury: a brief overview. *J Head Trauma Rehabil* 2006; **21**: 375–8.

2. **Brain Trauma Foundation**. American Association of Neurological Surgeons; Congress of Neurological Surgeons; Joint Section on Neurotrauma and Critical Care, AANS/CNS. Guidelines for the management of severe traumatic brain injury. *J Neurotrauma* 2007; **24** Suppl. 1: S1–95.

3. **M. R. Bullock, R. Chesnut, J. Ghajar** *et al*. Surgical Management of Traumatic Brain Injury Author Group. Guidelines for the surgical management of traumatic brain injury. *Neurosurgery* 2006; **58**: S2.

4. **N. D. Tomycz, B. G. Chew, Y. F. Chang** *et al*. MRI is unnecessary to clear the cervical spine in obtunded/comatose trauma patients: the four-year experience of a level I trauma center. *J Trauma* 2008; **64**: 1258–63.

5. **J. Sahuquillo, F. Arikan**. Decompressive craniectomy for the treatment of refractory high intracranial pressure in traumatic brain injury. *Cochrane Database Syst Rev* 2006; **25**: CD003983.

Traumatic brain injury

Elevated intracranial pressure

Richard Bowers and George A. Mashour

Intracranial pressure (ICP) is an important parameter guiding the management of patients in the intensive care unit (ICU) with intracranial pathology. Prompt and effective interventions in the event of elevated ICP are necessary to reduce ischemic neuronal loss and improve long-term neurologic outcomes.

Case description

A 57-year-old male presented following a fall down a flight of stone stairs. He had consumed a significant quantity of alcohol prior to the fall and was later found unresponsive. Paramedics secured his cervical spine and the trachea was intubated at the scene. Following transfer to hospital he underwent a noncontrast head computed tomography (CT) scan, which revealed a thin left-sided subdural hemorrhage and diffuse petechial parenchymal hemorrhage. The subdural hemorrhage was evacuated and a right frontal intraventricular ICP catheter was inserted under general anesthetic. The patient was subsequently transferred to the ICU where his ICP was measured continuously. Initial treatment of the patient consisted of infusions of sedatives and ventilation to a target $PaCO_2$ of 35 mmHg, but persistent spikes of his ICP were recorded. Acute treatment of these ICP increases consisted of an intravenous bolus of mannitol and additional boluses of sedation. Treatment was escalated with the commencement of an infusion of neuromuscular blocking agents, which improved ICP control. In addition to these treatments, the patient had a nasogastric feeding tube inserted, blood glucose was kept <150 mg/dL, full-length lower limb compression stockings fitted, and normothermia was ensured.

He began to demonstrate poor intracranial elastance approximately 12 hours later, with frequent ICP spikes that persisted. These spikes were treated with hypertonic saline and a repeat head CT found gross cerebral edema with evidence of hemorrhage. Treatment was escalated further to include active cooling to a core temperature not lower than 34 °C. Cooling was achieved by the use of a large-bore femoral vein cooling catheter. Shivering was prevented by the continued administration of neuromuscular blocking drugs.

Further episodes of elevated ICP occurred once the core temperature target had been achieved and it was therefore decided to institute a barbiturate infusion. The patient's electroencephalogram was monitored during barbiturate therapy, allowing dose titration of the barbiturates to achieve burst suppression. Additional neuroimaging revealed no further changes.

Therapy continued in this manner for several days with little sustained improvement of the patient's ICP, although acute elevations were less common.

Hypernatremia had become an increasingly difficult problem over the period in the ICU. Laboratory tests had begun to show evidence of acute renal failure after 8 days due to the combination of critical illness, hyperosmotic treatments, and an incipient respiratory tract infection. A decision was made with the patient's family to withdraw active treatment after 10 days and he died shortly thereafter.

Discussion

Why treat

Brain injuries from multiple etiologies consist of a primary insult that may be surgically amenable, as well as subsequent secondary insults that are the focus of intensive care management. The loss of neurons from secondary insults may be significantly greater than that of the primary insult. Appropriate and timely management may allow survival of these neurons and, hopefully, improvement in a patient's neurologic outcome and functional status.

Who to treat

There are many causes of increased ICP, both intracranial and extracranial (see Table 90.1). Treatment of

Table 90.1. Causes of intracranial hypertension.

Mass effects
    Tumor
    Hemorrhage – extradural, subdural, subarachnoid
    Intracerebral abscess

Vascular
    Hypercarbia, hypoxemia
    Hyperemia
    Pyrexia
    Cerebral venous sinus thrombosis

Excess cerebrospinal fluid
    Obstructive – Arnold–Chiari malformation, meningocele,
        meningitis, tumors, hemorrhage
    Excess production – choroid plexus tumor, subarachnoid
        hemorrhage
    Failed resorption – meningitis, subarachnoid hemorrhage

Edema
    Diffuse axonal injury
    Infection – encephalitis, meningoencephalitis

Miscellaneous
    Acute liver failure
    Idiopathic intracranial hypertension

the underlying cause may allow rapid resolution of intracranial hypertension, although most will initiate a cascade cycle of increasing ICP, reducing cerebral perfusion, further intracerebral inflammation, edema, and ICP rises.

Why intracranial pressure

Intracranial pressure has become central to the critical care management of neurologic patients. The reasons for this approach are several-fold, but primarily include the Monro–Kellie hypothesis of intracranial elastance, the relative ease of ICP measurement, quantifiable neurologic change based on ICP manipulation, such as the recovery of pupil reactivity following ICP reduction, and the association between maintenance of cerebral perfusion pressure (CPP) and improved patient outcomes, which relies on ICP measurement [1]. The Monroe–Kellie hypothesis suggests that since three noncompressible components (brain, blood, and CSF) are housed within a nondistensible vault (the cranium); changing the volume of one component of necessity means that either (1) the volume of another must change or (2) ICP must increase.

There are caveats to the use of ICP measurement that must be borne in mind. First, ICP is not uniform throughout the brain and the measured ICP may not fully reflect the area of intracranial injury. Other sources of inaccuracy may include catheter position,

catheter type, or a separate issue such as clotting of manometer tubing. There are also direct risks associated with the use of monitoring catheters including infection (approximate rate 10%) and hemorrhage [2, 3].

When to treat

Intracranial pressure is considered abnormal once it rises above 20 mmHg [1, 4]. Once this threshold has been passed, a methodical and thorough assessment of the patient should be instituted to (1) search for any reversible causes of the new deterioration, (2) maximize cerebral perfusion and oxygenation, and (3) reduce the volume of intracranial contents.

What to treat

Control of intracranial pressure in the ICU depends on the manipulation of a variety of factors with the aim of minimizing secondary insults. These factors involve:

- optimizing cerebral blood flow and oxygenation
- reducing cerebral oxygen consumption
- reducing volume of intracranial contents including:

    · blood – arterial and venous
    · cerebrospinal fluid
    · brain parenchyma – edema, mass lesions.

How to treat 1 – initial management

Initial management of raised ICP is straightforward, and may appear to consist of little more than "routine" ICU management. The following are, however, important points.

Optimizing cerebral blood flow and oxygenation

Normotension and cerebral perfusion pressure. Maintenance of CPP is essential. Frequency and duration of hypotension are associated with increasing mortality and morbidity in neurologically impaired patients [1]. Cerebral perfusion pressure is indirectly dependent on ICP:

$$CPP = Mean\ Arterial\ Pressure - ICP$$

A CPP of <60 mmHg is associated with a poor outcome and it is recommended that CPP be maintained >60 mmHg at all times [1]. This target is best achieved through both fluid resuscitation and vasopressor use.

There may be some advantage to the use of hypertonic saline in patients with traumatic brain injury as it significantly improved blood pressure when compared with resuscitation with normal saline [1] and it may also reduce cerebral edema. Failure to maintain adequate CPP despite fluid resuscitation should prompt use of vasopressor support as swiftly as possible. Norepinephrine is preferable to other vasopressors due to the relative cerebrovascular sparing of alpha-adrenergic receptors and its predictability of action. An escalating dose of norepinephrine causes concern and should prompt investigation for causes of intravascular fluid loss or poor cardiac output. Patients with nontraumatic etiology may display systemic hypertension as a reflex to maintain cerebral perfusion. This should not be treated until CPP can be calculated, i.e., after ICP monitoring is instituted.

Oxygenation and ventilation. All patients treated for traumatic brain injury should have a PaO_2 of greater than 11 kPa (approx 80 mmHg) [1]. It is reasonable to extend this goal to all patients treated for intracranial hypertension as hypoxia may exacerbate ICP rises. The use of positive end expiratory pressure (PEEP) to accomplish this goal is not contraindicated and, in general, improved cerebral oxygenation will give better control of ICP and should outweigh any concerns regarding reduced intracranial venous return from excessive intrathoracic pressure.

Cerebral blood vessels vasodilate as $PaCO_2$ rises, reaching maximal dilatation at approximately 90–100 mmHg (12–13 kPa) and ICP will consequently rise. Therefore, $PaCO_2$ should be controlled to approximately 35 mmHg (4.5 kPa). Further reductions of $PaCO_2$ should be avoided as vasoconstriction may induce ischemia, particularly in the early stages following traumatic head injury when cerebral blood flow is reduced [1, 4]; the long-term outcome is worsened with chronic hyperventilation [2]. The effect of hyperventilation is time-limited to cerebrospinal fluid pH buffering and so may only be of use as a temporizing measure while other strategies are being employed.

Reducing cerebral oxygen consumption and demand

Sedation and analgesia should be provided to prevent agitation and distress, thus reducing cerebral oxygen consumption. The selection of drugs depends mainly on the expected duration of sedation and any potential side effects such as hypotension. There is no intrinsic advantage of one drug over another for adequate sedation provided it is performed well. A bolus of sedation in the context of a longer-term infusion may also be used to acutely reduce ICP for ICU interventions e.g., tracheal suctioning, but caution should be paid to avoiding hypotension in this setting.

Avoidance of hyperthermia is also essential. Hyperthermia causes vasodilatation and increases metabolic rate [2]. Regular acetaminophen should be provided to all patients and cooling blankets used if necessary to restore normothermia.

*Hyper*glycemia has been shown to have a detrimental effect in other types of critical-care patients and should be generally avoided; however, *hypo*glycemia must absolutely be avoided due to the reliance of neuronal metabolism on glucose.

Reducing volume of intracranial contents

Mass lesions of the brain such as tumors or abscesses may be surgically evacuated with subsequent improvement of intracranial elastance. These processes also initiate edema formation, which may subsequently worsen ICP.

Cerebrospinal fluid may be drained via an intraventricular catheter to provide control for ICP. This process requires patent ventricles to allow aspiration or passive drainage of CSF. No benefit is present once ventricles are effaced [2].

How to treat 2 – subsequent management

Failure to control ICP to <20 mmHg with the above management requires further treatment. It is important to consider follow-up brain imaging in order to ensure that no further surgically amenable lesions have developed.

Maintenance of cerebral perfusion and oxygenation

A trial of elevated CPP may be attempted to examine whether ICP control is improved. There is however growing evidence that excessively elevated CPP is also associated with adverse cardiorespiratory and intracranial effects [1, 4]. Once a CPP is achieved that is adequate for cerebral perfusion and avoidance of ischemia, no benefit exists for further elevation.

Reducing cerebral oxygen consumption and demand

Seizures may be both a consequence and cause of raised ICP. Seizures produce significant increases in cerebral blood flow, cerebral anaerobic metabolism, cytotoxic edema, hypercarbia, and hypoxia, all of which contribute to ICP increases. Seizure prophylaxis

Addenbrooke's NCCU: ICP/CPP management algorithm

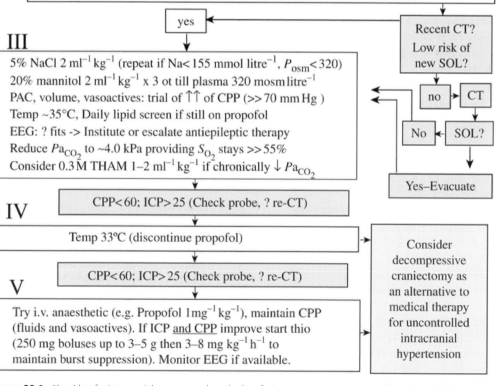

All patients with or at risk of intracranial hypertension must have invasive arterial monitoring, CVP line, ICP monitor, and Rt Sv_{O_2} catheter at admission to NCCU.

This algorithm should be used in conjunction with the full protocols for patient management.

Aim to establish multimodality monitoring within the first 6 h of NCCU stay.

Interventions in stage III to be targeted to clinical picture and multimodality monitoring.

CPP 70 mm Hg set as initial target, but CPP>> 60 mm Hg is acceptable in most patients.

If brain chemistry monitored, $Pt_{O_2} > 1$ kPa and LPR< 25 are 2° targets (see full protocol)

Evacuate significant SOLs and drain CSF before escalating medical Rx.

Rx in italics and Grades IV and V only after approval by NCCU Consultant.

I

10 –15° head up, no venous obstruction

CPP> 70 (CVP 6–10; + PAC); 2° targets: $Pt_{O_2} > 1$ kpa; LPR< 25

$Sp_{O_2} \geq 97\%$; $Pa_{O_2} \geq 11$ kpa, Pa_{CO_2} 4.5–5.0 kPa

Temp≤ 37°C; $S_{O_2} > 55\%$; blood sugar 4–7 mmol litre^{-1}

Propofol 2–5 mg kg^{-1} h^{-1}; Fentanyl 1–2 µg kg^{-1} h^{-1}; atracurium 0.5 mg kg^{-1} h^{-1} (consider indications for midazolam, remifentanil)

Ranitidine 50 mg 8° i.v. (or sucralfate 1 g 6° NG if enteral access)

Phenytoin 15 mg kg^{-1} if indicated (fits, depressed # etc.)

yes

ICP< 20
CPP>> 60

no

II — Drain CSF via EVD if possible and evacuate significant SOLs

yes

Recent CT?
Low risk of new SOL?

III

5% NaCl 2 ml^{-1} kg^{-1} (repeat if Na< 155 mmol litre^{-1}, $P_{osm} < 320$)

20% mannitol 2 ml^{-1} kg^{-1} x 3 ot till plasma 320 mosm litre^{-1}

PAC, volume, vasoactives: trial of ↑↑ of CPP (>> 70 mm Hg)

Temp ~35°C, Daily lipid screen if still on propofol

EEG: ? fits -> Institute or escalate antiepileptic therapy

Reduce Pa_{CO_2} to ~4.0 kPa providing S_{O_2} stays >> 55%

Consider 0.3 M THAM 1–2 ml^{-1} kg^{-1} if chronically ↓ Pa_{CO_2}

no — CT

No — SOL?

Yes–Evacuate

IV — CPP< 60; ICP> 25 (Check probe, ? re-CT)

Temp 33°C (discontinue propofol)

V — CPP< 60; ICP> 25 (Check probe, ? re-CT)

Try i.v. anaesthetic (e.g. Propofol 1mg^{-1} kg^{-1}), maintain CPP (fluids and vasoactives). If ICP and CPP improve start thio (250 mg boluses up to 3–5 g then 3–8 mg kg^{-1} h^{-1} to maintain burst suppression). Monitor EEG if available.

Consider decompressive craniectomy as an alternative to medical therapy for uncontrolled intracranial hypertension

Figure 90.1. Algorithm for intracranial pressure and cerebral perfusion pressure management. Reproduced with permission from Helmy et al. Br J Anaesth 2007; 99: 32–42 [4].

is recommended for the first week following traumatic brain injury [1, 4]. A diagnosis of occult seizures must always be considered in the event of an acute ICP rise and treated aggressively.

Reducing volume of intracranial contents

Osmotic diuretics produce a shift of water from the intracellular and interstitial spaces into the intravascular space. An intact blood–brain barrier is required for this process. Mannitol can be used in a dose of 0.25–1 g/kg and may reduce ICP for up to 6 hours [4]. The initial effects of mannitol include plasma volume expansion and improved small vessel flow characteristics. Cerebral blood flow increases and consequently vasoconstriction ensues if cerebral autoregulation is intact. Thereafter, its effects as an osmotic agent predominate. Chronic usage has been associated with rebound cerebral edema due to mannitol accumulation in the interstitium and intravascular dehydration. Hypertonic saline is an alternative that will also provide intravascular replacement [2, 4]. Maintenance of high serum osmolarity will also help reduce cellular swelling. Use of 0.9% sodium chloride as intravenous fluid increases serum osmolarity, though it is associated with some electrolyte abnormalities [4]. Osmolarity should be kept between 310–320 mOsm/L, and following treatment should be returned slowly to baseline to guard against rebound cerebral edema.

How to treat 3 – final options

The following options may offer control of ICP when all the above have failed. A sequential progression through these steps is suggested.

- Neuromuscular paralysis may be useful if high doses of sedation fail to control ICP particularly during ICU interventions such as suctioning and turning. Long-term use should be avoided, especially the steroid-based drugs, due to the risks of neuropathy and myopathy.
- The use of active hypothermia is more controversial, but it has shown some benefit for the control of ICP in otherwise refractory intracranial hypertension following traumatic brain injury [4]. It can be undertaken by ice packing of the head, groin, and axillae, covering the patient with cold wet blankets, or with intravascular cooling catheters. Hypothermia has significant side effects and core temperature should not be lower than 34 °C.

- Barbiturate coma involves intravenous infusion of barbiturates to achieve burst suppression (periods of low-voltage activity interspersed by shorter periods of higher amplitude complexes) on electroencephalogram. While in general ICP is more likely to be controlled, outcomes following barbiturate coma are not improved. Side effects are significant including hypotension, electrolyte abnormalities, infection and hepatorenal dysfunction [2]. It should only be considered in the event of failure of all other treatment.
- Decompressive craniectomy may be effective in the reduction of ICP when refractory to medical management [2]. It does offer the prospect of improved ICP control by effectively removing the constraints to intracranial volume. However, this may be at the cost of further intracranial complications and the overall benefit of the procedure is not yet known. Studies are comparing this treatment with barbiturate coma for outcomes in refractory intracranial hypertension.

Most management for ICP is standardized by use of protocols. An example of such a protocol is shown in Figure 90.1.

The management of intracranial hypertension in the ICU requires a multifaceted stepwise approach, with particular care and attention to avoidable complications such as hypoxia, hypercarbia, and hypotension that may dramatically worsen outcome. Rapid control of ICP and resumption of adequate CPP are the focus of a management strategy, which requires a systematic approach.

References

1. **Brain Trauma Foundation**. American Association of Neurological Surgeons; Congress of Neurological Surgeons; Joint Section on Neurotrauma and Critical Care, AANS/CNS. Guidelines for the management of severe traumatic brain injury. *J Neurotrauma* 2007; **24** Suppl. 1: S1–95.

2. **L. Rangel-Castillo, S. Gopinath, C. Robertson**. Management of intrcranial hypertension. *Neurol Clin* 2008; **26**: 521–41.

3. **O. L. Cremer**. Does ICP monitoring make a difference in neurocritical care? *Eur J Anaesthesiol Suppl* 2008; **42**: 87–93.

4. **A. Helmy, M. Vizcaychipi, A. K. Gupta**. Traumatic brain injury: intensive care management. *Br J Anaesth* 2007; **99**: 32–42.

91

Succinylcholine in the patient with increased intracranial pressure

Andrew Zura

The use of succinylcholine in a patient with increased intracranial pressure is still a controversial issue. In this case we highlight the benefits and the relative contraindications for using succinylcholine in these patients.

Case description

The patient was a 79-year-old female who fell and hit her head on the floor, after leaning back in her chair while eating dinner. Her mental status had progressively deteriorated since that time and she was brought to the emergency department (ED) by ambulance approximately 1 hour after the event.

Her past medical history included hypertension and atrial fibrillation, for which she was on coumadin. Incidentally, her international normalized ratio was checked by her primary care physician the day prior to the incident and found to be 2.2. On physical examination she appeared stuporous and did not answer any questions, but she reacted to painful stimuli. Vital signs were heart rate 42 beats per minute, blood pressure 200/110 mmHg, respirations 30 breaths per minute and temperature 37.0 °C. A computed tomography scan in the ED showed a massive subdural hematoma with a 2-cm midline shift. The anesthesiology team had been called to the ED to emergently intubate this patient prior to taking her to the operating room. The endotracheal intubation was performed using sodium pentothal and succinylcholine. After end-tidal CO_2 and bilateral breath sounds were confirmed, the resident asked the anesthesiology attending whether another agent such as rocuronium should have been used due to the patient's increased intracranial pressure (ICP).

Discussion

The question "Does succinylcholine increase intracranial pressure in patients with neurologic injury?" has concerned clinicians since it was first described in the 1950s [1]. When researchers tried to replicate the initial study they found that they obtained different results depending on the species studied and anesthetic technique used. Animal studies in cats and dogs have demonstrated reliable increases in ICP with succinylcholine [2, 3], but a study in monkeys failed to demonstrate this effect [4].

Two studies have demonstrated that succinylcholine will increase ICP in humans and that this effect can be attenuated by a "defasciculating" dose of a nondepolarizing muscle relaxant [5, 6]. More recent studies, also done in human patients with neurologic injury, have failed to demonstrate the increase in ICP. They concluded that succinylcholine in itself does not increase ICP or cerebral blood flow velocity [7, 8]. It is important to note that they also mentioned that other factors such as light anesthesia and tracheal intubation, which are often found together with the administration of succinylcholine, can and do significantly contribute to increases in ICP in patients with neurologic injury [7].

Conclusion

At this time, the data remain equivocal. There has never been a randomized controlled trial conducted to answer this question conclusively. Until more definitive recommendations are made, the clinician must continue to be aware of the risks and benefits of the drugs administered when deciding how to best treat the patient.

References

1. **M. Halldin, A. Wahlin**. Effect of succinylcholine on the intraspinal fluid pressure. *Acta Anaesthesiol Scand* 1959; **3**: 155–61.

2. **J. E. Cottrell, J. Hartung, J. P. Giffin** *et al.* Intracranial and hemodynamic changes after succinylcholine administration in cats. *Anesth Analg* 1983; **62**: 1006–9.

3. W. L. Lanier, P. A. Iaizzo, J. H. Milde. Cerebral function and muscle afferent activity following intravenous succinylcholine in dogs anesthetized with halothane: the effects of pretreatment with a defasciculating dose of pancuronium. *Anesthesiology* 1989; **71**: 87–95.

4. J. D. Haigh, E. M. Nemoto, A. M. DeWolf *et al.* Comparison of the effects of succinylcholine and atracurium on intracranial pressure in monkeys with intracranial hypertension. *Can Anaesth Soc J* 1986; **33**: 421–6.

5. M. D. Minton, K. Grosslight, J. A. Stirt *et al.* Increases in intracranial pressure from succinylcholine: prevention by prior nondepolarizing blockade. *Anesthesiology* 1986; **65**: 165–9.

6. J. A. Stirt, K. R. Grosslight, R. F. Bedford *et al.* "Defasciculation" with metocurine prevents succinylcholine-induced increases in intracranial pressure. *Anesthesiology* 1987; **67**: 50–3.

7. W. D. Kovarik, T. S. Mayberg, A. M. Lam *et al.* Succinylcholine does not change intracranial pressure, cerebral blood flow velocity, or the electroencephalogram in patients with neurologic injury. *Anesth Analg* 1994; **78**: 469–73.

8. M. M. Brown, M. J. Parr, A. R. Manara. The effect of suxamethonium on intracranial pressure and cerebral perfusion pressure in patients with severe head injuries following blunt trauma. *Eur J Anaesth* 1996; **13**: 474–7.

92

Pharmacologic management of status epilepticus

Alaa A. Abd-Elsayed, George K. Istaphanous and Ehab Farag

The management of status epilepticus is both challenging and costly. The annual incidence is estimated to be about 78 per 100 000 population in the USA [1]. The designation of status epilepticus may vary amongst clinicians, but it generally describes a cluster of frequent clinical seizures or a single unremitting seizure that lasts longer than 5–10 minutes without return to baseline or interictal state [2]. Historically, the International League against Epilepsy in 1981 defined status epilepticus as a seizure that persists for a sufficient length of time or is repeated frequently without recovery between attacks [3]. The duration of what is accepted as status epilepticus has varied according to different classifications. It has been changed from 30 min to 20 min, according to the guidelines of the Epilepsy Foundation of America's Working Group on Status Epilepticus. The Veterans Affairs Status Epilepticus Cooperation Study stipulated 10 min and, most recently, the duration of only 5 min has been proposed. Most seizures cease within a minute or two and if the seizure is prolonged beyond a few minutes, it is unlikely to be self-remitting [4]. The lack of a specific duration of the seizures has made this definition difficult to use.

Status epilepticus historically has been categorized into two main groups, convulsive and nonconvulsive. Convulsive status epilepticus can be further classified into (a) tonic–clonic status epilepticus, (b) tonic status epilepticus, (c) clonic status epilepticus, and (d) myoclonic status epilepticus. Nonconvulsive status epilepticus refers to a continuous or near-continuous generalized electrical seizure activity lasting for at least 30 min, but without convulsions (see Case 93). Nonconvulsive status epilepticus can be accompanied by abnormal mental status, unresponsiveness, ocular motor abnormalities, and persistent subclinical seizures. Nonconvulsive status epilepticus has long been divided into two main categories: absence status epilepticus and complex partial status epilepticus. Here we present the pharmacologic management of a case of convulsive status epilepticus.

Case description

A 12-year-old right-handed male with a history of cortical dysplasia, 3–4 tonic–clonic seizures a week and language/cognitive regression presented for placement of seizure-focus-localization grids via craniotomy. After cessation of antiepileptic drugs and a successful procedure, he was admitted to the intensive care unit (ICU) for monitoring. The patient experienced a tonic–clonic seizure on postoperative day 2 that continued despite administration of two doses of intravenous (IV) lorazepam 0.2 mg/kg (10 minutes apart) and fosphenytoin 20 mg/kg. On examination the patient was found to be unresponsive with increased muscle tone. Laboratory workup was grossly normal with no metabolic aberrations. Following intubation of the airway, pentobarbital 5 mg/kg IV bolus was given and then infused at a rate of 1 mg/kg/hour (general anesthesia) until burst-suppression was achieved, as assessed by electroencephalogram (EEG).

Computed tomography (CT) scans did not reveal any intracranial hemorrhage, masses, or midline shift. The patient was monitored by a continuous EEG to assist with pharmacologic management. The patient had a resection of the seizure focus 1 week later and he was discharged home in stable neurologic condition 1 week after the procedure.

Discussion

Status epilepticus is a life-threatening condition that requires immediate identification and treatment. Common causes of seizures include, but are not limited to, discontinuation of antiepileptic drugs, acute or longstanding brain injury, hemorrhage or infections, alcohol or drug withdrawals (benzodiazepines, barbiturates, baclofen), metabolic abnormalities (hypo/hyperglycemia, uremia, hyponatremia, hypocalcemia, hypomagnesemia) or drug overdose (penicillin G, theophylline, flumazenil, lidocaine, bupivacaine). Publication of the Veterans Affairs Cooperative Trial in 1998 [5] and the San Francisco Emergency Medical Services Study in 2001 [6] allowed for an evidence-based approach to the choice of the first-line agent to be used in terminating status epilepticus; current evidence indicates that lorazepam administered intravenously in out-of-hospital settings by paramedics or in emergency room settings is superior to diazepam and phenytoin in abolishing status epilepticus in a short period of time.

Fosphenytoin is second-line therapy in status epilepticus and offers several advantages over phenytoin. First, it can be infused with different standard intravenous solutions, whereas phenytoin can only be mixed with non-dextrose fluids. Fosphenytoin can be infused at a faster rate with decreased risk of cardiac arrhythmia and hypotension, especially in the elderly, and may be given intramuscularly.

Intravenous valproate is another therapeutic option for those patients with cardiorespiratory impairment and myoclonic status epilepticus. It is a nonsedative drug with an attractive safety profile and it is easy to use. Levetiracetam is a relatively new antiepileptic drug that has a potentially important role in the management of refractory status epilepticus. It is available as an intravenous preparation that can be infused rapidly without the necessity of ventilator assistance.

Topiramate is also another new antiepileptic drug with a mechanism of action that is different from that of the benzodiazepines and other first-line antiepileptic drugs. It can be administered by nasogastric tube in doses ranging from 300–1600 mg/day for the management of refractory status epilepticus.

Patients with refractory status epilepticus who have not responded to the first-line treatment will require admission to the ICU for more aggressive management. Tracheal intubation and controlled mechanical ventilation with the use of muscle relaxants are the first steps in intensive care management of refractory status epilepticus. It is necessary in this setting to use continuous EEG monitoring in order to guide infusions of phenobarbital, midazolam, propofol, or pentobarbital; arterial and central venous access may also be

required. The EEG endpoint of therapy is the burst-suppression pattern, which needs to be continued for 12 hours after the last seizure. Infusion of the sedative agent can be reduced every 3 hours with EEG monitoring and if there is no EEG evidence of seizures, then the patient can be weaned off the ventilator [7].

Phenobarbital is found to be effective in patients who have failed lorazepam or fosphenytoin, with or without valproate. Propofol is an alkyl phenol with a global central nervous system depressant effect. It directly activates the gamma-aminobutyric acid (GABA) receptors [8], modulates calcium influx through slow calcium ion channels, and has antioxidant activity. The pharmacokinetics and favorable adverse effect profile make propofol an excellent drug to treat refractory status epilepticus. The two main advantages of propofol are a rapid onset and short duration of action. Propofol is a highly lipophilic agent with a large volume of distribution that leads to its rapid uptake and elimination from the central nervous system. The main disadvantage of prolonged propofol infusion in the ICU is the development of propofol infusion syndrome. The main presentation of this syndrome is unexplained metabolic acidosis.

Midazolam is a fast-acting, water-soluble benzodiazepine with a half life of 4–6 hours. It acts by binding to GABA-A receptors. Midazolam is an alternative to propofol. It is typically started after securing endotracheal intubation and ventilator assistance. Inhalational anesthetics offer an alternative approach to the treatment of refractory status epilepticus. Isoflurane and desflurane are the two agents that have been tried in the treatment of refractory status epilepticus because of the safety associated with their long-term administration.

Surgical intervention can be considered as a last resort in patients who failed medical treatment and have a lesion amenable to surgery. Management of the underlying causes of status epilepticus such as noncompliance with antiepileptic drug therapy, acute infections, high fever, hypoglycemia, electrolyte imbalance, organ dysfunction, drug intoxication, poisoning, alcohol withdrawal, excess use of alcohol, stroke, trauma, and hypertensive encephalopathy is essential. Rhabdomyolysis can be a consequence of convulsive status epilepticus; the clinician should also be vigilant for the development of pneumonia in patients who are maintained in burst suppression for prolonged periods of time.

Conclusion

The management of status epilepticus is both challenging and costly. Prognosis depends both on the underlying condition and expeditious treatment. Therefore a thorough neurologic examination is critical, along with EEG to guide the management.

There are different strategies to treat status epilepticus, such as (1) lorazepam 0.02–0.03 mg/kg intravenously repeated as needed up to 0.1 mg/kg as a first-line agent, followed by (2) fosphenytoin or phenytoin 20 mg/kg, then (3) propofol or phenobarbital infusions to achieve burst suppression on the EEG.

References

1. **R. J. DeLorenzo, J. M. Pellock, A. R. Towne** *et al.* Epidemiology of status epilepticus. *J Clin Neurophysiol* 1995; **12**: 316.

2. **H. Gastaut**. A propos d' une classification symptomatologique des etats de mal epileptiques. In **Gastaut H, Roger J., Lob H.**, eds. *Les etats de mal epileptiques.* Paris: Masson, 1967; 1–8.

3. Proposal for revised clinical and electroencephalographic classification of epileptic seizures: from the Commission on Classification and Terminology of the International League against Epilepsy. *Epilepsia* 1981; **22**: 489–501.

4. **W. H. Theodore, R. J. Porter, P. Albert** *et al.* The secondarily generalized tonic-clonic seizure: a videotape analysis. *Neurology* 1994; **44**: 1403–7.

5. **D. M. Treiman, P. D. Meyers, N. Y. Walton**. A comparison of four treatments for generalized convulsive status epilepticus: Veterans Affairs Status Epilepticus Cooperative Study Group. *N Engl J Med* 1998; **339**: 792–8.

6. **B. K. Alldredge, A. M. Gelb, S. M. Isaacs** *et al.* A comparison of lorazepam, diazepam, and placebo for the treatment of out-of-hospital status epilepticus. *N Engl J Med* 2001; **345**: 631–7.

7. **Indian Epilepsy Society**. Indian Guidelines for the Management of Epilepsy: GEMIND. Available from: http://www.epilepsyindia.org/gemind-main.asp [cited in 2008].

8. **M. Hara, Y. Kai, Y. Ikemoto**. Propofol activates GABA-A receptor-chloride ionophore complex in dissociated hippocampal pyramidal neurons of the rat. *Anesthesiology* 1993; **79**: 781–8.

93

Nonconvulsive status epilepticus

Sheron Beltran

Nonconvulsive status epilepticus (NCSE) is an under-recognized cause of mental status decline. As implied by the name, it represents prolonged seizure activity or repeated seizures without a return to baseline mental status, in the absence of the classic motor symptoms commonly associated with seizure activity. It may be the sole cause of altered cognition or may be coupled with an underlying central nervous system abnormality resulting in seizure activity. The dysregulation of excitatory central nervous system (CNS) pathways results in suppression or impairment of normal consciousness. Diagnosis can prove difficult, and may not even be considered, as many clinicians are unaware of the existence of NCSE. Given the wide spectrum of clinical presentations, a high index of suspicion must be maintained for prompt diagnosis and treatment.

Case description

A 55-year-old male with a history of shunted hydrocephalus, seizure disorder, and hypothyroidism presented to the emergency department with complaints of nausea, vomiting, headache, and confusion persisting for several days. He had been seizure-free for several years on levetiracetam and lamotrigine. Over the preceding days he had been disoriented to the point of being lost a few blocks from his home and, according to family members, he had difficulties communicating with them on several occasions. On neurologic examination he was alert and oriented only to person and place. His speech was intact, however, he was found to be repetitive and to perseverate during conversation. On cranial nerve exam he had some difficulty with upgaze. Imaging revealed a dysmorphic ventricular system with enlarged fourth, third, and lateral ventricles (Figure 93.1). Additionally, there was a space-occupying mass deemed likely to be an arachnoid cyst.

The patient was then taken to the operating room for an uneventful revision of a right frontal ventriculoperitoneal shunt. During the immediate postopera-

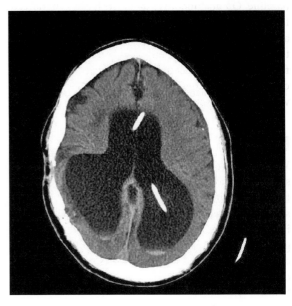

Figure 93.1. Enlarged and dysmorphic ventricular system.

tive period, the patient was alert and conversant. He had no focal neurologic findings and seemed to be improving. However, during an overnight neurologic examination he was noted to be hemiparetic and unresponsive. Imaging revealed a large frontoparietal subdural hematoma along with intraventricular hemorrhage. The hematoma was subsequently evacuated in the operating room.

Over the next 2 days the patient remained stably hemiparetic, but his mental status waxed and waned. He continued to have periods of disorientation and speech disturbances. He had difficulty following directions and was unable to complete multistep tasks. His repeat imaging studies were unchanged, he was hemodynamically stable without electrolyte abnormalities, and there was no witnessed seizure activity. He continued on his pre-admission anticonvulsant agents; however, the possibility of NCSE was entertained. An electroencephalogram (EEG) was performed showing diffuse slowing of activity suggestive of encephalopathy with intermittent rhythmic activity representing possible seizures. The patient was placed on continuous EEG monitoring and lorazepam was administered. Fosphenytoin was also added to his antiseizure regimen. The seizure activity subsequently stopped after the addition of fosphenytoin and the patient's neurologic status stabilized.

By postoperative day 6, the patient remained hemiparetic but had full return of his cognitive status to baseline. On postoperative day 7, he had a generalized tonic–clonic seizure and was treated with lorazepam and a loading dose of fosphenytoin, as his free phenytoin level was subtherapeutic. His seizure activity was rapidly terminated after administration of the benzodiazepine. The patient was thereafter seizure-free and was able to participate in rehabilitation.

Discussion

When seizure activity presents with classic motor symptoms and loss of consciousness, there is often little debate as to the diagnosis. In this case, however, seizure activity presented subtly with waxing and waning of mental status. Diagnosing NCSE may be elusive given the variety of possible presenting features. Nonconvulsive status epilepticus may present with nonspecific neurologic deficits such as impaired attention, difficulties with complex tasks, or simply as a headache [1]. Nonconvulsive status epilepticus may also be preceded by motor activity with prolonged postictal confusion. At the opposite end of the spectrum, NCSE may be the cause of coma [2]. The diagnostic criteria for NCSE are not universally accepted; it has been suggested that an altered state of consciousness coupled with EEG evidence of seizure activity are sufficient for diagnosis, however, some believe that a response to antiepileptic agents is necessary to prove the diagnosis.

There is no universally accepted classification scheme for NCSE, although it may be subdivided based on clinical features or EEG characteristics. Electroencephalogram patterns may be generalized, as in absence or petit mal status epilepticus, or focal as in complex partial status epilepticus (CPSE). Focal seizures may progress to secondary generalization, further complicating the classification system.

It is difficult to determine whether NCSE, in and of itself, causes permanent neurologic deficits. Absence seizures are generally considered benign, whereas CPSE may lead to prolonged impairment. Additionally, seizure activity is often a symptom of underlying CNS disease, and ongoing seizures may lead to secondary injury and prolonged cognitive deficits. Thus, NCSE is an important entity to recognize and treat. Nonconvulsive status epilepticus often responds to initial intervention strategies, but it may prove refractory and the benefits of treating a condition in which the outcome is controversial must be weighed against the risk of more aggressive treatment.

Initial measures should include management of underlying CNS disorders and metabolic derangements, as well as administration of anticonvulsant agents. Continuous EEG monitoring during treatment allows for ongoing evaluation of drug administration. Benzodiazepines are considered the first-line treatment for NCSE and may lead to a rapid termination of seizure activity. However, resistance to benzodiazepines and barbiturates may occur in patients with prolonged status epilepticus necessitating secondary treatment. Care must be taken as benzodiazepine treatment may result in respiratory depression.

Antiepileptic agents such as phenytoin, valproate, and levetiracetam have all been used in the treatment of NCSE. Intravenous phenytoin has been associated with hypotension, respiratory depression, and cardiac arrhythmias. Fosphenytoin is a water-soluble prodrug that is better tolerated than phenytoin. Valproate has been shown to be more effective than phenytoin in controlling seizures in generalized convulsive status epilepticus with no serious side effects. Case reports have suggested that valproate is also effective in the setting of NCSE; however, it has also been implicated as a cause of NCSE [3]. Levetiracetam has been reported to be effective in a small case series without significant side effects [4].

Ketamine, a glutamate receptor (NMDA) antagonist, has been shown to be effective at terminating seizure activity in animals, particularly in refractory cases. This may be explained by evidence that as a seizure progresses to status, receptor trafficking occurs as gamma-aminobutyric acid (GABA) receptors become internalized and NMDA receptors are recruited to the synaptic membrane. Thus, agents acting on GABA receptors may become ineffective while NMDA antagonists may terminate the seizure activity [5].

General anesthesia has been used in refractory cases of NCSE; however, hemodynamic support may be required to maintain adequate perfusion pressure. Performing general anesthesia in an intensive care setting is often logistically difficult requiring specialized equipment and personnel; mortality may be significant.

Conclusion

In our case, NCSE presented subtly with waxing and waning of mental status in a patient with underlying central nervous system pathology (subdural hematoma) and a known seizure disorder. A high level of suspicion for NCSE prompted evaluation and an early diagnosis was made. Treatment with benzodiazepines and fosphenytoin was initiated while monitoring continuous EEG activity to evaluate the patient's response to therapy. The patient's neurologic status improved and EEG evidence of seizure activity resolved possibly sparing the patient further prolonged cognitive deficits.

References

1. **M. Ghofrani, F. Mahvelati, H. Tonekaboni** et al. Headache as a sole manifestation in nonconvulsive status epilepticus. *J Child Neurol* 2007 May; **22**: 660–2.

2. **A. R. Towne, E. J. Waterhouse, J. G. Boggs** et al. Prevalence of nonconvulsive status epilepticus in comatose patients. *Neurology* 2000; **54**: 340–5.

3. **S. K. Velioğlu, S. Gazioğlu.** Non-convulsive status epilepticus secondary to valproic acid-induced hyperammonemic encephalopathy. *Acta Neurol Scand* 2007; **116**: 128–32.

4. **S. Rupprecht, K. Franke, S. Fitzek** et al. Levetiracetam as a treatment option in non-convulsive status epilepticus. *Epilepsy Res* 2007; **73**: 238–44.

5. **D. J. Borris, E. H. Bertram, J. Kapur.** Ketamine controls prolonged status epilepticus. *Epilepsy Res* 2000; **42**: 117–22.

94

Rhabdomyolysis

Mauricio Perilla and Jerome O'Hara

Although not a disease of the nervous system itself, rhabdomyolysis can significantly complicate the care of patients presenting with neurologic disorders. Early diagnosis and aggressive management are key to avoiding major adverse events such as renal failure.

Case description

A 53-year-old patient was scheduled for L2–S1 spine revision and new instrumentation. The patient was admitted the day before surgery after being found unconscious on the floor at home. At hospital admission, the patient was sleepy but arousable and complained of severe back pain. Magnetic resonance imaging of the spine showed L3–L4 compression facture with spinal stenosis. The patient had a history of seizure disorder, postlaminectomy syndrome, diabetes, morbid obesity, and drug abuse. After 8 hours of uneventful surgery in prone position, the trachea was extubated and the patient was transferred to the postanesthesia care unit in stable condition. On postoperative day 1, the patient reported generalized muscle pain (chest and back), nausea, and vomiting. The patient was hypotensive, tachycardic, dehydrated, oliguric, and "dark tea-colored" urine was noted.

The patient's initial differential diagnosis included but was not restricted to: hypovolemia, sepsis, rhabdomyolysis, acute coronary syndrome, allergic reaction, hemolytic reaction, acute renal failure, disseminated intravascular coagulation, thromboembolism, diabetic ketoacidosis, hyperosmolar hyperglycemia, nonketotic coma, drug withdrawal/toxicity, hypernatremia, hypokalemia, hypophosphatemia, myoglobinuria, sickle cell crisis.

The following abnormal laboratory values were found: urea 98 mg/dL, creatinine 3.1 mg/dL, potassium 6.2 mmol/L and lactic acid 4.1 mmol/L. Creatine kinase (CK) was reported to be 16 000 U/L (normal 30–220 U/L), MB isoenzyme <0.1%. Urinalysis was positive for hemoglobin but no red blood cells. Electrocardiogram showed a sinus tachycardia and a chest X-ray showed left basilar atelectasis.

Discussion

Rhabdomyolysis is a potentially life-threatening clinical syndrome caused by damage of the muscle fibers, which results in necrosis and disintegration of the striated muscle. The initial injury triggers the release of muscular cell constituents (electrolytes, myoglobin, and creatine kinase) into the extracellular fluid and the bloodstream. Extracellular calcium activates sustained contraction of myofibers with increase of adenosine triphosphate consumption and further depletion.

The escalation of proteases and phospholipase activity and the discharge of vasoactive molecules with production of free radicals magnify the damage [1]. Cell leakage increases the interstitial fluid with the rise of compartmental pressures, producing arterial, venous occlusion, and nerve compression (compartment syndrome). Massive release of myoglobin to the circulation is filtered through the glomerular basement membrane. As water is reabsorbed the concentration of myoglobin rises promoting precipitation and cast formation. Tubular flow declines with dehydration and renal vasoconstriction. Degradation of intratubular myoglobin results in the release of free iron, which catalyzes free radical production aggravating ischemic injury. Uric acid contributes to tubular obstruction by decreasing urine pH and favoring myoglobin precipitation and uric acid casts formation [2].

Rhabdomyolysis is most common in situations of extreme muscle activity like seizures, trauma, crush injuries, prolonged lying down on the ground (patient unconscious for several hours), burns, drugs, toxins, hyperthermia, infections, and inflammatory or ischemic processes. Metabolic, autoimmune, and genetic causes also have been identified [3]. Some clinical features include fever, myalgia, stiffness, weakness, nausea, vomiting, confusion, delirium, and coma. The physical examination should focus on areas of muscle trauma, limb weakness, or just myalgias. Hypotension and dehydration are common due to extensive cellular lysis. Clinical signs and symptoms might not be evident and mild forms can be underdiagnosed. Acute renal failure is a common complication that might be prevented with an early diagnosis. Other complications include cardiac arrhythmias and cardiac arrest due to hyperkalemia, hepatic dysfunction, and diffuse intravascular coagulation. Compartment syndrome can both be a cause or a consequence of rhabdomyolysis. In this case the patient was lying on the floor unconscious for several hours; his further history of seizures suggested an etiology of the initial fall and a risk factor for rhabdomyolysis.

Diagnosis

Myoglobin in plasma: After an extensive release, myoglobin overcomes plasma globulin's binding capacity and is filtrated to the renal tubules. Visible myoglobinuria is seen when its excretion exceeds 250 mcg/ml. The short life of myoglobin in plasma (3–6 hours) limits its diagnostic capacity.

Creatine kinase (CK): Increased levels five times normal are strongly suggestive of rhabdomyolysis. Creatine kinase levels should be tested after any evidence of extensive muscle injury. Creatine kinase levels peak in 24–36 hours [4] and can reach levels up to 100 000 U/L. Sustained levels are associated with compartment syndrome and relate to the severity of the muscle damage. Typical isoenzymes from skeletal muscle CK-MM can be differentiated from cardiac enzymes CK-MB.

Urine dipstick: This test characteristically shows a large amount of blood but the orthotoluidine portion of the dipstick is unable to distinguish myoglobinuria from hematuria or hemoglobinuria. Urine sediment may show minimal or total absence of red blood cells. Casts are often present and immunochemistry is required for myoglobin identification.

Electrolyte abnormalities: Hyperkalemia, hypocalcemia, hyperphosphatemia, hypoalbuminemia, and hyperuricemia are frequently present.

Toxicology screen: Ethanol, cocaine, and other illicit drug utilization have been associated with this syndrome and a toxicology screen is recommended with the initial assessment.

Management

The treatment of this condition should be to (1) rapidly recognize the initial trigger, (2) restore intravascular volume, (3) prevent acute renal failure, and (4) monitor the development of common complications. Patients should be treated in an intensive care unit where fluid balance can be continuously evaluated. Early fluid resuscitation includes initial administration of high rates of normal saline (1.5 liters per hour) in order to maintain urine output around 300 mL/hour [5]. Invasive hemodynamic monitoring may be required in patients with limited cardiovascular reserve or previous renal impairment. Urine alkalinization prevents myoglobin protein binding and cast precipitation; a urine pH >6.5 promotes myoglobin cast elimination. Mannitol is an osmotic diuretic that produces renal vasodilation and possibly acts as a free radical scavenger. Mannitol increases urine flow and may prevent tubular obstruction; its use in rhabdomyolysis is still controversial. Loop diuretics should not be used because they acidify urine. Renal replacement therapy should be considered in patients who develop oliguric acute tubular necrosis. Hyperkalemia is a common complication that should be treated promptly due to its fatal arrhythmogenic effect when it is associated with hypocalcemia. Hypocalcemia should be corrected in symptomatic patients; hypercalcemia is commonly present during the recovery phase of rhabdomyolysis. Muscle swelling and pain should be regularly evaluated and fasciotomies may be needed in case of compartment syndrome. Succinylcholine is contraindicated due to a life-threatening potassium elevation. Disseminated intravascular coagulation and liver failure should be suspected in rhabdomyolysis cases.

Conclusion

Rhabdomyolysis can be associated with life-threatening complications in neurologic patients. Rapid diagnosis, aggressive hydration, and correction of electrolyte abnormalities are key features of management.

References

1. F. G. O'Connor, P. A. Deuster. Rhabdomyolysis. In Goldman L., Ausiello D. A., eds. *Cecil Medicine*, 23rd edition. Philadelphia, PA: Saunders Elsevier, 2008; 798–802.

2. **R. Vanholder, M. S. Sever, E. Erek** *et al.* Rhabdomyolysis. *J Am Soc Nephrol* 2000; **11**: 1553–61.

3. **J. D. Warren, P. C. Blumbergs, P. D. Thompson**. Rhabdomyolysis: a review. *Muscle Nerve* 2002; **25**: 332–47.

4. **W. Tan, B. C. Herzlich, R. Funaro** *et al.* Rhabdomyolysis and myoglobinuric acute renal failure associated with classic heat stroke. *South Med J* 1995; **88**: 1065–8.

5. **M. S. Slater, R. J. Mullins**. Rhabdomyolysis and myoglobinuric renal failure in trauma and surgical patients: a review. *J Am Coll Surg* 1998; **186**: 693–716.

Neuromuscular disease

Myasthenic crisis

Wael Ali Sakr Esa

Myasthenia gravis (MG) is an autoimmune disease with antibodies directed against the nicotinic acetylcholine receptor or other muscle membrane proteins. Myasthenic crisis is usually associated with infection and is characterized by respiratory failure requiring invasive or noninvasive mechanical ventilation [1].

Case description

A 46-year-old African–American female with a 9-year history of MG developed a progressive bilateral lower extremity numbness and pain from a bulging lumbar disc. The patient was admitted for a two level lumbar discectomy. Her daily medications were pyridostigmine 60 mg every 8 hours, levothyroxine 175 mcg daily, esmoperazole 20 mg daily. Her past medical history included hypothyroidism and gastroesophageal reflux disease. She had one myasthenic crisis 5 years ago associated with a pulmonary infection that required intubation and mechanical ventilation.

In the operating room, standard ASA monitors were placed on the patient and a left radial arterial line was placed. Remifentanil infusion was then started at 0.05 mcg/kg/minute. Anesthesia was induced with propofol and lidocaine, then an endotracheal tube was placed without the use of any muscle relaxant. Anesthesia was maintained with inhalational anesthesia, hydromorphone 1 mg and remifentanil infusion 0.05–0.3 mcg/kg/minute. No muscle relaxant was used during the whole 2-hour surgery. At the end of the case, inhalational anesthesia and remifentanil infusion were stopped but the patient remained weak and was not achieving adequate tidal volume.

The patient was transferred to the intensive care unit (ICU), intubated, and sedated with a propofol infusion. A 10 mg intravenous dose of edrophonium was given and 60 mg pyridostigmine was administered through the nasogastric tube with partial improvement in motor power and tidal volume. Plasmapheresis was performed and then the patient was weaned

successfully from the mechanical ventilation after she regained her motor strength on the second day after the surgery.

Discussion

The clinical hallmark of MG is skeletal muscle weakness. Eighty-five percent of patients with MG have identifiable anti-acetylcholine receptor antibodies. Anti-acetylcholine receptor antibodies damage the postsynaptic muscle membrane via a complement-mediated reaction, causing an increased degradation and decreased formation of acetylcholine receptors. Many myasthenic patients also have antinuclear and antithyroid antibodies and other autoimmune diseases such as systemic lupus erythematosus, rheumatoid arthritis, pernicious anemia, and thyroiditis. Myasthenic crisis is defined as respiratory failure requiring mechanical ventilation in the MG patient. Myasthenic crisis is a common life-threatening complication that occurs in approximately 15–20% of patients with MG during their lifetime [2].

Myasthenic crises are often precipitated by pulmonary infections and result in respiratory failure requiring mechanical ventilation. Potential cardiac manifestations of MG include focal myocarditis, atrial fibrillation, atrioventricular conduction delay, and left ventricular diastolic dysfunction. Many conditions such as viral infections, stress, surgery, and extreme heat may exacerbate the symptoms of myasthenia. The Osserman staging system is based on the severity of the disease. Type I: Ocular signs and symptoms only; Type II A: generalized muscle weakness; Type II B: generalized moderate weakness and/or bulbar dysfunction; Type III: acute fulminant presentation and/or respiratory dysfunction; and Type IV: severe, generalized myasthenia [3].

The primary concern in anesthesia for the patient with myasthenia gravis is the use of muscle relaxants. Patients tend to be resistant to succinylcholine and

Table 95.1. Comparison of Myasthenic syndrome and myasthenia gravis.

	Myasthenic syndrome	Myasthenia gravis
Manifestations	Proximal limb weakness (arms >legs) Exercise improves strength Reflexes absent or decreased Myalgia common	Extraocular, bulbar, and facial muscle weakness Fatigue with exercise Reflexes normal No myalgia
Response to muscle relaxants	Sensitive to succinylcholine and nondepolarizing muscle relaxants No improvement with acetylcholinesterase inhibitors	Resistant to succinylcholine. Sensitive to nondepolarizing muscle relaxants Improvement with acetylcholinesterase inhibitors
Gender	Male > female	Female > male
Pathogenesis	IgG autoantibodies directed against prejunctional voltage-sensitive calcium channels Associated with small cell carcinoma of the lung, sarcoidosis	Destruction of postsynaptic acetylcholine receptors, usually by autoimmune antibodies Associated with thymoma
Treatment	Aminopyridines that increase presynaptic release of acetylcholinesterase	Acetylcholinesterase inhibitors, steroids, thymectomy, immunosuppressants

have increased sensitivity to nondepolarizing relaxants, necessitating caution with their use. As in our case, an anesthetic technique that eliminated the use of a muscle relaxant is preferred. Conditions suitable for tracheal intubation can be obtained with a standard induction technique using propofol and the inhalation of volatile halogenated agents such as isoflurane or sevoflurane with the addition of an opioid infusion such as remifentanil. Sevoflurane, isoflurane, and desflurane depress neuromuscular transmission and may provide enough muscle relaxation so that tracheal intubation can be performed without neuromuscular blocking drugs after an adequate depth of anesthesia has been attained. Adjuvant drugs that blunt responses to laryngoscopy such as propofol, opioids, and lidocaine may be useful as seen in our case.

In this case, remifentanil infusion was maintained during the surgery to avoid the use of any muscle relaxants. Acetylcholinesterase inhibitors such as pyridostigmine and edrophonium enhance neuromuscular function by preventing synaptic degradation of acetylcholine and thereby increasing the amount of acetylcholine available in the synapse. Excess pyridostigmine may cause a cholinergic crisis, in which weakness and muscarinic signs (bradycardia, miosis, salivation, diarrhea) also develop from excess acetycholine. Conversely, too little pyridostigmine may cause a myasthenic crisis, in which weakness also results from too little acetylcholine. To distinguish a cholinergic crisis from a myasthenic crisis, muscarinic signs that are consistent with a cholinergic crisis should be considered. In addition, the adminis-

tration of 10 mg edrophonium intravenously results in persistent weakness if the patient is experiencing a cholinergic crisis, but improvement in strength if the patient is experiencing a myasthenic crisis. The other important diagnostic point is to differentiate between myasthenic syndrome and MG as shown in Table 95.1.

In the approach to the patient with myasthenic crisis, (1) the diagnosis of MG should be confirmed; (2) respiratory failure should be evaluated and treated in the ICU, while potential precipitating factors are identified and managed; (3) immunomodulatory treatment should be initiated; and (4) complications should be avoided or managed promptly. The general criteria for intubation are vital capacity of <15–20 mL/kg, peak inspiratory pressure <−40 cmH$_2$O, peak expiratory force of <40 cmH$_2$O, and evidence of respiratory muscle fatigue, hypercapnia, or hypoxia [4]. Plasma exchange may be more effective than intravenous immunoglobulin in the treatment of myasthenic crisis involving respiratory failure. In the acute setting, the role of immunosuppression and intravenous/intramuscular pyridostigmine and the newer agents such as tacrolimus remains limited and at times controversial [5]. Since the advent of these immune interventions and improved methods of mechanical ventilation in specialized ICUs, mortality rates in MG and myasthenic crisis have substantially decreased. Also, patients in myasthenic crisis should undergo careful cardiac monitoring and equipment for external cardiac pacing or the insertion of a temporary pacemaker should be provided at all times for the critically ill patient.

Conclusion

In conclusion, the recent improvements in prognosis for a patient with myasthenic crisis can be attributed to improved respiratory care during the crisis, admission to an ICU, substitution of endotracheal intubation for tracheostomy, and improvements in monitoring, tracheal toilet, and antibiotics.

References

1. **J. Palace, A. Vincent, D. Becson**. Myasthenia gravis: diagnostic and management dilemmas. *Curr Opin Neurol* 2001; **14**: 583.

2. **A. Alshekhlee, J. D. Miles, B. Katirji** *et al.* Incidence and mortality rates of myasthenia gravis and myasthenic crisis in US hospitals. *Neurology* 2009; **72**: 1548–54.

3. **S. F. Dierdorf, J. S. Walton**. Anesthesia for patients with rare and coexisting disease. In **Barash P. G., Cullen B. F., Stoelting R. K.**, eds. *Clinical Anesthesia*, 5th edition. Philadelphia, PA: Lippincott Williams & Wilkins, 2006; 507–8.

4. **J. Senerviratne, J. Mandrekar, E. F. Wijdicks** *et al.* Predictors of extubation failure in myasthenic crisis. *Arch Neurol* 2008; **65**: 929–33.

5. **S. Ahmed, J. F. Kirmani, N. Janjua** *et al.* An update on myasthenic crisis. *Neurology* 2005; **7**: 129–41.

Neuromuscular disease

Guillain-Barré syndrome

Anupa Deogaonkar and Ehab Farag

Guillian-Barré syndrome (GBS) is an acute inflammatory demyelinating polyradiculoneuropathy affecting approximately 1–2/100 000 each year. Typical clinical manifestations include progressive ascending motor weakness, areflexia and autonomic instability, with severe cases progressing to respiratory failure. Usually patients have a history of infection 1–3 weeks prior to onset of the disease.

Case description

A 50-year-old, 75 kg, 166 cm male ASA physical status 2E was scheduled to undergo emergent exploratory laparotomy. He had a history of tingling, numbness and progressive ascending weakness in both hands and feet for 2 days. Two weeks previously, he had seen his primary-care physician for a viral illness with fever, skin rash, and arthralgias. On admission, the neurologic examination revealed bilateral facial palsy, quadriparesis (distal more than proximal), and areflexia. A lumbar puncture performed on admission revealed albuminocytologic dissociation and increased cerebrospinal fluid protein content compared with white cells. Nerve conduction studies indicated GBS. The patient was started on immunoglobulin therapy. On arrival to the preoperative holding area, intravenous metoclopramide, glycopyrrolate 0.2 mg and hydrocortisone were administered. A preinduction radial arterial catheter was placed on the right side and the patient was transferred to the operating table with full body warming blanket. After preoxygenation with 100% oxygen for 3 minutes, rapid sequence induction with cricoid pressure was performed. After securing the endotracheal tube, a nasogastric tube and esophageal stethoscope were placed. Isoflurane in 50% oxygen and air was used for maintenance. Intraoperatively, blood pressure was labile and phenylephrine infusion was used to maintain systolic blood pressure within 20% of the patient's baseline. The patient was transported to the intensive care unit (ICU) intubated

and mechanically ventilated. Immunoglobulin therapy was continued in the postoperative period and the patient was weaned to extubate on postoperative day 2. He developed deep venous thrombosis of the left lower extremity on postoperative day 9, which was further complicated by pulmonary embolism. He was discharged home on postoperative day 18. His neurologic examination after 6 months was normal.

Discussion

There are no specific guidelines available for anesthetic management for patients presenting with GBS; multidisciplinary care is necessary in the perioperative period to avoid fatal complications. Preoperative evaluation including history, physical examination, electrocardiogram and laboratory data such as cerebrospinal fluid and nerve conduction studies will help identify patients who will require postoperative mechanical ventilation. Stress-dose steroids should be administered to all patients who have been on steroids to reduce risk of cardiovascular collapse due to inhibition of endogenous cortisol production. Autonomic instability can cause severe hypotension/hypertension intraoperatively necessitating the use of invasive intra-arterial blood pressure monitoring. Succinylcholine should not be used in order to avoid hyperkalemic response and cardiac arrest [1]. Nondepolarizing agents with a minimal cardiovascular side-effect profile are considered safe. Sudden changes in positioning intraoperatively should be avoided to prevent fluctuations of blood pressure. Alpha and beta agonist and antagonists medications should be drawn and kept ready to use. These patients are believed to be more sensitive to local anesthetics and overall the use of regional anesthesia is controversial. Profound sympathectomy due to regional anesthesia in the setting of autonomic instability is not desirable and may lead to cardiac arrest [2]. Worsening of neurologic symptoms may occur after epidural anesthesia for labor in pregnant patients presenting with GBS [3] or due to direct nerve root damage during regional technique [4]. Opioids may be used to treat pain in the perioperative period in the ICUs [5]. In nonambulatory patients, subcutaneous heparin and compression stockings should be used to prevent deep vein thrombosis. Plasmapheresis and immunoglobulins may have to be continued in the perioperative period besides conservative management.

Conclusion

Early preoperative assessment, adequate monitoring, appropriate selection of anesthetic technique and postoperative intensive care treatment can lead to uneventful anesthetic management in GBS patients.

References

1. **J. M. Feldman**. Cardiac arrest after succinylcholine administration in a pregnant patient recovered from Guillain-Barré syndrome. *Anesthesiology* 1990; **72**: 942–4.

2. **A. Perel, A. Reches, J. T. Davidson**. Anaesthesia in the Guillian-Barré syndrome. A case report and recommendations. *Anaesthesia* 1977; **32**: 257–60.

3. **S. Wiertlewski, A. Magot, S. Drapier** *et al.* Worsening of neurologic symptoms after epidural anesthesia for labor in a Guillain-Barré patient. *Anesth Analg* 2004; **98**: 825–7.

4. **I. Steiner, Z. Argov, C. Cahan** *et al.* Guillain-Barré syndrome after epidural anesthesia: direct nerve root damage may trigger disease. *Neurology* 1985; **35**: 1473–5.

5. **D. S. Johnson, M. J. Dunn**. Remifentanil for pain due to Guillain-Barré syndrome. *Anaesthesia* 2008; **63**: 676–7.

End-of-life issues

97 Conducting a family meeting to decide withdrawal of care

Marc J. Popovich

Conducting a family meeting to decide withdrawal of care can be a very difficult process. Both experience and understanding is necessary for effective communication with the patient's family. The following case discussion elucidates one approach to this delicate situation.

Case description

A 79-year-old male was found unconscious in his home by his wife. Upon arrival at the home, emergency medical services began full cardiopulmonary resuscitation including intubation of the airway. There was return of spontaneous circulation after about 5 minutes of resuscitation. The patient was taken to the emergency department, where a head computed tomography (CT) scan demonstrated a large stroke in the left middle cerebral artery territory. Cardiac enzymes were positive for acute myocardial infarction. The patient was breathing spontaneously, but was otherwise unresponsive. He was admitted to the intensive care unit and over the course of the next 12 hours became progressively febrile, hypotensive, and oliguric. He remained unresponsive and required ongoing resuscitation and vasopressor support. The patient's wife and two sons had been informed of the patient's stroke and myocardial infarction, but were now at the bedside requesting an update on the patient's condition and prognosis.

The intensivist explained to the family that a meaningful outcome (independent existence at home) would be extremely unlikely given the large stroke, myocardial infarction, and multisystem organ failure. The intensivist then asked the family about how the patient would feel about being dependent on nursing care in an extended care facility, perhaps indefinitely. When presented with this prognosis, it was clear to the family that such a treatment course would be inconsistent with the patient's previously stated wishes. The intensivist offered the option of providing care primarily directed towards comfort, including extubation. After a discussion, the family agreed to this treatment course. One hour after extubation and withdrawal of vasopressor support, the patient expired peacefully in the presence of his family.

Discussion

One of the more difficult situations a critical care physician faces is a discussion regarding withdrawal of care or limitation of support with family members whose loved one has developed medical problems from which he or she clearly cannot recover. This discussion is meant to aid in the management of the subset of patients who do *not* meet brain death criteria, but who are clearly moribund, have developed irreversible organ failures, or where the medical opinion is that the chance of meaningful recovery is nil, despite extraordinary efforts. Family discussions for these situations require a great deal of forethought, as well as experience in answering questions that typically arise. Entering into discussions with families for these types of problems without prior consideration and expertise can be fraught with difficulty, negative emotions, and may lead to prolongation of suffering of an otherwise dying patient.

The first thing that the intensivist must establish before engaging in a withdrawal-of-life-support discussion with a family is that the medical opinion is unanimous. In critical care, it is very common to have a multitude of physicians or consultants who may be asked to offer their opinion to family members during the patient's clinical course. When there is clear evidence for need of a withdrawal-of-support discussion, the intensivist should review the situation with the physicians involved to make sure their opinions are consistent, *prior* to engaging the family. It is particularly important, if the patient has undergone a surgical procedure, that the surgeon is in agreement. Entering into a family discussion without unanimity of the medical and surgical opinions will almost assuredly be counterproductive [1].

Second, since frequently in these situations physicians are reluctant to declare that the outcome of death is 100% guaranteed, it is important for the intensivist to be prepared to describe the most realistic outcome scenario in real-world terminology. The intensivist should additionally prepare to frame the discussion in terms of how the patient would feel about, for example, indefinite ventilator dependency, dialysis, chronic long-term care placement, constant nursing attention including bathing and toileting, or the unlikelihood of regaining functional independence.

Third, the intensivist should not fear using open, honest, and definitive words regarding the dying process. What's more, the intensivist should be prepared to offer a care plan individualized to the primary goal of ensuring the patient's comfort. For example, the intensivist may decide that comfort relative to the patient's respiratory status will be impossible if extubated. In that situation, maintaining ventilator support (albeit with minimal settings) may be necessary.

Most families appreciate an open, honest approach when discussing withdrawal of life supportive measures. It is important that the intensivist feel comfortable engaging in these types of discussions, because although difficult, they are a necessary component of an intensivist's practice [2, 3].

References

1. **M. D. Siegel**. End-of-life decision making in the ICU. *Clin Chest Med* 2009; **30**: 181–94.

2. **D. Wiegand**. In their own time: the family experience during the process of withdrawal of life-sustaining therapy. *J Pall Med* 2008; **11**: 1115–21.

3. **H. M. Delisser**. A practical approach to the family that expects a miracle. *Chest* 2009; **135**: 1643–7.

Brain death

98

Venkatakrishna Rajajee

Unfortunately, catastrophic events such as stroke or brain trauma can lead to the cessation of neural function. Understanding the precise diagnosis of brain death is therefore of importance to the neurointensivist.

Case description

A 21-year-old male was brought to the neurosurgical intensive care unit (ICU) following evacuation of a large right-sided traumatic subdural hematoma. Immediately prior to evacuation his Glasgow Coma Scale (GCS) was 3T with absent pupillary and corneal reflexes but with intact cough and spontaneous respiratory effort. His vital signs appeared stable – blood pressure (BP) 126/80 mmHg, heart rate 99, respiratory rate 16 and oxygen saturation 100% on Assist Control ventilation. The intracranial pressure was 18 mmHg. His GCS was 3T. His pupils were both 6 mm and unreactive. There was no cough, gag, corneal, or oculocephalic reflex. The anesthesiologist reported that the last use of neuromuscular blockade (4 mg vecuronium) was 45 minutes prior to admission. Brain death evaluation was therefore deferred. Four hours later a train-of-four evaluation revealed four twitches. The GCS remained 3T and the intracranial pressure was 57 mmHg. The patient's family was counseled that his prognosis was very poor and that a brain death evaluation was in progress. They were counseled by the representative of the regional organ donation agency, who was notified of the patient's condition at the time of his arrival in the neurosurgical ICU. The parents asked that the patient's organs be donated and agreed with completion of the brain death evaluation rather than choose immediate withdrawal of care. The first brain death evaluation was performed, by a senior neurosurgical resident physician. The patient's temperature was 35 °C, so a warming blanket was applied. The sodium was 150 meq/L and the potassium was 3.2 meq/L; other laboratory values were normal. On clinical examination, the corneal, pupillary, gag, cough, and oculocephalic ("doll's-eye" – when the brainstem is intact in the comatose patient, the eyes do not turn with the head when it is passively turned from side to side) reflexes were absent. Ice-water injection into the ears (following an otoscopic examination) resulted in no eye movement (vestibulo-ocular reflex). On applying pain to the toes, dorsiflexion of the foot was noted. The resident physician documented his evaluation as revealing "no signs of brainstem function at this time." The patient's blood pressure (BP) then dropped to 70/40 mmHg and heart rate increased to 130, following output of 3 liters of dilute-looking urine over a 2-hour period. Normal saline was administered with a pressure-bag and 3 liters infused before the BP returned to 100/60 mmHg. The urine specific gravity was 1.002, and a 2 mcg intravenous therapy dose of desmopressin was administered. Repeat doses of desmopressin were used as necessary and a norepinephrine infusion was started. A bedside nuclear medicine cerebral perfusion scan was obtained, which revealed no evidence of blood flow in the brain. A second brain death evaluation was then performed by an attending neurologist. Brainstem reflexes were again absent and an apnea test was performed. The patient was preoxygenated at FiO_2 100% for 15 minutes and a baseline arterial blood gas (ABG) test obtained. The $PaCO_2$ was 40 mmHg. The ventilator was disconnected and a tracheal cannula passed through the endotracheal tube, connected to 6 L/minute flow of oxygen. The patient's chest was uncovered to observe for respiratory excursions and vital signs were closely monitored. After 10 minutes, an ABG was drawn and the ventilator connected back. The repeat $PaCO_2$ was 75 mmHg, with no evidence of respiratory function. Brain death was declared; the patient's lungs, kidneys, and liver were successfully transplanted.

Discussion

Brain death is the irreversible cessation of all brain function, including brainstem function. Brain death is widely, although not universally, considered equivalent to cardiovascular death. In the USA, brain death is considered to represent legal death, although different states have very different criteria for the determination of brain death. It is important to be aware of the specific criteria used in one's institution, which are generally guided by local laws. The most common primary neurologic diseases that result in brain death are traumatic brain injury and subarachnoid hemorrhage. Several other conditions including hypoxic-ischemic injury and fulminant hepatic failure can result in brain death. Although criteria vary, certain basic requirements are fundamental to its determination. The American Academy of Neurology (AAN) has published practice parameters for the diagnosis of brain death [1]. Certain prerequisites must be met before the evaluation proceeds. First, there must be clear clinical or neuroimaging evidence of a central nervous system catastrophe compatible with the diagnosis of brain death – in this case the known traumatic brain injury with computed tomography evidence of intracranial hemorrhage and herniation. Metabolic confounders that might mimic brain death must be excluded with a basic metabolic and electrolyte panel. Although the sodium level was mildly elevated and the potassium level was low in this case, neither of these values was likely to confound the determination of brain death. Significant hypothermia should be excluded (temperature above 32 °C in the AAN summary statement). No confounding medications or drugs should be in the patient's system. At the time of this patient's arrival in the neurosurgical ICU, brain death evaluation was postponed because he had received a dose of vecuronium prior to transfer. The evaluation commenced only after an adequate period (several half lives) was allowed for drug elimination and train-of-four testing was performed.

The three cardinal features of brain death are coma, absence of brainstem reflexes, and apnea. A clinical examination is performed to confirm the patient's comatose state and to evaluate brainstem reflexes. This includes the pupillary reflex, corneal reflex, jaw jerk, oculocephalic reflex, gag reflex, and cough reflex. The vestibulo-ocular reflex is also tested, with injection of 50 mL iced water in each ear at least 5 minutes apart (after otoscopic examination to confirm patency of the external auditory canal and exclude tympanic injury).

No ocular movement should be seen with injection. It is important to note that while movements originating from the brain (including decerebrate posturing, decorticate posturing, and seizures) are incompatible with the diagnosis of brain death, both spontaneous and evoked movements originating often from spinal reflexes may be observed [2]. These include deep tendon reflexes, triple flexion, Babinski reflex, and neck and upper body tonic reflexes. Hence, the finding of dorsiflexion of the toes in this patient did not exclude the diagnosis of brain death.

Apnea testing has certain prerequisites – the AAN summary statement specifies a core temperature >36.5 °C, a systolic BP ≥90 mmHg, euvolemia, $PaCO_2$ ≥40 mmHg and preoxygenation (usually with FiO_2 100% for 10–15 minutes) preferably to PaO_2 >200 mmHg. Oxygenation is maintained following ventilator disconnection, typically with O_2 flow at 6 L/minute. The next critical step is to observe closely for any respiratory movement. A repeat blood gas after 10 minutes that demonstrates a $PaCO_2$ of 60 mmHg (or a rise of 20 mmHg) is considered evidence of adequate stimulus for respiration. If no respiratory movement was seen with an adequate $PaCO_2$ stimulus, the test is positive for apnea. If the patient demonstrates hemodynamic instability or oxygen desaturation prior to completion of the 10 minute period, an arterial blood gas is drawn and the test terminated. If the blood gas analysis confirms an adequate CO_2 stimulus with no observed respiratory effort, the test is positive despite an observation period of <10 minutes.

A waiting period followed by a second evaluation is often required by institutional protocols, although several institutions do not consider this essential when clear evidence of devastating brain injury is present. The AAN practice parameter recommends a 6-hour waiting period for the adult patient. Longer intervals are recommended for children, particularly neonates. With regards to this patient, the institutional protocol specified a 12-hour waiting period, with the option of eliminating this waiting period with the use of confirmatory testing. A confirmatory test – a nuclear medicine scan – was therefore performed.

Confirmatory testing is generally not a requirement for the diagnosis of brain death, although there is considerable variation in international and state law with regards to the role of such testing and the type of testing accepted. Confirmatory testing is useful when a full clinical evaluation cannot be performed, such as

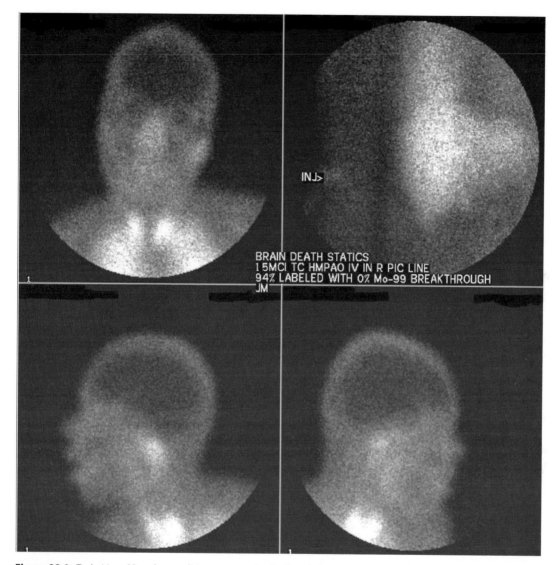

BRAIN DEATH STATICS
15MCI TC HMPAO IV IN R PIC LINE
94% LABELED WITH 0% Mo-99 BREAKTHROUGH
JM

Figure 98.1. Technitium-99 nuclear medicine scan reveals a "hollow skull" with no isotope uptake in brain.

in the patient with severe facial and orbital injury and patients in coma from long-acting medications such as pentobarbital. Also, as in the case discussed, specific institutional protocols may allow for reduction or elimination of the waiting period when confirmatory testing is done. Confirmatory testing can be done using electroencephalography, cerebral angiography, nuclear medicine (Technitium-99) scanning, transcranial Doppler (TCD) and somatosensory evoked potential testing. Specific stringent electroencephalographic criteria exist to confirm "electrocerebral silence" in brain death [3]. Electroencephalography

is prone to interference from medication use and to artifact that mimics brain activity. Cerebral angiography must demonstrate the complete absence of intracranial blood flow. Somatosensory evoked potential testing also must meet specific brain death testing criteria and must demonstrate bilateral absence of the N20–P22 responses with stimulation of the median nerve. Transcranial Doppler testing is complicated by the fact that 10–20% of patients do not have an acoustic window to permit TCD evaluation. Initial absence of detectable Doppler signal (a common consequence of true brain death) is therefore not an acceptable diagnostic criterion. Transcranial Doppler may demonstrate an absence of flow where flow was previously demonstrated or may demonstrate short systolic peaks with absent or reversed diastolic flow. The bedside Technitium-99 nuclear medicine scan, performed in this case, demonstrates complete absence of isotope uptake by the brain (Figure 98.1 – "hollow skull") in the brain-dead patient [4].

Institutional protocols may also specify the individuals qualified to perform a brain death evaluation. Some institutions require that a neurologist or neurosurgeon perform the evaluation, others permit nurses to perform the evaluation, followed by physician certification. Other common requirements include that at least one of the evaluations be performed by an attending physician and that at least one evaluation be performed by a physician who is not part of the treating team. Members of the organ transplant team are generally not permitted to perform the brain death evaluation. In the case discussed, the first exam was performed by a neurosurgical resident (from the treating team) and the second by a neurology attending physician.

The brain-dead patient usually, but not always, develops diabetes insipidus, caused by injury to the hypothalamic–pituitary axis. This manifests by polyuria and dilute urine (specific gravity <1.004) and, as seen in this case, can very rapidly lead to hypovolemia and hypotension. Diabetes insipidus is managed with aggressive volume replacement and use of either intermittent desmopressin injections or a vasopressin infusion. Loss of brainstem vasomotor tone in the brain-dead patient often necessitates the use of a vasopressor infusion.

The key impetus to the accurate and timely diagnosis of brain death is the critical shortage of organs available for transplantation. Neurosurgical ICUs should have a policy of early notification of the local organ donation agency, when a critically ill patient is admitted, prior even to initiation of the brain death evaluation. Typically, the representative of the organ donation agency then counsels the family. Donation following brain death is considered preferable to donation after cardiac death (performed when organ donation is planned without declaration of brain death), which generally limits the organs available for transplantation. A sensitive, respectful, and supportive approach to communication with the family is absolutely essential. Every reasonable accommodation of family wishes must be made following the declaration of brain death, including waiting for out-of-town family members prior to discontinuation of mechanical ventilation. Should a family refuse to accept the diagnosis of death, every effort is usually made to gain their understanding and acceptance, despite there being legal precedent for discontinuation of mechanical ventilation from a brain-dead individual against family wishes [5].

References

1. Practice parameters for determining brain death in adults (summary statement). The Quality Standards Subcommittee of the American Academy of Neurology. *Neurology* 1995; **45**: 1012–14.

2. **G. Saposnik, J. A. Bueri, J. Maurino** *et al.* Spontaneous and reflex movements in brain death. *Neurology* 2000; **54**: 221–3.

3. Guideline three: minimum technical standards for EEG recording in suspected cerebral death. American Electroencephalographic Society. *J Clin Neurophysiol* 1994; **11**: 10–13.

4. **H. Wieler, K. Marohl, K. P. Kaiser** *et al.* Tc-99m HMPAO cerebral scintigraphy. A reliable, noninvasive method for determination of brain death. *Clin Nucl Med* 1993; **18**: 104–9.

5. **R. E. Cranford**. Discontinuation of ventilation after brain death. Policy should be balanced with concern for the family. *Br Med J* 1999; **318**: 1754–5.

Index